Management of Hand Fractures

Editor

JEFFREY N. LAWTON

HAND CLINICS

www.hand.theclinics.com

Consulting Editor
KEVIN C. CHUNG

November 2013 • Volume 29 • Number 4

ELSEVIER

1600 John F. Kennedy Boulevard • Suite 1800 • Philadelphia, Pennsylvania, 19103-2899

http://www.theclinics.com

HAND CLINICS Volume 29, Number 4
November 2013 ISSN 0749-0712, ISBN-13: 978-0-3231-8605-6

Editor: Jennifer Flynn-Briggs

Hand Clinics (ISSN 0749-0712) is published quarterly by Elsevier Inc., 360 Park Avenue South, New York, NY 10010-1710. Months of publication are February, May, August, and November. Business and Editorial Offices: 1600 John F. Kennedy Blvd., Ste. 1800, Philadelphia, PA 19103-2899. Customer Service Office: 3251 Riverport Lane, Maryland Heights, MO 63043. Periodicals postage paid at New York, NY and at additional mailing offices. Subscription price is $390.00 per year (domestic individuals), $606.00 per year (domestic institutions), $194.00 per year (domestic students/residents), $445.00 per year (Canadian individuals), $691.00 per year (Canadian institutions), $530.00 per year (international individuals), $691.00 per year (international institutions), and $256.00 per year (international and Canadian students/residents). Foreign air speed delivery is included in all *Clinics* subscription prices. All prices are subject to change without notice. **POSTMASTER:** Send address changes to *Hand Clinics*, Elsevier Health Sciences Division, Subscription Customer Service, 3251 Riverport Lane, Maryland Heights, MO 63043. Customer Service (orders, claims, online, change of address): Elsevier Health Sciences Division, Subscription Customer Service, 3251 Riverport Lane, Maryland Heights, MO 63043. Tel: 1-800-654-2452 (U.S. and Canada); 314-447-8871 (outside U.S. and Canada). Fax: 314-447-8029. E-mail: journalscustomerservice-usa@elsevier.com (for print support); journalsonlinesupport-usa@elsevier.com (for online support).

Reprints. For copies of 100 or more of articles in this publication, please contact the Commercial Reprints Department, Elsevier Inc., 360 Park Avenue South, New York, New York 10010-1710. Tel.: 212-633-3874; Fax: 212-633-3820; E-mail: reprints@elsevier.com.

Hand Clinics is covered in *MEDLINE/PubMed (Index Medicus), Current Contents/Clinical Medicine, EMBASE/Excerpta Medica,* and *ISI/BIOMED.*

Printed and bound by CPI Group (UK) Ltd, Croydon, CR0 4YY

Transferred to digital print 2012

Contributors

CONSULTING EDITOR

KEVIN C. CHUNG, MD, MS
Charles B.G. de Nancrede Professor of
Surgery, Section of Plastic Surgery,
Department of Surgery, Assistant Dean for
Faculty Affairs, Associate Director of Global
REACH, University of Michigan Medical
School, University of Michigan Health System,
Ann Arbor, Michigan

EDITOR

JEFFREY N. LAWTON, MD
Associate Professor, Chief, Division of Elbow,
Hand and Microsurgery, Department of
Orthopaedic Surgery, University of Michigan,
Ann Arbor, Michigan

AUTHORS

JULIE E. ADAMS, MD
Department of Orthopaedic Surgery,
The University of Minnesota, Minneapolis,
Minnesota

PAUL C. BALDWIN, MD
Resident Physician, Department of
Orthopaedic Surgery, New England
Musculoskeletal Institute, University of
Connecticut Health Center, Farmington,
Connecticut

SHANNON CARPENTER, MD
Resident, Department of Orthopaedic Surgery,
Oakland University William Beaumont School
of Medicine, Beaumont Health System, Royal
Oak, Michigan

KEVIN C. CHUNG, MD, MS
Charles B.G. de Nancrede Professor of
Surgery, Section of Plastic Surgery,
Department of Surgery, Assistant Dean for
Faculty Affairs, Associate Director of Global
REACH, University of Michigan Medical
School, University of Michigan Health System,
Ann Arbor, Michigan

MICHAEL DAROWISH, MD
Assistant Professor, Department of
Orthopaedic Surgery, Penn State Milton
S. Hershey Medical Center, Hershey,
Pennsylvania

RAFAEL DIAZ-GARCIA, MD
House Officer, Section of Plastic Surgery,
Department of Surgery, University of Michigan
Health System, Ann Arbor, Michigan

SCOTT F.M. DUNCAN, MD, MPH, MBA
Department of Orthopedic Surgery, Ochsner
Health System, New Orleans, Louisiana

STEVEN C. HAASE, MD, FACS
Associate Professor, Section of Plastic
Surgery, Department of Surgery, University
of Michigan Health System, Ann Arbor,
Michigan

PEYTON L. HAYS, MD
Orthopaedic Hand Fellow, Beth Israel
Deaconess Medical Center, Department of
Orthopaedic Surgery, Boston, Massachusetts

TARIK HUSAIN, MD
Hand Surgery Fellow, Department of Plastic
Surgery, University of Texas Southwestern
Medical School, Dallas, Texas

RYOSUKE KAKINOKI, MD, PhD
Department of Orthopedic Surgery, Graduate
School of Medicine, Kyoto University,
Sakyo-ku, Kyoto, Japan

JEFFREY N. LAWTON, MD
Associate Professor, Chief, Division of Elbow,
Hand and Microsurgery, Department of
Orthopaedic Surgery, University of Michigan,
Ann Arbor, Michigan

KEVIN MALONE, MD
Assistant Professor, Case Western Reserve
University School of Medicine, Department of
Orthopaedic Surgery, MetroHealth Medical
Center, Cleveland, Ohio

ANDREW D. MARKIEWITZ, MD
Volunteer Clinical Professor, Department of
Orthopaedic Surgery, University of Cincinnati,
Cincinnati, Ohio; Assistant Professor,
Department of Surgery, Uniformed Services
University of the Health Services, Bethesda,
Maryland

THOMAS MILLER, BS
Department of Orthopaedic Surgery,
The University of Minnesota, Minneapolis,
Minnesota

KATE W. NELLANS, MD, MPH
Hand Fellow, Section of Plastic Surgery,
University of Michigan Health System,
University of Michigan, Ann Arbor, Michigan

NIKHIL OAK, MD
Senior Resident Orthopaedic Surgeon,
Department of Orthopaedic Surgery, University
of Michigan, Ann Arbor, Michigan

KAGAN OZER, MD
Associate Professor, Department of
Orthopaedic Surgery, University of Michigan,
Ann Arbor, Michigan

SURBHI PANCHAL-KILDARE, MD
Cary, Illinois

REY RAMIREZ, MD
Hand Surgery Fellow, Department of Plastic
Surgery, University of Texas Southwestern
Medical School, Dallas, Texas

MARCO RIZZO, MD
Department of Orthopedic Surgery, The Mayo
Clinic, Rochester, Minnesota

RACHEL S. ROHDE, MD
Assistant Professor of Orthopaedic Surgery,
Oakland University William Beaumont School
of Medicine, Beaumont Health System, Royal
Oak, Michigan

TAMARA D. ROZENTAL, MD
Assistant Professor, Harvard Medical
School - Beth Israel Deaconess Medical
Center, Department of Orthopaedic Surgery,
Boston, Massachusetts

DAVID RUTA, MD
Department of Orthopaedic Surgery, University
of Michigan, Ann Arbor, Michigan

DOUGLAS M. SAMMER, MD
Assistant Professor, Program Director Hand
Surgery Fellowship, Department of Plastic
Surgery, University of Texas Southwestern
Medical School, Dallas, Texas

CAITLIN E. SARACEVIC
York University, Toronto, Ontario, Canada

VIKRAM SATHYENDRA, MD
Chief Resident, Department of Orthopaedic
Surgery, Penn State Milton S. Hershey Medical
Center, Hershey, Pennsylvania

JENNIFER F. WALJEE, MD, MS
Assistant Professor, Section of Plastic
Surgery, Department of Surgery, University
of Michigan Health System, Ann Arbor,
Michigan

JENNIFER MORIATIS WOLF, MD
Associate Professor, Department of
Orthopaedic Surgery, New England
Musculoskeletal Institute, University of
Connecticut Health Center, Farmington,
Connecticut

Contents

nonoperative treatment options. Unfortunately, the scientific evidence to help guide decision making is not of high quality. Because of this, the surgeon must rely on a few basic principles to guide treatment. This article provides an overview of the scientific evidence, and discusses the principles and rationale used to treat hand fractures.

Metacarpal fractures are common, and many can be managed nonoperatively with appropriate reduction and immobilization. As with any hand fracture, the primary goals are to achieve anatomic and stable reduction, bony union, and early mobilization to minimize disability. Appropriate treatment requires a keen understanding of the types of fractures, their inherent stability, and the available treatment options. Functional outcomes depend on appropriate treatment and early range of motion whenever possible.

Treatment of phalangeal fractures depends on the characteristics of the fracture, condition of the soft tissue envelope, associated injuries, patient functional requirements, and surgeon familiarity and comfort with various techniques. Most phalangeal fractures can be treated successfully with nonoperative means. Surgery is considered to treat unstable injuries, articular incongruity, concomitant soft tissue damage, or other situations in which restoration of anatomy and preservation of function are achieved only via operative stabilization. Careful soft tissue handling and early mobilization are premises on which surgical phalangeal fracture treatment is based.

Fractures of the hand are common injuries and in particular, fractures involving the articular surfaces can present difficulties to the orthopedic surgeon in practice. Although the treatment of these fractures needs to be individualized based on fracture pattern and location, the goals for these fractures are to restore the alignment, stability, and congruity and to allow for early motion to prevent stiffness and traumatic arthritis. This article classifies the various types of intra-articular hand fractures as well as the workup and management of these injuries.

The evaluation, initial treatment, and definitive reconstruction of open fractures of the hand with associated soft tissue loss are reviewed. Specific attention is given to the literature on open fracture antibiotic prophylaxis in the hand; the timing of bone and soft tissue reconstruction; and options for soft tissue coverage, including local, regional, and distant tissue transfer. Factors that have shown association with outcomes in these injuries are also discussed, and the authors' preferred management is summarized.

Pediatric hand fractures are common childhood injuries. Identification of the fractures in the emergency room setting can be challenging owing to the physes and incomplete ossification of the carpus that are not revealed in the radiographs. Most simple fractures can be treated with appropriate immobilization through buddy taping, finger splints, or casting. If correctly diagnosed, reduced, and immobilized, these fractures usually result in excellent clinical outcomes.

Pathologic fractures occur in bone weakened by a disease process. In the hand, the most common cause of pathologic fracture is a solitary enchondroma, although many other less common causes exist, including bone cysts, benign and malignant tumors, and other rarer entities. Arriving at a correct diagnosis is the key to successful treatment. If the fracture seems the result of a benign process, the fracture can be allowed to heal prior to definitive treatment of the underlying lesion. Fractures associated with aggressive or malignant lesions require more urgent treatment, although the overall prognosis for pathologic fracture due to malignancy is poor.

The importance of rehabilitation in the management of hand fractures cannot be overstated. The breadth of rehabilitative strategies ranges from heat and range-of-motion exercises to more complex splinting and tendon gliding modalities. The goals, however, are clear: control pain; limit soft tissue swelling; provide support for fracture healing; restore motion, strength, and function; and enable the return to work and daily activities.

Regardless of the clinician's technical skill, the results of hand fracture treatment may not be optimal. Tissue planes are damaged by the initial trauma, and surgical approaches to restore bony anatomy or develop tendon gliding further violate them with scarring producing adhesions and motion deficits. Close communication with therapists may help reduce complications. Identification and prompt treatment of these complications may allow improved function. However, repeat surgery may be necessary to improve the results. It is critical to work with the patient to match expectations and to minimize frustration of both the patient and the surgeon.

There is no outcome measure designated as the gold standard when assessing the treatment results following fractures of the hand. Numerous measures have been described in the literature, but only a limited number have been validated to specifically evaluate functional recovery with respect to hand fractures. Of the outcome measures validated for use with hand fractures, few have been studied in comparative trials designed to analyze their ability to predict functional recovery. This review article provides an evidence-based description of the validated scales and scores frequently used in assessing the functional outcomes and their ability to predict recovery.

HAND CLINICS

HAND CLINICS

Preface

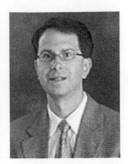

Jeffrey N. Lawton, MD
Editor

I am particularly proud of this issue of *Hand Clinics* regarding the care of Hand Fractures. As with other issues of *Hand Clinics*, we are able to go in-depth on a single important topic. In this case, something that we can all relate to—the care of hand fractures. Rarely, in one source, is one able to summarize all facets of a specific entity like Hand Fractures the way that *Hand Clinics* can. We look at the anatomy, basic science, biomechanics, soft tissue injuries, bone and joint involvement, pediatric-related issues, pathologic fractures, and various techniques for treatments. In addition, as more and more emphasis is made on the outcomes of our treatment and evidence-based medicine, we thought it would be helpful to evaluate the current state of outcomes research as it relates to hand fractures. Alas, much of our knowledge, reviewed and summarized in this edition of *Hand Clinics*, is based on level III and IV evidence. Finally, we address what happens and what to do when things don't go so well—evaluating our complications associated with hand fractures.

I am quite proud of the assembled work that we have put together. Representing some of the finest centers of hand care throughout America,

this group of authors has made a substantial contribution. I appreciate the significant amount of work that my colleagues have put into this *Hand Clinics* collection in contributions of time and their academic and clinical experience in this field. In addition, I would like to thank Jennifer Flynn-Briggs at Elsevier for her professional assistance. Last, I would like to thank Kevin Chung, my consulting editor, for his guidance and for giving me the opportunity to put this collection together for you.

Thank you,
Jeff

Jeffrey N. Lawton, MD
Associate Professor
Chief, Division of Elbow, Hand, and Microsurgery
University of Michigan
Department of Orthopaedic Surgery
1500 East Medical Center Drive TC 2912
Ann Arbor, MI 48109, USA

E-mail address:
jeflawto@med.umich.edu

Hand Clin 29 (2013) xi
http://dx.doi.org/10.1016/j.hcl.2013.09.003

Skeletal Anatomy of the Hand

Surbhi Panchal-Kildare, MD[a], Kevin Malone, MD[b],*

KEYWORDS

• Hand anatomy • Phalanges • Metacarpals • Carpals

KEY POINTS

- Hand function is result of intricate interaction between the skeletal anatomy and the intrinsic and extrinsic hand musculature.
- Hand capable of performing precise fine motor tasks as well as tasks that require force and endurance.
- Knowledge of normal anatomy will allow for better understanding of the injured or abnormal hand.
- Anatomy knowledge is essential element in framework of constructing a treatment plan for patient care.

With the possible exception of our brain, the hand is truly man's greatest tool (**Figs. 1–3**).[1] Our evolution into upright biped creatures has allowed the continued development and refinement of this tool over time. Its function is a product of the complex interactions between the power provided by the intrinsic and extrinsic musculature, the stability provided by the ligaments, and the structure provided by the bones, which serve as insertion and attachment sites for the muscles and ligaments. This article provides a detailed description of the skeletal anatomy of the human hand.

The skeletal anatomy of the hand is composed of phalanges, metacarpal bones, and carpal bones. The metacarpal and phalanges move relative to each other and the carpal bones in primarily flexion and extension, allowing for both precise and powerful grasping.[2] Traditionally the carpal bones are considered part of the wrist joint, and contribute to stability and wrist motion in the sagittal and coronal planes. In addition, motion between the carpal bones contributes to forearm rotation and allows for the complex "dart-thrower's motion" (radial and ulnar deviation).[3] The thumb is structurally different from the other fingers because of the position it holds relative to the hand, the mobile carpometacarpal (CMC) articulation that allows for motion in 2 planes to allow prehension, and the fact that it has 1 fewer phalanx than the other digits.

PHALANGES

Phalanx and metacarpal fractures are the most common upper extremity fracture in an active/athletic population.[4] These fractures can result in restricted activity and days missed from work. Because of the economic consequences of these injuries, it is important to understand the anatomy of each of these bones so that the postinjury function can be fully maximized.

The distal phalanx has a base, shaft, and distal tuft. The base has the same width as the adjacent head of the middle phalanx at the distal interphalangeal (DIP) joint. The dorsal aspect of the distal phalanx base contains a central flare and a dorsal tubercle that serves as the insertion site for the terminal extensor tendon. On each side of the dorsal tubercle sit the lateral tubercles for attachment of the collateral ligaments of the DIP joint.[5] The palmar lip is known as the volar tubercle, and is the insertion site for the volar plate. The flexor digitorum profundus (FDP) tendon inserts onto a flat area just distal to the volar plate. The distal phalanx tuft is a wide ridge of bone that is crescent

[a] 1346 Collins Drive, Cary, IL 60013, USA; [b] Case Western Reserve University School of Medicine, Department of Orthopaedic Surgery, MetroHealth Medical Center, Cleveland, OH 44109, USA
* Corresponding author.
E-mail address: kmalone@metrohealth.org

Hand Clin 29 (2013) 459–471
http://dx.doi.org/10.1016/j.hcl.2013.08.001
0749-0712/13/$ – see front matter © 2013 Elsevier Inc. All rights reserved.

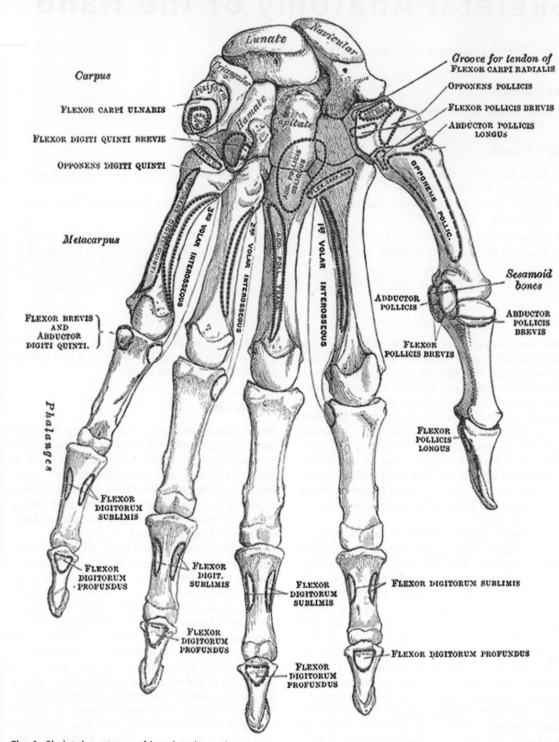

Fig. 1. Skeletal anatomy of hand, palmar view.

shaped. This structure supports the fingernail complex. Numerous septa connect the skin to the tuft and provide support for the pulp of the digit. The germinal matrix of the fingernail complex lies on the dorsal surface of the distal phalanx distal to the insertion site of the extensor tendon, and is the tissue responsible for the development and generation of the nail plate. The sterile matrix lies on the dorsal surface of the distal tuft and provides support and adherence for the fingernail.[6]

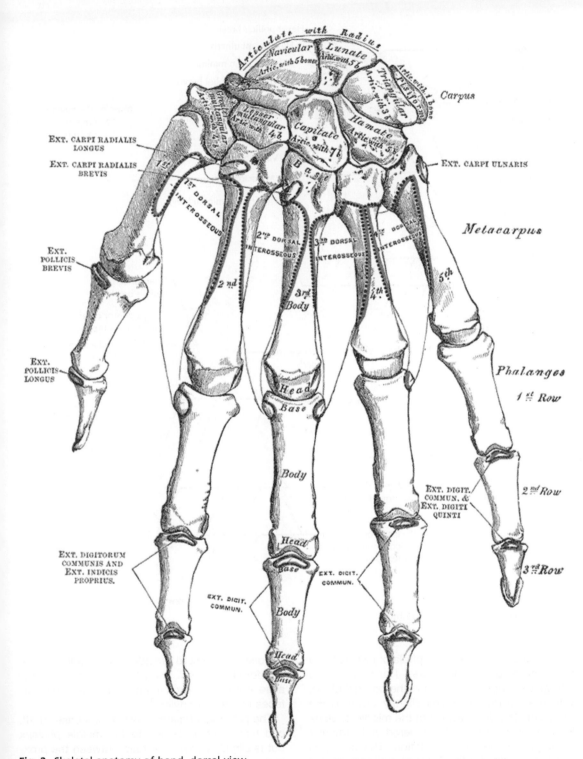

Fig. 2. Skeletal anatomy of hand, dorsal view.

The middle and proximal phalanges are similar in osteology, although there are particular distinct differences. On the middle phalanx the central slip of the extensor mechanism attaches to the proximal portion on the dorsal aspect. Along the sides

of this tubercle are ridges where the collateral ligaments of the proximal interphalangeal (PIP) joint insert. Just distal to this are multiple foramina for nutrient vessels. The flexor digitorum superficialis (FDS) tendon attaches to a flat area on the volar

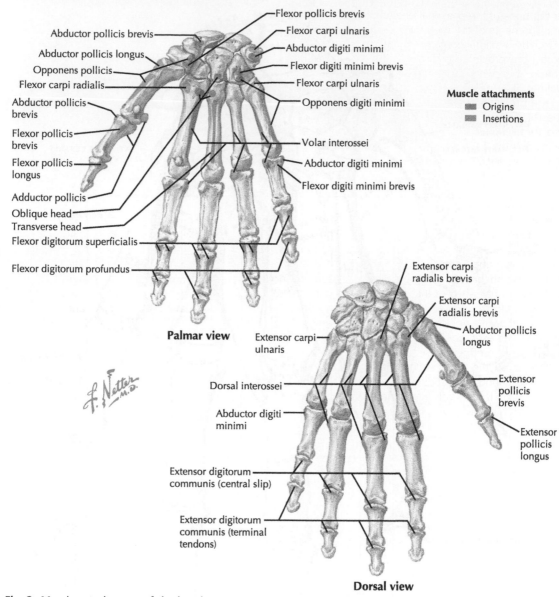

Abductor pollicis brevis
Abductor pollicis longus
Opponens pollicis
Flexor carpi radialis
Abductor pollicis brevis
Flexor pollicis brevis
Flexor pollicis longus
Adductor pollicis
Oblique head
Transverse head
Flexor digitorum superficialis
Flexor digitorum profundus

Flexor pollicis brevis
Flexor carpi ulnaris
Abductor digiti minimi
Flexor digiti minimi brevis
Flexor carpi ulnaris
Opponens digiti minimi
Volar interossei
Abductor digiti minimi
Flexor digiti minimi brevis

Muscle attachments
■ Origins
■ Insertions

Palmar view

Extensor carpi ulnaris
Dorsal interossei
Abductor digiti minimi
Extensor digitorum communis (central slip)
Extensor digitorum communis (terminal tendons)

Extensor carpi radialis brevis
Extensor carpi radialis brevis
Abductor pollicis longus
Extensor pollicis brevis
Extensor pollicis longus

Dorsal view

Fig. 3. Muscle attachments of the hand.

aspect of the middle of the phalanx just distal to the insertion of the volar plate.[7] The shaft has an hourglass shape when seen in the coronal plane, with the narrowest portion slightly distal to the midpoint. The distal aspect of the middle phalanx is composed of condyles covered with articular cartilage for the DIP articulation. The condyles provide stability for the PIP joint, which is important to note in the instability a unicondylar fracture provides. The joint surface extends further palmarly than dorsally, which allows for more flexion than extension. There is a groove between the 2 condyles of the middle phalanx head that corresponds to a ridge on the articular base of

the distal phalanx to provide stability and orientation for DIP motion. The DIP collateral ligaments arise from bony prominences on the outer surfaces of the 2 condyles.[5]

The proximal phalanx consists of a base, shaft, and head, and is similar to the middle phalanx but is slightly larger. The ratio between the proximal and middle phalanges is often 2:1 as seen on a radiograph. The proximal phalanx shaft has a slight convexity on the dorsal surface and slight concavity on the palmar surface. Along the base, the palmar surface contains a groove that supports the floor of the flexor tendon sheath. There are insertion sites on the radial and ulnar aspects of the base of the proximal phalanx for the collateral ligaments of the metacarpophalangeal (MCP) joint. The proximal phalanx shaft is smooth and tapers from proximal to distal. The shaft is oval in shape, but with the long axis from dorsal to palmar. The general shape of the articular head of the proximal phalanx and location of origin of the PIP collateral ligaments are similar to that of the middle phalanx, and the PIP joint motion is similar to the DIP joint motion. In contrast to the middle phalanx, there are no direct tendinous insertions onto the proximal phalanx. The extensor system's sagittal bands that insert onto the volar plate and flexor tendon sheath drive extension of the proximal phalanx at the MCP joint. Flexion at the MCP joint is driven primarily by the lumbrical and interosseus muscle tendinous insertions into the extensor apparatus.[8]

The thumb has only 2 phalanges, compared with the 3 phalanges of the fingers. The proximal phalanx of the thumb resembles the proximal phalanx of the remaining digits, but in general is shorter. The extensor pollicis brevis (EPB) tendon inserts onto a ridge on the dorsal base. There is a groove on the volar surface to accommodate the flexor tendon of the thumb. The distal phalanx of the thumb is markedly larger than the distal phalanges of the other digits; however, the characteristics of this bone are similar to those of other digits. The extensor pollicis longus (EPL) inserts on the dorsal base while the flexor pollicis longus (FPL) inserts on the volar base.[9]

The length of the proximal phalanges helps to provide the arch and function of the hand in actions such as pinch and grip. The thumb proximal phalanx is shorter than the rest of the digits, and resembles the length of the proximal phalanx of the small finger. The proximal phalanx of the middle finger is usually the longest, followed by the ring, index, and small. The same relationship is true for the middle phalanges. The distal phalanges are often similar in length, with the middle and ring fingers similarly followed by the index and small fingers.[5]

METACARPALS

The metacarpals' axis is parallel when looking at a lateral projection of the hand, but looking at the hand axially the metacarpals form an arch (**Fig. 4**). Because of this relationship, oblique radiograph views are important to adequately visualize the MCP and CMC joints. This spatial orientation is also important when fixing the skeleton of the hand.[7] Each metacarpal is unique in its articulations with the respective carpal bones as well as muscle attachments.[10]

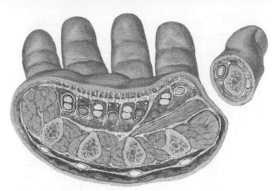

Fig. 4. Skeletal anatomy of hand, transverse arch created by the metacarpals.

The thumb metacarpal is distinctive in that the pronated position relative to the other metacarpals means the anatomic dorsal cortex actually faces laterally. This metacarpal is short and thick, and also differs anatomically from the rest of the metacarpals. The base of the thumb metacarpal is important in that it is saddle shaped to fit into the articulation with the trapezium. The base has a prominent palmar lip while also having expansions radially and ulnarly to form this saddle-shaped joint. When viewed in the sagittal plane this joint appears concave, and when viewed in the coronal plane it appears convex. This saddle joint is important in allowing the mobility of the thumb in 2 planes. Unlike the other metacarpals, the thumb metacarpal does not articulate with any of the adjacent metacarpals. **Fig. 5** illustrates the articulations and the shape of the metacarpal.[5]

The shaft of the thumb metacarpal is short and thick with a small canal. The dorsal portion is flat and wide, and somewhat triangular. Lengthwise, the shaft is mildly convex along the dorsal surface while it is concave along the palmar surface. There is a ridge along the radial cortex for insertion of the opponens pollicis muscle. There also is a smaller ridge along the ulnar cortex, which gives rise to the dorsal interosseous muscle. The head of the thumb metacarpal is rounded but less spherical than the other metacarpals. Because of this anatomy, the thumb MCP joint is more suited for pure hinge motion, and is more stable when radial directed force is applied when pinching.[11] The articular surface extends further palmarly than dorsally.

Four muscles attach to the thumb metacarpal: abductor pollicis longus (APL), opponens pollicis, first dorsal interosseous, and a small portion of flexor pollicis brevis (FPB). The APL inserts into a tubercle on the dorsal surface. The opponens inserts into an oval area on the radiopalmar surface

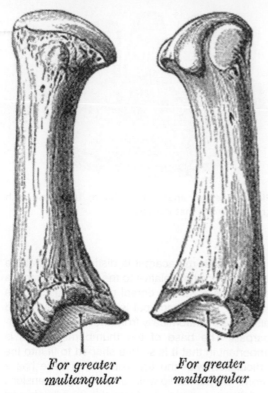

For greater multangular   *For greater multangular*

Fig. 5. Dorsal and palmar views of thumb metacarpal.

of the shaft. The first dorsal interosseous muscle is bipennate and partially originates on the thumb along the dorsomedial aspect. The FPB originates mainly on the transverse carpal ligament, trapezoid, and trapezium, but often there is a small slip that arises from the palmar, medial aspect of the base.[11]

The index metacarpal (**Fig. 6**) often is the longest metacarpal, with the largest base for articulation with the trapezoid and trapezium. Because this bone articulates with 2 carpal bones, it has more of a Y shape than an oval shape. The fork is larger medially and proximally. At the base of this metacarpal, the flexor carpi radialis (FCR) tendon attaches on the palmar surface and the extensor carpi radialis longus (ECRL) attaches on the dorsal surface. There are strong interosseous ligaments that hold the index metacarpal to the long metacarpal. Three interosseous muscles originate from the index metacarpal shaft. The MCP collateral ligaments arise from prominences on the radial and ulnar condyles. The articular head of the metacarpal is more prominent volarly. The added width of the volar aspect of the condyles relative to the dorsal width results in tightening of the collateral ligament and enhances MCP joint stability in flexion.[6]

The middle finger has the second longest metacarpal. The base of the third metacarpal articulates with the second and fourth metacarpals, as well as the carpal capitate (**Figs. 7** and **8**). The extensor carpi radialis brevis (ECRB) attaches on the dorsal surface. The adductor pollicis originates from the volar base along with the capitate. This metacarpal is unique in that there is a short projection that extends proximally from the radial side of the dorsal surface. This styloid process separates articular facets and serves as insertion for the intermetacarpal interosseous ligament. **Fig. 7** illustrates this styloid process and its location relative to the CMC articulations. The shaft of the third metacarpal is similar to the index metacarpal and is somewhat triangular in cross section. The dorsal surface is somewhat flat in comparison with the palmar surface, which allows for gliding of the extensor tendons. The head of this metacarpal is similar in morphology to the index finger. Finally, there are 2 dorsal interosseous muscles that originate on the shaft, which provide vascularity and connection to the surrounding bones.[5]

The ring-finger and small-finger metacarpals are noticeably shorter and thinner than the index-finger and long-finger metacarpals. It is essential to recognize this width to choose the correct plate when fixing a fracture.[4] Of note, the ring metacarpal most often has the smallest diameter, which may affect intramedullary fixation. Proximally, the fourth metacarpal articulates with the third and fifth metacarpals, and the capitate and hamate bones. Muscle attachments include the third and fourth dorsal interosseous muscles as well as the second palmar interosseous muscle. A minor ridge that is similar to those in other metacarpals separates these muscles.

The base of the fifth metacarpal is larger than that of the fourth metacarpal, and slopes proximally and ulnarly. Proximally, the fifth metacarpal articulates with the fourth metacarpal and hamate. The articulation between the fifth metacarpal and hamate is somewhat saddle shaped (**Fig. 9**). Because of this orientation, the small-finger CMC joint is more mobile so as to manipulate and grasp objects of different size.[12] This mobility can be seen when forming a fist into a power grip. The metacarpals go from a straighter alignment to a more rounded alignment to create more power. The mobility at the fourth and fifth CMC joints allow for this function and movement, sometimes termed encompassment.[5]

Attachments to the small finger are most notable for the extensor carpi ulnaris and opponens digiti minimi. The fourth dorsal interosseous muscle also attaches to the shaft of the fifth metacarpal. The foramina for the nutrient vessels of these

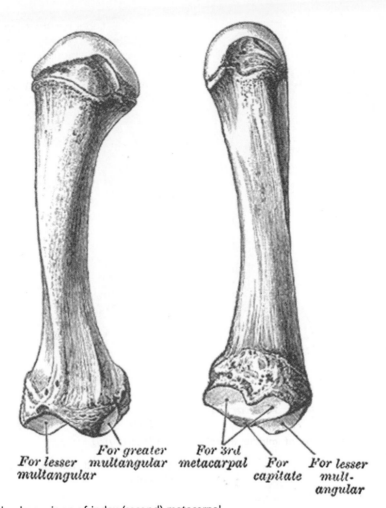

For lesser multangular   *For greater multangular*   *For 3rd metacarpal*   *For capitate*   *For lesser multangular*

Fig. 6. Dorsal and palmar views of index (second) metacarpal.

metacarpals are located at the base and head/neck regions.[6]

The index-finger and middle-finger CMC joints are very stable, with little observed motion. This stability derives from the shape of these joints and the ligamentous structure, and is useful for power pinch and precision. Conversely, the ring-finger and small-finger CMC joints demonstrate more motion in the sagittal plane because of the shape of these joints. This additional motion allows the hand to accommodate differently shaped objects and affords the ability for power grasp. However, like the thumb CMC joint, this additional motion and inherent less stability puts these joints at greater risk for fracture dislocation injuries.[13]

Metacarpal shaft fractures can often result in shortening. Because of the mobility of the hamate saddle joint, up to 20° of angulation is acceptable for transverse shaft fractures of the small and ring metacarpals. Owing to the lack of mobility of the index and long metacarpals at the carpal metacarpal joint, only 5° to 10° of angulation may be accepted in the index and long metacarpals,[10] thus demonstrating the importance of the bone's articulations in determining the functionality. A study demonstrated that 2 mm of shortening in the metacarpal can result in a 7° extensor lag[14]; this is a good example of the relationship between the bone and surrounding soft tissue and their resultant interaction in the function of the hand.

CARPALS

There are 8 carpal bones. The hamate, capitate, trapezoid, and trapezium make up the distal carpal row. The triquetrum, lunate, and scaphoid make up the proximal row. The pisiform, though considered one of the carpal bones, does not contribute significantly to the stability or function of the wrist joint. The carpus is contained entirely within the wrist capsule, and there are no muscle

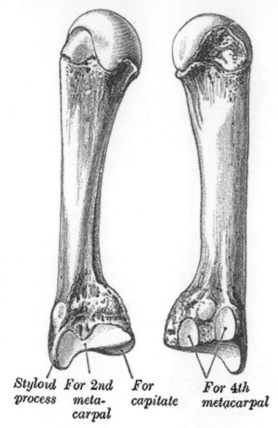

Styloid For 2nd   For   For 4th
process meta-   capitate   metacarpal
         carpal

Fig. 7. Dorsal and palmar views of middle (third) metacarpal.

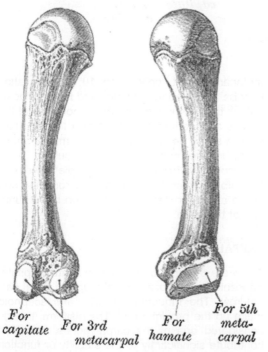

For   For 5th
capitate   For 3rd   For meta-
           metacarpal hamate carpal

Fig. 8. Dorsal and palmar views of ring (fourth) metacarpal.

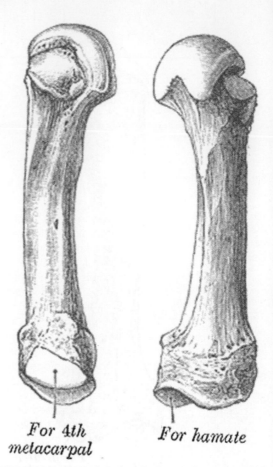

For 4th   For hamate
metacarpal

Fig. 9. Dorsal and palmar views of small (fifth) metacarpal.

or tendon insertions onto any of these bones except for the pisiform, which lies partially within the flexor carpi ulnaris tendon. Tendons that cross the wrist joint power the motion of these bones through the intercarpal and radiocarpal joints.[2] The proximal and distal rows tend to move independently of each other, but are linked to each other by the scaphoid bone and the complex ligamentous anatomy.[15]

The hamate consists of a body, a proximal pole, and a hook (**Fig. 10**). The name is derived from the Latin *hamatus*, which means "hooked." It articulates with the fourth and fifth metacarpals, capitate, and triquetrum. The hook is located on the distal portion of the palmar surface, and serves as an attachment of the transverse carpal ligament. There is a groove for the deep branch of the ulnar nerve around the ulnar and distal aspect of the hook at its base. The radial side of the hook is smooth, and the flexor tendons to the small finger glide along this surface. The close association of the ulnar motor nerve branch and the small-finger flexor tendon can affect the clinical

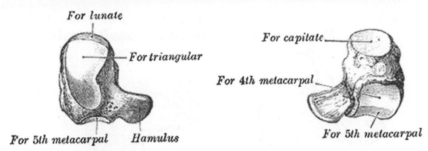

Fig. 10. Medial and lateral views of hamate.

scenario of a hook fracture/nonunion. The opponens digiti minimi and flexor digiti minimi originate from the palmar ulnar surface of the hook of hamate. The body of the hamate is triangular, and the surfaces are covered in roughened areas where carpal ligaments attach. Distally there are articulations for the fourth and fifth metacarpals, with the fifth finger metacarpal articulation being larger.[16] These articulations are concave and allow for movement within these joints. The arc of concavity is similar to that of the proximal phalanx base. For this reason, osteoarticular grafts have been harvested for reconstruction of unstable proximal phalangeal base fractures.[7]

The capitate is the largest and most central of all the carpal bones (**Fig. 11**). The name is derived from the Latin *capitatus*, which means "having a head." It articulates predominantly with the lunate, scaphoid, trapezoid, hamate, and third metacarpal.[5] There are also smaller articulations with the triquetrum, and second and fourth metacarpals. There is a slight waist that is created by a curve that is on the dorsal, radial, and ulnar surfaces. The capitate is larger distally. Vascular foramina exist on the capitate on the nonarticular surfaces of the dorsal and palmar aspects. These vessels course proximally within the bone and supply the body and head in a retrograde fashion.[17] The dorsal

surface is roughened for the attachment of the dorsal carpal ligaments, which can be seen in the corresponding figure.

The trapezoid is the smallest bone of the distal row of the carpal bones (**Fig. 12**). The name is derived from the Greek *trapezion*, meaning "irregular quadrilateral." The trapezoid articulates with the scaphoid, trapezium, capitate, and second metacarpal. The palmar portion is smaller than the dorsal portion. The FPB and, occasionally, the oblique head of the adductor pollicis originate from the trapezoid. This bone is well protected; therefore, fracture of the trapezoid is rare.[15]

The trapezium sits at the base of the thumb metacarpal and is the most radially located carpal bone in the distal row. There are articulations with the scaphoid, trapezoid, and second and first metacarpals (**Fig. 13**). The dorsal surface is roughened and contains a groove for the radial artery. The palmar surface is comparatively narrow and contains a groove for the FCR, with the transverse carpal ligament spanning this groove. There is a ridge radial to the groove for the attachment of the transverse carpal ligament so that, although the FCR tendon lies below the transverse carpal ligament, it is not in the carpal tunnel. The abductor pollicis brevis, opponens pollicis, and FPB also originate from the palmar surface

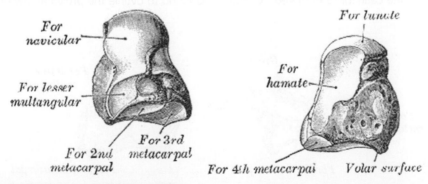

Fig. 11. Lateral and medial views of the capitate.

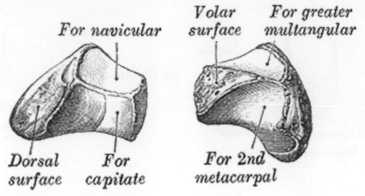

Fig. 12. Lateral and medial views of trapezoid.

of the trapezium. The lateral surface of the trapezium is roughened and provides attachment for the carpal ligaments. The proximal articulation with the scaphoid is smaller than the distal surface. This articulation is larger, oval shaped, and saddle shaped to allow for the circumduction movement of the thumb.[9] Although the trapezoid is supplied by branches from the dorsal and palmar blood sources, the main blood supply is from the dorsal supply. The dorsal surface is broad and flat to allow for 3 or 4 small vessels to enter the bone.

The axis of the trapezium-metacarpal allows for optimum functional positioning of the thumb. The axis sits in a pronated position and approximately 80° flexed relative to the rest of the metacarpals. The trapezium is approximately one-third smaller in size than the metacarpal. Because of the saddle-shaped nature of the trapezium-first metacarpal joint and the size differential between the metacarpal and the trapezium, there is little inherent osseous stability for the joint. Therefore, there are 16 ligaments that provide constraint to allow for pinch and grasp with the thumb.[9]

The triquetrum is pyramid shaped, the name being derived from the Latin for "3-cornered." Owing to its shape, the triquetrum has several surfaces: proximal, distal, lateral, dorsal, and palmar. The proximal surface lies medial and "articulates" with the triangular fibrocartilage complex.[3] The triquetrum articulates with 3 bones in total: the lunate, the pisiform, and the hamate (Fig. 14). The distal surface is smooth for articulation, and articulates with the medial surface of the hamate. It is the contour of this portion of the triquetral-hamate joint that creates an extension moment on the triquetrum. The dorsal surface is roughened for attachments of the carpal ligaments. The palmar surface is smooth and articulates with the pisiform. Vascularity of this bone comes from branches of the ulnar artery. There is usually a ridge on the dorsal surface of the triquetrum that contains the vascular foramina. Two to 4 vessels enter this ridge to supply about 60% of the bone, and this is the main blood supply. Although this bone is well placed beneath the ulnar styloid, it is the third most fractured carpal bone and should be visualized well on a radiograph.[3]

The pisiform's name is derived from the Latin *pisum*, which means pea. Most notably, the pisiform (Fig. 15) is a sesamoid bone and is within the flexor carpi ulnaris tendon sheath. The pisiform is found to overlie the proximal row of the carpus

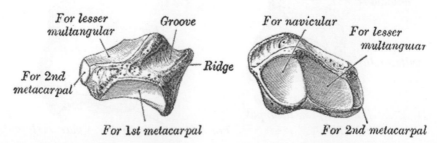

Fig. 13. Palmar and medial views of trapezium.

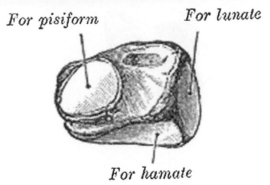

For pisiform   *For lunate*

For hamate

Fig. 14. Palmar view of triquetrum.

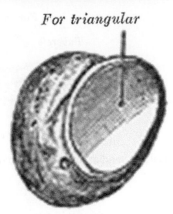

For triangular

Fig. 15. Palmar view of pisiform.

and articulates with the triquetrum, as this bone sits anterior to the rest of the carpal bones. Therefore, the dorsal surface is smooth for this articulation but the palmar surface is roughened for attachment of the transverse carpal ligament, flexor carpi ulnaris, and abductor digiti minimi.[5]

The lunate is a hemi-moon shape as seen on the lateral radiograph; the name comes from the Latin *luna*, which means moon (**Fig. 16**). The dorsal and palmar surfaces are roughened for the attachment of intrinsic and extrinsic carpal ligaments. The palmar surface is roughly triangular and is larger than the dorsal surface. The distal and proximal surfaces are covered with articular cartilage. The proximal surface articulates with the lunate fossa of the radius. The distal surface articulates with the capitate. The lateral surface articulates with the scaphoid, and the medial surface articulates with the triquetrum and hamate.[5]

In a majority of cases, the lunate receives its blood supplies from both the palmar and dorsal sources. In approximately 20% of cases the lunate receives its blood supply only from the palmar surface. The majority of the lunate is covered with articular cartilage and, therefore, no other vessels

enter the lunate.[7] The dorsal supply comes from the dorsal radiocarpal arch, dorsal intercarpal arch, and branches from the anterior interosseous artery. The palmar source includes the palmar intercarpal arch, palmar radiocarpal arch, and branches from the anterior interosseous artery and ulnar recurrent artery. The vessels that come from the palmar surface are larger and more prominent.

The scaphoid has been studied and illustrated since the 1500s and yet is still not completely understood. The name comes from the Greek *skaphos*, which means "boat" (**Fig. 17**). Often the scaphoid is called the navicular bone of the wrist, as there is also a similar bone in the ankle. The scaphoid bone is located proximally and radially, and is the largest bone of the proximal carpal row. The scaphoid is important in biomechanically linking the proximal and distal rows of the carpal bones.[18] Approximately 75% of the surface is covered in articular cartilage. It articulates proximally with the radius (the scaphoid fossa), medially with the capitate and lunate, and distally with the trapezium and trapezoid. The axis of the scaphoid is directed distally, laterally, and palmarly. It must be borne in

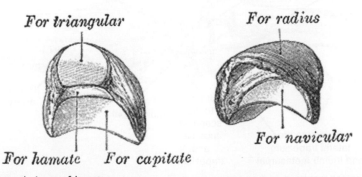

For triangular   *For radius*

For hamate   *For capitate*   *For navicular*

Fig. 16. Distal and lateral views of lunate.

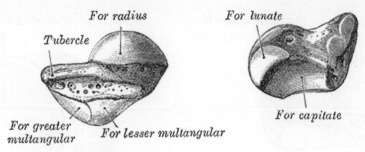

Fig. 17. Dorsal and medial views of scaphoid.

mind that the scaphoid sits in a plane at approximately 45° to the longitudinal axis of the wrist. The net force on the scaphoid is a flexion moment. There are significant insertions of carpal ligaments onto the scaphoid, including the radioscaphocapitate (RSC) ligament, scaphotrapezium-trapezoid (STT) ligament, and radioscapholunate (RSL) ligament, among others.[5] The scapholunate interosseous ligament is U-shaped and extends from the palmar, proximal, and dorsal aspect of the ulnar base to the lunate. The dorsal limb is the thickest and strongest. The scaphoid consists of a tuberosity, body, and proximal pole.[19]

The scaphoid primarily receives its blood supply from the radial artery. The scaphoid is like the lunate and has an extensive articular cartilage surface. The dorsal blood supply accounts for 70% to 80% of the vascularity of the scaphoid.[20] The dorsal supply enters the bone through the small foramina located on the dorsal ridge in the region of the waist. The radial artery splits into 2 branches, with 1 branch going to the dorsum of the wrist; the other is palmar and runs up the second metacarpal. The proximal pole of the scaphoid gets its blood supply, in a dependent fashion, from this source and, therefore, the blood supply is retrograde and needs to be protected.[20] Fig. 18 illustrates the radial artery projection and dorsal blood supply to the carpus.

Appreciation and knowledge of the skeletal anatomy of the hand is crucial in properly providing a framework to the treatment of hand disorders. Understanding of each bone, its attachments, and its articulations is important in recognizing pathologic, degenerative, and traumatic conditions of the hand. The interactions between these bones, the power provided by forearm and hand musculature, and the stability of the ligamentous structures result in the vast array of tasks that this tool can accomplish. With 27 bones, interaction among those bones allows for the smooth motion of the hand that provides alignment for various grips such as power, cylindrical, spherical, and hook, as well as the differing types of pinch. An understanding of this functional anatomy allows fuller comprehension of the daily use of the hand.

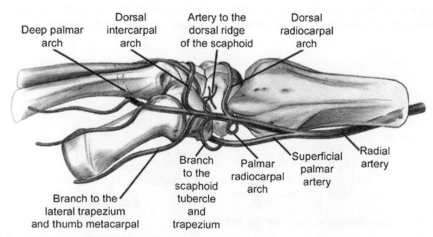

Fig. 18. Vascular tree for scaphoid and carpus.

REFERENCES

1. Alemohammad AM, Nakamura K, El-Sheneway M, et al. Incidence of carpal boss and osseous coalition: an anatomic study. J Hand Surg 2009;34(1):1–6.

2. Kjima Y, Viegas SF. Wrist anatomy and biomechanics. J Hand Surg 2009;34(8):1555–63.

3. Vezeridis PS, Yoshioka H, Han R, et al. Ulnar-sided wrist pain. Part I: anatomy and physical examination. Skeletal Radiol 2010;39(8):733–45.

4. Geissler WB. Operative fixation of metacarpal and phalangeal fractures in athletes. Hand Clin 2009; 25(3):409–21.

5. Landsmeer J. Atlas of anatomy of the hand. Edinburgh (United Kingdom): Churchill Livingstone; 1976.

6. Doyle JR, Botte MJ. Surgical anatomy of the hand and upper extremity. Philadelphia: Lippincott Williams and Wilkins; 2003.

7. Wiesel SW. Operative techniques in orthopaedic surgery. Philadelphia: Wolters Kluwer and Lippincott Williams and Wilkins; 2011.

8. Liss FE. The interosseous muscles: the foundation of hand function. Hand Clin 2012;28:9–12.

9. Leversedge FJ. Anatomy and pathomechanics of the thumb. Hand Clin 2008;24:219–29.

10. Green DP. Green's operative hand surgery. 5th edition. Philadelphia: Elsevier Churchill Livingstone; 2005.

11. Boden ND, Spangler R, Thoder JJ. Interposition arthroplasty options for carpometacarpal arthritis of the thumb. Hand Clin 2010;26(3): 339–50.

12. Slutsky DJ. Arthroscopic reduction and percutaneous fixation of fifth carpometacarpal fracture dislocations. Hand Clin 2011;27(3):361–7.

13. Nakamura K, Patterson RM, Viegas SF. The ligament and skeletal anatomy of the second through fifth carpometacarpal joints and adjacent structures. J Hand Surg 2001;26(6):1016–29.

14. Strauch RJ, Rosenwasser MP, Lunt JG. Metacarpal shaft fractures: the effect of shortening on the extensor tendon mechanism. J Hand Surg 1998; 23(3):519–23.

15. Cohen MS. Fractures of carpal bones. Hand Clin 1997;13(4):587–99.

16. Yoshida R, Shah MA, Patterson RM, et al. Anatomy and pathomechanics of ring and small finger carpometacarpal joint injuries. J Hand Surg 2003;28(6): 1035–43.

17. Cardoso R, Szabo RM. Wrist anatomy and surgical approaches. Hand Clin 2010;26:1–19.

18. Buijze GA, Lozano-Calderon SA, Strackee SD, et al. Osseous and ligamentous scaphoid anatomy: part I. A systematic literature review highlighting controversies. J Hand Surg 2001;36:1926–35.

19. Slade JF 3rd, Milewski MD. Management of carpal instability in athletes. Hand Clin 2009;25(3):395–408.

20. Buijze GA, Othman L, Ring D. Management of scaphoid nonunion. J Hand Surg 2012;37(5): 1095–100.

Basic Science of Bone Healing

Vikram Sathyendra, MD, Michael Darowish, MD*

KEYWORDS

- Fracture healing • Primary healing • Secondary healing

KEY POINTS

- Fracture healing is impacted by both biology and the mechanical environment.
- Mesenchymal stem cells can be attracted locally and systemically to a fracture site and undergo differentiation into chondrocytes or osteoblasts.
- Multiple growth factors can influence fracture healing.
- Angiogenesis, blood supply, and high oxygen tension is required for new bone to form.
- Mechanical stability enhances angiogenesis.
- Nonsteroidal anti-inflammatory drugs, bisphosphonates, smoking, diabetes, and age can negatively impact fracture healing.

INTRODUCTION

Bone can be injured from a variety of mechanisms, including trauma, infection, tumors, and compromised blood supply. Bone healing is a physiologic process that replaces the injured bone with new bone, thereby renewing the biologic and mechanical properties to the preinjured state.[1] This process involves a complex interplay of events playing out in the biologic environment proximal to the site of injury coupled with the impact of mechanical forces on this local milieu.

Immediately following injury, a physiologic process is triggered in which cells are attracted to the site of injury to mediate the inflammatory process and contribute to the replacement of necrotic bone with new bone matrix. In the setting of trauma, the inherent stability of the bone and the vascular supply are both disrupted. Restoration of absolute stability at the fracture site will result in healing through intramembranous ossification or primary bone healing, with minimal callus formation.[2] This involves reestablishing blood supply at the site of the fracture by establishing new Haversian systems, and eventually replacing any necrotic bone by osteoclastic excavation and osteoblastic deposition of new bone in a process similar to physiologic homeostatic remodeling.[3] Similar to healing that occurs after rigid plating, in the setting of infection, tumors, and avascular necrosis, bone heals through mechanisms resembling intramembranous ossification.[1]

In the case in which significant motion at the injury site is caused by unavoidable mechanical force, restoring the bone to a state of relative stability at the fracture site will be driven by the formation of an intermediate cartilaginous callus that ultimately becomes ossified. This process is referred to as enchondral ossification and it entails attraction of stem cells, the formation of a cartilage scaffold, conversion of this cartilage scaffold (ie, callus) into woven bone (primary remodeling), and finally remodeling of the woven bone callus into the anatomically correct lamellar structure (secondary remodeling). Most fractures heal with a combination of both intramembranous and enchondral ossification.[1,4,5] To adequately understand both processes, we must understand the basics of host biology and the influence of the external mechanical environment.

The authors have no financial disclosures.
Department of Orthopaedic Surgery, Penn State Milton S. Hershey Medical Center, 30 Hope Drive, PO Box 859, Hershey, PA 17033, USA
* Corresponding author.
E-mail address: mdarowish@hmc.psu.edu

Hand Clin 29 (2013) 473–481
http://dx.doi.org/10.1016/j.hcl.2013.08.002
0749-0712/13/$ – see front matter © 2013 Elsevier Inc. All rights reserved.

hand.theclinics.com

HOST BIOLOGY

For any tissue in the human body to regenerate, basic requirements must be met. These include the presence of progenitor cells, the creation of a scaffold or extracellular matrix (ECM) produced by these cells, growth factor–mediated differentiation of progenitor cells into the desired cell type (chondrocyte, vascular endothelial cell, osteoblast, osteoclast), and an adequate blood supply to provide oxygen tension, nutrients, energy, and minerals.

PROGENITOR CELLS

When a fracture occurs, mesenchymal stem cells (MSCs) both from local surrounding tissue and systemic circulation enter the fracture site, proliferate, and differentiate into chondrocytes, osteoblasts, or osteoclasts. We know from studies more than a century ago that osteoprogenitor cells exist in bone marrow. When heterotopic bone marrow autograft was injected into tissue, bone formation occurred.[6] Current thinking suggests that the periosteum provides a major source of osteoblast precursor cells. Additional studies have shown that osteoblast precursors can also be found in the endosteum and Haversian canals of bone, as well as the cambial layer of periosteum and stromal portion of bone marrow.[1,6] In rodents, cells from the endosteum and marrow stroma proliferate to produce more than 50% of the new bone after the implantation of cancellous allografts. Additionally, endosteal cells have been found to stain for alkaline phosphatase and respond to parathyroid hormone (PTH), 2 markers of osteoblast activity.[6]

In addition to local sources of progenitor cells, osteoblast precursors can be recruited from the systemic circulation. Shirley and colleagues[7] used a rabbit ulnar osteotomy model to show that fluorescently labeled bone marrow MSCs injected into remote bone marrow would still repopulate the fracture site. Shen and colleagues[8] showed in a murine model that pluripotent MSCs injected into tail veins preferentially locate to a fracture site. From these studies it is clear that recruitment of osteoblast precursors not only occurs locally, but also systemically. There are molecules produced at the fracture site that both attract progenitor cells and also bind them. This involves a complex interaction between osteoblasts, growth factors, and the ECM.

ECM

The major role of the ECM is to provide structural support and to serve as a scaffold for new bone formation after injury. The ECM is primarily composed of collagen, proteoglycans that contain glycosaminoglycans (GAGs), and glycoproteins. Bone is primarily made up of collagen types I and IV, whereas cartilage is made up of collagen types II, IX, X, and XI. There are numerous GAGs in bone and cartilage, such as chondroitin sulfate A, which bind hyaluronic acids. Finally there are numerous glycoproteins that serve to bind to other ECM components, such as fibronectin and vitronectin.[1,9,10]

Collagen is the main structural protein in bone as well as cartilage. Numerous studies in the tissue engineering field have investigated the use of recombinant collagen as a scaffold for bone growth to be used in the treatment of segmental bone defects. Engineered recombinant collagen scaffolds, when combined with bone marrow, have been shown to be efficient in the treatment of segmental bone defects in the rabbit model.[11]

In addition to serving as a scaffold for osteogenesis, multiple components of the ECM are involved in the migration, adhesion, and proliferation of MSCs. Ode and colleagues[9] examined 13 components of the ECM to determine their effects on cell migration, adhesion, and proliferation. They found that collagen types I to IV and fibronectin stimulated cell migration, adhesion, and proliferation. Although vitronectin, chondroitin sulfate, heparin, and hyaluronic acid all stimulated adhesion and proliferation, they had no effect on migration. Finally, they found laminins to have an inhibitory effect on cell adhesion.

GROWTH FACTORS

Fracture repair is regulated by a variety of growth factors, such as platelet-derived growth factor (PDGF), fibroblast growth factor (FGF), insulinlike growth factor-1 (IGF-1), members of the Wnt/beta-catenin signaling family, PTH, and the transforming growth factor-beta (TGF-β) superfamily, which includes bone morphogenetic proteins (BMPs).[1,5,12,13]

FGF

Immediately after a fracture occurs, an initial hematoma forms that contains numerous growth factors, including FGF. FGFs have been linked to osteoblast and chondrocyte proliferation, as well as angiogenesis. Numerous studies have examined the effects of basic FGF (bFGF) on the healing of fractures and callus strength in the animal model. The bFGF has been shown to increase callus size and significantly increase the strength of the repaired fracture. In addition, bFGF can induce MSCs to differentiate into prechondrocytes and preosteoblasts.[1,12]

PDGF

PDGF has a stimulating effect on fracture healing. Tibial osteotomy models in rabbits treated with PDGF showed a more robust and mechanically more stable fracture callus compared with controls. Additionally, histologic specimens from fractured tibiae showed more mature osteoblasts when compared with control specimens.[1,12]

IGF-1 and Growth Hormone

IGF-1 plays a role in normal development and achievement of maximal skeletal growth. Studies investigating the effects of IGF-1 on fracture healing have been mixed. Some studies have shown that high doses of human growth hormone, which in turn stimulates IGF-1 production, stimulates fracture healing, whereas other studies have shown no significant difference in fracture strength or callus size after injection of growth hormone.[1,12] For this reason, development of modalities to enhance fracture repair have not commonly involved IGF-1.

TGF-β

TGF-β has a positive effect on fracture healing. Systemic as well as locally injected TGF-β can increase fracture callus size and strength. Lind and colleagues[14] found that TGF-β increased bending strength and callus size in rabbits with mid-tibial osteotomies, whereas TGF-β had no effect on stiffness, bone mineral content, and Haversian canal diameter. Overall, the stimulating effects of TGF-β on fracture healing appears to be very minor and may be linked in part with a member of its superfamily of proteins: BMP.[1,12]

BMPs

BMPs were first described by Urist in 1965.[15] Since then, there have been multiple studies showing the stimulatory effects of BMPs on fracture healing and osteoinduction. Recombinant BMPs (rhBMP-2 and rhBMP-7) have been successfully used clinically in the treatment of open fractures, fracture nonunions, and spinal fusions.[5,12,13,16]

Numerous animal studies have examined the use of BMP-2 in the treatment of segmental defects. Kirker-Head and colleagues created a segmental defect in sheep femora and subsequently treated these defects with a copolymer of polylactic/glycolic acid augmented with 2 mg BMP-2, 4 mg BMP-2, or autologous blood. They found increased union rates in the groups treated with copolymers augmented with BMP-2 compared with the group treated with autologous blood.[17] Additionally, Cook and colleagues used a rabbit model to show the efficacy of BMP-7 in stimulating fracture healing. They created a segmental defect in the mid diaphysis of ulnae in rabbits that were filled with nothing, allograft, or allograft treated with BMP-7. Results showed the BMP-treated specimens to have mechanical strength equivalent to the nonfractured ulna at 8 weeks. The ulnae implanted with allograft or nothing showed no bridging of the fracture defect.[18]

There have been many clinical studies investigating the efficacy of BMPs in fracture healing. Jones and colleagues[19] randomly assigned patients with segmental tibial defects to receive treatment with either autograft or allograft augmented with BMP-2. Both groups had similar clinical as well as radiographic outcomes at all time points. A similar study showed the efficacy of rhBMP-7 in the treatment of segmental fibular defects in patients.[5,12,13]

β-Catenin/Wingless-Type Signaling

Wingless-type (Wnt) proteins are glycoproteins that are known to influence normal limb development. Recent studies have shown that they play a role in early fracture healing as well. There are several pathways through which Wnt proteins work. The most understood pathway involves stabilizing β-catenins. Wnt binds Frizzled (Fzd) receptor, which in turn recruits low-density lipoprotein receptor-related proteins (LRP5 or 6). This then inhibits the phosphorylation of β-catenin, which in turn inhibits the degradation of β-catenin by proteosomes. As intracellular β-catenin levels increase, β-catenin translocates into the nucleus, where it associates with transcription factors, T-cell factor, and lymphoid-enhancing factor.[20] The net effect of the Wnt/β-catenin signaling pathway is enhanced bone formation.

In the first 3 to 5 days after a fracture occurs, the levels of Wnt proteins, Fzd proteins, LRP5, LRP6, and β-catenin all increase. In mouse models, conditional knockouts of β-catenin from osteoblasts led to a reduction of callus and nonunion, whereas transgenic expression of β-catenins in osteoblasts led to increased fracture healing. In addition, inhibitors of the Wnt pathway, specifically Dkk1 and sclerostin, have been shown in animal models to have an inhibitory effect on fracture healing. Finally, stabilization of β-catenins and LRP-6 play crucial roles in PTH-induced bone formation.[20,21]

In addition to growth factors, the fracture hematoma and matrix produce factors that stimulate vascular ingrowth.

ANGIOGENESIS

Immediately after a fracture occurs, there is a disruption of the vascular supply to the surrounding bone. To regenerate bone and bridge the fracture site, new vessels must form. There are many molecules that enhance angiogenesis. Vascular endothelial growth factor (VEGF), in particular, has been the focus of much research. Prostaglandin E2 (PGE$_2$), a known stimulator of osteoblasts, increases the production of VEGF from osteoblasts. Additionally, IGF-1 has been shown to stimulate osteoblastic production of VEGF. Finally, the local mechanical environment directly affects the formation of new capillaries. Increasing strain in the fracture gap will result in the tearing of nascent vessels leading to a resultant decrease in capillary formation.[1,22,23] This is a primary driving force in the switch from intramembranous healing to enchondral healing in long bone fractures.

MECHANICAL ENVIRONMENT

The local forces surrounding a fracture are critical to bone regeneration and healing. We know from the Wolff law that bone remodels in response to stress and strain. Some amount of strain at the fracture site is beneficial to healing, whereas excess strain will result in formation of granulation tissue or fibrous tissue and eventually fracture nonunion.[1] In fact, the amount of strain influences the cellular response, the formation of capillaries, and the resultant tissue formed at a fracture site.[22,24,25]

Recently, there has been increased research looking into the effects of load on bone tissue from a cellular perspective. As bone is loaded, interstitial fluid flows through a 3-dimensional network of canaliculi, which is populated by osteocytes. It has been shown that exposing osteocytes to pulsating fluid flow results in a release of cell signaling molecules, specifically nitric oxide and prostaglandins (PGE$_2$ and PGI$_2$), and the Wnt family of proteins[24,25] from osteocytes and the subsequent formation of a callus.[24]

Grossly, increased strain can affect the ability to form capillaries and, as a result, tissues with high oxygen requirements, such as bone. In a sheep model, Claes and colleagues[22] demonstrated that vascularity and tissue formation is dependent on the amount of strain at the fracture site. They created an osteotomy in the sheep metatarsal, and using a dynamic external fixator, were able to vary the micro-motion at the fracture site. The resultant callus was analyzed for neovascularization and bone formation. They found significantly increased vessel and bone formation in fractures

that experienced low strain (<9%) compared with fractures experiencing high strain (>30%). A follow-up study by the same group created a finite element model to determine the strains and compressive pressures at which intramembranous ossification, enchondral ossification, and fibrous tissue formation occurred. They found that strains less than 5% with compressive or tensile pressures of 0.15 MPa or less were required for intramembranous ossification, strains of less than 15% with compressive pressures higher than 0.15 MPa were required for enchondral ossification, and any other conditions resulted in the formation of fibrous tissue.[26] Thus, gross instability at the fracture site leads to fibrocartilage formation, whereas increased stability results in increased vascularity and bone formation.

Understanding the basics of the biology and mechanical environment not only makes it easier to understand the fundamentals of fracture repair, but also provides insight into external factors that can effect fracture healing.

PRIMARY FRACTURE HEALING

Primary fracture healing, or intramembranous ossification, refers to healing that occurs without the formation of an intermediate cartilaginous callus. Immediately following a fracture, a hematoma forms and there is an inflammatory response. Platelets and macrophages enter the fracture site and begin to secrete inflammatory cytokines, such as interleukin 1 (IL-1) and IL-6, tumor necrosis factor alpha (TNF-α), and PGE$_2$.[2] These cytokines serve to attract progenitor cells that can differentiate into osteoblasts, endothelial cells, and osteoclasts. When the fracture ends are rigidly stabilized in contact with each other, the bridging of the fracture site occurs on a microscopic level and is mediated by the endosteal tissues, the Haversian systems, and the periosteum.[3]

In primary bone healing, the fracture ends are not resorbed, but rather new Haversian systems recannulate the fracture ends. When the ends are close enough in proximity, these Haversian systems can cross into the opposing fragment. The process of forming new Haversian systems, similar to physiologic bone remodeling, is thought to involve a close interaction between osteoclasts and osteoblasts. Once osteoclasts enter the fracture site, they form cutting cones, or canals through which osteoblasts can form osteons.[3] Once cutting cones are formed, there is an increase in VEGF, TGF-β, and BMPs (especially BMP-5 and 6).[27,28] This stimulates the production of new vessels by endothelial cells and new bone by osteoblasts. New lamellar bone is formed and the fracture is bridged primarily.

SECONDARY FRACTURE HEALING

Secondary fracture healing, or enchondral ossification, refers to healing that occurs via a cartilage callus. Enchondral ossification is observed when fracture ends do not directly contact one another or relative instability at the fracture exists, such as found in intramedullary nailing, bridge plating, or when external casting is used for stabilization. Just as in primary fracture healing, there is an inflammatory phase. After the inflammatory phase, new bone does not primarily bridge the fracture, but rather a cartilaginous callus forms, which is gradually replaced by bone.[1]

Inflammatory Phase

Similar to primary bone healing, the initial injury results in the formation of a fracture hematoma, which results in an inflammatory response. Again, platelets and macrophages enter the fracture site and begin to secrete inflammatory cytokines, such as IL-1 and IL-6, TNF-α, and PGE$_2$.[27,28] These cytokines recruit MSCs and chondroprogenitors/osteoprogenitors from various locations, including the marrow, muscle, peripheral blood, and periosteum. Additionally, the fracture hematoma serves as a demarcation zone for differentiating chondrocytes to begin creating a cartilage scaffold.[1]

Soft Callus Phase

Because of increased strain at the center of the fracture gap, new blood vessels cannot form, resulting in areas of low oxygen tension. Bone cannot form in areas of high strain or low oxygen tension; therefore, the formation of cartilage, which has low oxygen requirements, is favored.[22] MSCs have the ability to differentiate into osteoblasts as well as chondrocytes.[6] The local ischemia in the callus triggers the release of TGF-b2, TGF-b3, and growth differentiating factor (GDF-5) from degranulated platelets. This promotes differentiation of MSCs into chondrocytes.[27] Even more importantly, the low oxygen tension leads to activation of hypoxia inducible factor transcription factor, which is critical in the induction of VEGF production from chondrocytes.[29] Chondrocytes proliferate to create an initially cellular scaffold that is augmented by their secretion of type II collagen and proteoglycans. As the fracture gap fills with cartilage, mechanical stability increases, and chondrocytes undergo hypertrophic differentiation. This increased stability decreases strain, allowing neovascularization, which is modulated

by VEGF and other angiogenic factors (angiopoietins).[23] Macrophages and osteoclasts are attracted to the soft callus and remove the cartilage matrix. Finally, toward the end of the soft callus phase, there is an increase in the production of BMP-3, BMP-4, BMP-7, and BMP-8. These molecules serve to recruit osteoblasts, which eventually work to form woven bone.[27]

Hard Callus Phase

Following hypertrophy of the chondrocytes, primary callus remodeling begins. TNF-α, receptor-activated nucleated kinase ligand, macrophage colony-stimulating factor, and matrix mineralizing proteins are produced that activate osteoclasts, macrophages, and chondroclasts to resorb the callus. The cartilage is removed and chondrocytes undergo apoptosis.[27,30,31] Coordinated with the resorption of the cartilagenous callus is the osteoblast-driven creation of a woven bone callus that initiates at the peripheral regions and ultimately replaces the entire callus.

To reachieve the anatomically correct shape, secondary remodeling of the woven bone is initiated next. This is a gradual and continuous process that overlaps with the hard callus phase and can last for years. In this phase, woven bone is replaced by lamellar bone. IL-1 and IL-6 rise, and osteoblastic activity increases during remodeling. The callus remodels according to the Wolff law: increased bone formation in areas of high stress and resorption in areas of low stress. The entire phase is considered complete once a medullary cavity is reformed.[1,27,31]

DISTRACTION OSTEOGENESIS

Distraction osteogenesis is a process of bone regeneration in which a corticotomy is performed followed by gradual distraction, resulting in the formation of new bone. There are 3 stages in distraction osteogenesis: latency, distraction, and consolidation.[27]

Latency

The latency phase starts immediately after the creation of a minimally traumatic corticotomy and typically lasts between 3 and 10 days. Latency begins with an initial inflammatory response and culminates with the beginning of lengthening. The molecular response during this stage is similar to the inflammatory stage of enchondral ossification.[27,32]

Distraction

As the bone ends are distracted, angiogenesis is directly stimulated by mechanical forces. BMP-2 and BMP-4 expression is increased and osteo-blasts begin to lay down osteoid parallel to the vector of the line of tension, forming a regenerate. Similar to intramembranous ossification, there is no intermediate cartilage callus.[27,32] The distraction process is very sensitive to the velocity of distraction. Ilizarov[33] found that distracting at a rate of less than 0.5 mm per day resulted in premature consolidation of the regenerate and inability to achieve the desired lengthening, whereas lengthening at a rate greater than 2 mm resulted in less than ideal bone formation of the regenerate. The optimal distraction rate has been established to be 0.7 to 1.3 mm per day.[13]

Consolidation

Once the desired amount of distraction is achieved, the osteoid is mineralized and the bone formed undergoes remodeling similar to the final stage of enchondral ossification.[27]

PATIENT-RELATED FACTORS

There are numerous extrinsic factors and systemic factors in addition to intrinsic biology and the mechanical environment that can affect fracture healing.

Nonsteroidal Anti-Inflammatory Drugs

Nonsteroidal anti-inflammatory drugs (NSAIDs) inhibit the inflammatory response by directly inhibiting the enzyme cyclooxygenase-2 (COX-2). This in turn dramatically decreases the production of prostaglandins, including PGE_2, which are produced during the inflammatory stage of fracture repair and play a key role in cell migration and differentiation. COX-2 knockout mice showed a significantly delayed healing response when compared with wild-type mice. Additionally, histology from the nonunion site revealed undifferentiated MSCs. When MSCs from the bone marrow of the COX-2 knockout mice were cultured in vitro to form osteoblasts, the addition of PGE_2 or BMP stimulated osteoblastogenesis comparable to control MSCs.[34]

Clinical studies found an increased rate of delayed union and nonunion in patients taking NSAIDs shortly after developing a fracture.[5,30] Administration of even a single dose of NSAIDs in patients with tibial fractures have shown a delay in union of, on average, 7 weeks when compared with patients not receiving NSAIDs during treatment.[35]

Smoking

The effects of smoking have been investigated in both animal and clinical models. Nicotine administration slows cartilage differentiation and results in delayed hard callus formation. In a clinical study, smokers were found to be 37% more likely to develop a fracture nonunion after sustaining an open tibia fracture.[27] Additionally, the time to union in smokers with open tibia fractures was found to be on average 4 weeks longer.[5,30] Finally, nicotine has been implicated in the development of nonunion. Donigan and colleagues[36] found that rabbits treated with transdermal nicotine had a higher incidence of nonunion and weaker callus when compared with controls.

Diabetes

According to the National Diabetes Fact Sheet, there are 25.8 million patients with diabetes in the United States, approximately 8.3% of the population. Macey and colleagues[37] found that untreated diabetic rats had a 29% decrease in tensile strength and a 50% decrease in stiffness compared with controls 2 weeks after sustaining a fracture. Additionally, the collagen content of the callus in the untreated diabetic rats during the first 2 weeks after fracture was almost half as much as control rats. Interestingly, treating diabetic rats with insulin to normalize the blood sugar levels restored the mechanical and histologic properties of the callus to that of control rats. Clinically, studies have shown an increased risk of nonunion (38% in diabetic vs 27% in nondiabetic individuals) and a significantly increased time (163%–187%) to achieve union in diabetic patients.[38,39] Given these risks, it is imperative to tightly control blood glucose levels especially during the early phases of fracture healing, as well as to consider prolonged immobilization due to the expected slower rate of healing in these patients.

Age

As the average life span of our population increases, we are seeing an increasing number of fractures in elderly patients. Although there are numerous factors that can contribute to impaired healing in elderly patients, there is evidence that age is an independent factor that can delay fracture healing. Studies in rats have shown a decreased expression of BMP-2 in older rats, whereas levels of the BMP inhibitor (Noggin) remain the same. Additionally, serum from older donors was found to be a less potent stimulator of osteoblastic differentiation when compared with serum from younger patients.[5,37] Finally, there is an association with age and COX-2 production. Naik and colleagues[40] found a decrease of 75% in the expression of COX-2 in aged (52–56-week-old) mice when compared with young (7–9-week-old) mice.

Bisphosphonates

With an aging population, we are now treating an increasing rate of osteoporotic fractures. Many of these patients are concurrently being treated with bisphosphonates. Bisphosphonates decrease the rate of osteoclastic bone resorption. Although bisphosphonates have been a mainstay in the treatment of osteoporosis, Paget disease, and osteogenesis imperfecta, bisphosphonates delay fracture healing due to the inhibition of bone tunneling in intramembranous ossification and re-modeling in enchondral ossification by osteo-clasts.[30] Furthermore, because of half-lives that range from 1.5 to 10 years, bisphosphonates can remain in the skeleton for a prolonged period of time even after discontinuation.[41]

Radiographic studies have shown an in-creased rate of nonunion in proximal humerus fractures and delayed union with surgically treated distal radius fractures.[30] In younger pa-tients, we see similar effects of bisphosphonates on delayed healing. In children being treated for osteogenesis imperfecta, patients on bisphosph-onates experienced delayed union of osteotomy sites.[42]

Teriparatide

In 2002, the Food and Drug Administration approved teriparatide (Forteo) for use in osteopo-rosis. Forteo is a recombinant form of the initial 34 amino acids of PTH. PTH has a crucial role in bone metabolism. PTH serves to increase serum calcium levels in part by releasing stores from bone. PTH receptors are found on osteoblast membranes. Continuous exposure to PTH causes osteoblasts to secrete IL-1, which in turn stimu-lates osteoclasts to resorb bone. Intermittent exposure to PTH, however, causes stimulation of osteoblasts and formation of new bone.[30]

Intermittent PTH has been used to treat osteo-porosis. In a clinical study, investigators found a statistically significant increase in bone mineral density in patients treated with Forteo compared with patients not receiving Forteo. Additionally, there was decreased risk of vertebral fractures and long bone fractures in the Forteo-treated group. These results have led to investigators re-searching the effects of Forteo on the healing of long bone fractures.

In animal studies, mice treated with intermittent Forteo exhibited increased strength, stiffness, bone mineral content, and bone mineral density, while exhibiting a significant decrease in total cartilage callus volume.[43] In a case report, Rubery and colleagues[44] reported on 3 cases of painful odontoid fracture nonunions treated with Forteo that went on to heal. Additionally, Aspenberg and colleagues[45] found a statistically significant short-ened time to healing distal radius fractures in pa-tients treated with 20 μg of teriparatide when compared with placebo. These results support an enhanced fracture-healing rate in response to intermittent Forteo.[37] It is important to note that endogenous PTH levels must be normal for teri-paratide treatment to be effective; elevated PTH levels (which may be seen in Vitamin D deficiency, hyperparathyroidism, and other conditions) mask the intermittent peaks caused by the dosing, and render treatment ineffective.

Bone Stimulators (Electrical and Ultrasound)

External stimulation in the form of electrical signals or acoustic signals has been shown to stimulate fracture healing. The basis behind the enhanced healing rate is in part due to Wolff law and piezo-electric charges in bone. According to Wolff law, bone remodels in response to stress. In addition, bone is a piezoelectric tissue in that as it experi-ences stress, it builds an electrical charge. The compression side of bone is electronegative and stimulates osteoblasts, whereas the tension side of bone in electropositive and stimulates osteo-clasts. Because of the intrinsic charges present in bone, we can extrinsically manipulate these charges to enhance healing.[1]

Electrical stimulation occurs in many forms, including inductive coupling, capacitive coupling, and direct current. All methods generate an elec-tric field in bone. In inductive coupling, current pro-duces a magnetic field that in turn generates an electric field at the fracture site. In capacitive coupling, electrodes are placed on the skin and alternating current produces an electric field at the fracture site. In direct current stimulation, an electric field is generated by invasively placing a cathode at the fracture and an anode in soft tissue. The electric field generated, in turn, stimulates angiogenesis, chondrogenesis, and osteogenesis by upregulating the production of previously mentioned growth factors. Studies have shown that electrical stimulation enhances healing in known fracture nonunions.[1]

Ultrasound stimulates bone in a more mecha-nical manner. Low-intensity pulsed ultrasound (LIPUS) transmits energy to bone and enhances healing. The exact mechanism by which this oc-curs is yet to be elucidated. However, clinical studies have shown ultrasound to decrease the healing time of tibial and distal radius fractures when treated with closed reduction and cast immobilization.[1]

Future Directions

Recent animal studies have shown the importance of the Wnt signaling pathway in fracture healing. Sclerostin is a protein secreted by osteocytes that binds and antagonizes the LRP5/6 complex, thereby inhibiting the Wnt pathway. This in turn inhibits bone formation. Therefore, inhibition of sclerostin would increase fracture healing. Ominsky and colleagues[21] found that rats treated with sclerostin antibodies showed a statistically significant increase in callus area, bone mineral content, peak load (60% increase) and stiffness (149% increase). Similar results were also found in nonhuman primate models. These results support the use of sclerostin antibodies as an adjunct to enhance fracture healing.

SUMMARY

Bone regeneration is a complex process that involves several interacting biologic mechanisms and is a critical component of many aspects of musculoskeletal care, including fracture healing, spinal fusion, and osteointegration of implants. It is estimated that of the approximately 7.9 million fractures that occur in the United States each year, impaired healing complicates as many as 10% of all fractures. As we further understand the biologic and mechanical science behind fracture healing, and just as important, fracture nonunion, we can target therapies to enhance fracture repair.

ACKNOWLEDGMENTS

The authors would like to thank Michael Zuscik, PhD, for his thoughtful insights and comments on this article.

REFERENCES

1. Buckwalter JA, Einhorn TA, O'Keefe RJ, American Academy of Orthopaedic Surgeons. Orthopaedic basic science: foundations of clinical practice. 3rd edition. Rosemont (IL): American Academy of Orthopaedic Surgeons; 2007. p. 331–46.
2. Shapiro F. Bone development and its relation to fracture repair. The role of mesenchymal osteoblasts and surface osteoblasts. Eur Cell Mater 2008;15: 53–76.
3. McKibbin B. The biology of fracture healing in long bones. J Bone Joint Surg Br 1978;60-B(2):150–62.
4. Aro HT, Chao EY. Bone-healing patterns affected by loading, fracture fragment stability, fracture type,
5. and fracture site compression. Clin Orthop Relat Res 1993;(293):8–17.
5. Kwong FN, Harris MB. Recent developments in the biology of fracture repair. J Am Acad Orthop Surg 2008;16(11):619–25.
6. Wlodarski KH. Properties and origin of osteoblasts. Clin Orthop Relat Res 1990;(252):276–93.
7. Shirley D, Marsh D, Jordan G, et al. Systemic recruitment of osteoblastic cells in fracture healing. J Orthop Res 2005;23(5):1013–21.
8. Shen FH, Visger JM, Balian G, et al. Systemically administered mesenchymal stromal cells transduced with insulin-like growth factor-I localize to a fracture site and potentiate healing. J Orthop Trauma 2002;16(9):651–9.
9. Ode A, Duda GN, Glaeser JD, et al. Toward biomimetic materials in bone regeneration: functional behavior of mesenchymal stem cells on a broad spectrum of extracellular matrix components. J Biomed Mater Res A 2010;95(4):1114–24.
10. Musgrave DS, Fu FH, Huard J. Gene therapy and tissue engineering in orthopaedic surgery. J Am Acad Orthop Surg 2002;10(1):6–15.
11. Thibault RA, Mikos AG, Kasper FK. Scaffold/extracellular matrix hybrid constructs for bone-tissue engineering. Adv Healthc Mater 2012;2(1):13–24.
12. Bostrom MP, Saleh KJ, Einhorn TA. Osteoinductive growth factors in preclinical fracture and long bone defects models. Orthop Clin North Am 1999;30(4): 647–58.
13. Einhorn TA, Lee CA. Bone regeneration: new findings and potential clinical applications. J Am Acad Orthop Surg 2001;9(3):157–65.
14. Lind M, Schumacker B, Soballe K, et al. Transforming growth factor-beta enhances fracture healing in rabbit tibiae. Acta Orthop Scand 1993;64(5): 553–6.
15. Urist M. Bone: Formation by Autoinduction. Science 1965;150(3698):893–9.
16. Gazit D, Turgeman G, Kelley P, et al. Engineered pluripotent mesenchymal cells integrate and differentiate in regenerating bone: a novel cell-mediated gene therapy. J Gene Med 1999;1(2):121–33.
17. Gerhart TN, Kirker-Head CA, Kriz MJ, et al. Healing segmental femoral defects in sheep using recombinant human bone morphogenetic protein. Clin Orthop Relat Res 1993 Aug;(293):317–26.
18. Cook SD, Baffes GC, Wolfe MW, et al. The effect of recombinant human osteogenic protein-1 on healing of large segmental bone defects. J Bone Joint Surg Am 1994 Jun;76(6):827–38.
19. Jones AL, Bucholz RW, Bosse MJ, et al. Recombinant Human BMP-2 and Allograft Compared with Autogenous Bone Graft for Reconstruction of Diaphyseal Tibial Fractures with Cortical Defects: A Randomized, Controlled Trial. J Bone Joint Surg Am 2006 Jul;88(7):1431–41.

20. Secreto FJ, Hoeppner LH, Westendorf JJ. Wnt signaling during fracture repair. Curr Osteoporos Rep 2009;7(2):64–9.

21. Ominsky MS, Li C, Li X, et al. Inhibition of sclerostin by monoclonal antibody enhances bone healing and improves bone density and strength of nonfractured bones. J Bone Miner Res 2011;26(5):1012–21.

22. Claes L, Eckert-Hubner K, Augat P. The effect of mechanical stability on local vascularization and tissue differentiation in callus healing. J Orthop Res 2002; 20(5):1099–105.

23. Glowacki J. Angiogenesis in fracture repair. Clin Orthop Relat Res 1998;(Suppl 355):S82–9.

24. Huang C, Ogawa R. Mechanotransduction in bone repair and regeneration. FASEB J 2010;24(10): 3625–32.

25. Santos A, Bakker AD, Klein-Nulend J. The role of osteocytes in bone mechanotransduction. Osteoporos Int 2009;20(6):1027–31.

26. Claes LE, Heigele CA. Magnitudes of local stress and strain along bony surfaces predict the course and type of fracture healing. J Biomech 1999; 32(3):255–66.

27. Castillo RC, Bosse MJ, MacKenzie EJ, et al. Impact of smoking on fracture healing and risk of complications in limb-threatening open tibia fractures. J Orthop Trauma 2005;19(3):151–7.

28. Tsiridis E, Upadhyay N, Giannoudis P. Molecular aspects of fracture healing: which are the important molecules? Injury 2007;38(Suppl 1):S11–25.

29. Cramer T, Schipani E, Johnson RS, et al. Expression of VEGF isoforms by epiphyseal chondrocytes during low-oxygen tension is HIF-1 alpha dependent. Osteoarthritis Cartilage 2004;12(6):433–9.

30. Dimitriou R, Tsiridis E, Giannoudis PV. Current concepts of molecular aspects of bone healing. Injury 2005;36(12):1392–404.

31. Kon T, Cho TJ, Aizawa T, et al. Expression of osteoprotegerin, receptor activator of NF-kappaB ligand (osteoprotegerin ligand) and related proinflammatory cytokines during fracture healing. J Bone Miner Res 2001;16(6):1004–14.

32. Jacobsen KA, Al-Aql ZS, Wan C, et al. Bone formation during distraction osteogenesis is dependent on both VEGFR1 and VEGFR2 signaling. J Bone Miner Res 2008;23(5):596–609.

33. Ilizarov GA. The Tension-Stress Effect on the Genesis and Growth of Tissues: Part I. The Influence of Stability of Fixation and Soft-Tissue Preservation. Clin Orthop Relat Res 1989;(238):249–81.

34. Zhang X, Schwarz EM, Young DA, et al. Cyclooxygenase-2 regulates mesenchymal cell differentiation into the osteoblast lineage and is critically involved in bone repair. J Clin Invest 2002;109(11):1405–15.

35. Butcher CK, Marsh DR. Nonsteroidal anti-inflammatory drugs delay tibial fracture union. Injury 1996;27(5):1.

36. Donigan JA, Fredericks DC, Nepola JV, et al. The effect of transdermal nicotine on fracture healing in a rabbit model. J Orthop Trauma 2012;26(12):724–7.

37. Macey LR, Kana SM, Jingushi S, et al. Defects of early fracture-healing in experimental diabetes. J Bone Joint Surg Am 1989;71(5):722–33.

38. Perlman MH, Thordarson DB. Ankle fusion in a high risk population: an assessment of nonunion risk factors. Foot Ankle Int 1999;20(8):491–6.

39. Loder RT. The influence of diabetes mellitus on the healing of closed fractures. Clin Orthop Relat Res 1988;(232):210–6.

40. Naik AA, Xie C, Zuscik MJ, et al. Reduced COX-2 expression in aged mice is associated with impaired fracture healing. J Bone Miner Res 2009; 24(2):251–64.

41. Lin JT, Lane JM. Bisphosphonates. J Am Acad Orthop Surg 2003;11(1):1–4.

42. Munns CF, Rauch F, Zeitlin L, et al. Delayed osteotomy but not fracture healing in pediatric osteogenesis imperfecta patients receiving pamidronate. J Bone Miner Res 2004;19(11):1779–86.

43. Kaback LA, Soung do Y, Naik A, et al. Teriparatide (1-34 human PTH) regulation of osterix during fracture repair. J Cell Biochem 2008;105(1): 219–26.

44. Rubery PT, Bukata SV. Teriparatide may accelerate healing in delayed unions of type III odontoid fractures: a report of 3 cases. J Spinal Disord Tech 2010;23(2):151–5.

45. Aspenberg P, Genant HK, Johansson T, et al. Teriparatide for acceleration of fracture repair in humans: a prospective, randomized, double-blind study of 102 postmenopausal women with distal radial fractures. J Bone Miner Res 2010;25(2):404–14.

Biomechanics of the Hand

Scott F.M. Duncan, MD, MPH, MBA[a],*, Caitlin E. Saracevic[b],
Ryosuke Kakinoki, MD, PhD[c]

KEYWORDS

- Hand • Biomechanics • Thenar • Hypothenar • Interosseous • Lumbrical

KEY POINTS

- Ideally digits need sensation and freedom of motion to enable patients to use them effectively. The patients' perception of sensations and level of pain determines the eventual functional use and agility of the hand.
- Understanding how patients used their hand in daily living and employment will assist the surgeon in determining which procedure will be most effective to allow patients to return to their active pre-injury lifestyle and employment.
- Effective surgery ideally restores the biomechanical motions so that patients have optimum use.
- Optimum use can be restored through (1) existing anatomy or (2) tendon transfers, fusions, and even amputation.

INTRODUCTION

In its most simplified form, the hand is made up of a stable wrist with 2 digits, at the minimum, that are able to oppose against each other with some power. Ideally one or both of the digits are capable of motion so grasping can be performed. In its minimal form, one digit can be stable with one digit having motion to move against that stable post. Digits benefit from having sensation and from being pain free so that their usage is facilitated. In regard to biomechanical motion, the hand has 7 maneuvers that make up most hand functions.

1. The precision pinch, otherwise known as the terminal pinch, involves flexion of the interphalangeal (IP) joint of the thumb and the distal IP (DIP) joint of the index finger. The fingernail tips are brought together so that a small item, such as a pen, can be picked up (**Fig. 1**).
2. The next basic function is the oppositional pinch, otherwise known as the subterminal pinch. This pinch is where the pulp of the thumb and index finger are brought together with the IP and DIP joints in extension, which allows for increased forces to be generated through thumb opposition. It also relies on the first dorsal interosseous contracting while, simultaneously, the index profundus flexion is occurring (**Fig. 2**).
3. Key pinch maneuvering, in this situation, is when the thumb is adducted to the radial aspect of the index finger's middle phalanx. The key pinch maneuver does require a stable post, which in this situation is really the index finger. It also requires adequate length of the digit and a metacarpal phalangeal joint (MCP), which is capable of resisting thumb adduction (**Fig. 3**).
4. The chuck grip, otherwise known as the directional grip, allows the index finger, long finger, and thumb to come together to envelop a cylindrical object. A rotational and axial force is usually applied to the object when using this type of grip (**Fig. 4**).

[a] Department of Orthopedic Surgery, Ochsner Health System, 1514 Jefferson Highway, New Orleans, LA 70121, USA; [b] York University, 4700 Keele Street, Toronto, Ontario M3J 1P3, Canada; [c] Department of Orthopedic Surgery, Graduate School of Medicine, Kyoto University, 54 Shogoin Kawahara-cho, Sakyo-ku, Kyoto 606-8570, Japan
* Corresponding author.
E-mail address: Duncan.academic@gmail.com

Hand Clin 29 (2013) 483–492
http://dx.doi.org/10.1016/j.hcl.2013.08.003
0749-0712/13/$ – see front matter © 2013 Elsevier Inc. All rights reserved.

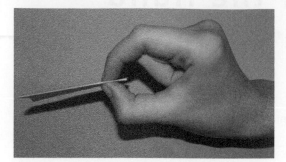

Fig. 1. Terminal pinch/precision pinch.

5. The hook grip requires finger flexion at the IP joints and extension at the MCP joints. This grip is used, for example, when one picks up a suitcase or a briefcase. It does not require thumb function (**Fig. 5**).
6. In the power grasp position, the fingers are flexed and the thumb is flexed and opposed relative to the other digits such as gripping a club or bat (**Fig. 6**).
7. The span grasp maneuver is when the DIP joints and the proximal IP (PIP) joints flex to approximately 30° and the thumb is palmarly abducted such that forces are generated between the thumb and fingers. This maneuver differs from the power grasps maneuver whereby forces are generated between the fingers and the palm. Stability is needed at the thumb, MCP, and IP joints. This type of grip is used, for example, to grab a ball (**Fig. 7**).

After surgery, the hand's ability to accommodate these various positions and exert the appropriate biomechanical forces through them determines how well patients recover from the injuries and procedures. For this reason, it is important to obtain a thorough history of patients to be able to emphasize which functions are mostly needed in order for patients to resume activities of daily living as well as previous employment.

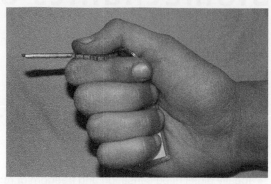

Fig. 3. Key pinch.

THE THUMB

The thumb is a unique aspect of humans (and higher primates), and this is related to its position on the hand. The thumb axis has its foundation at the trapeziometacarpal joint and is normally pronated and flexed approximately 80° with respect to the other metacarpals of the hand.[1] This unique position allows for circumduction of the thumb, which then facilitates opposition of the thumb to the digits.

Thumb opposition is required for all useful prehension, and its preservation is needed as the basis for many hand surgical procedures. Thumb opposition results from the angular and rotatory motion produced via palmar abduction at the trapeziometacarpal joint as well as flexion and rotation of the trapeziometacarpal and the MCP joints.[2]

Functional opposition requires recruitment of multiple muscle groups. These muscles include the abductor pollicis brevis, opponens pollicis, and the superficial head of the flexor pollicis brevis. These muscles work simultaneously on the trapeziometacarpal joint and the MCP joint. The major force of opposition comes from the abductor pollicis brevis, with the opponens pollicis and flexor pollicis brevis providing secondary motors for opposition maneuvering. The extensor

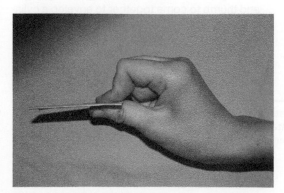

Fig. 2. Opposition pinch.

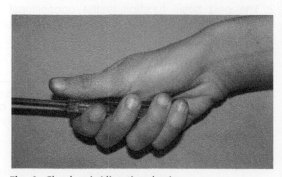

Fig. 4. Chuck grip/directional grip.

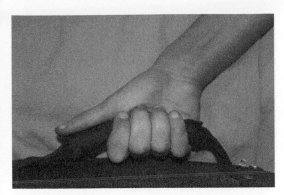

Fig. 5. Hook grip.

pollicis longus and the adductor pollicis are antagonistic to thumb opposition and provide supination, extension, and adduction forces to thumb maneuvering.

The complex motions of the thumb are facilitated by the coordination of intrinsic thenar and extrinsic muscle groups. The thumb muscles allow for precision pinching and power gripping, and its stability is maintained actively by muscles and not by articular constraints. Opposition of the thumb involves the combined motions of flexion, pronation, and palmar adduction of the thumb metacarpal. The opposite of opposition (reposition) is performed by extension, supination, and adduction of the thumb metacarpal.

The abductor pollicis brevis is a subcutaneous muscle that lies radial to the flexor pollicis brevis. It originates primarily from the transverse carpal ligament, with some fibers coming from the scaphoid tubercle and the trapezium. The muscle then inserts onto the radial base of the thumb proximal phalanx, with some fibers also going to the radial side of the MCP joint. It should be noted that its fibers do blend with those of the flexor pollicis brevis. The recurrent branch of the median nerve innervates this muscle. The vascular supply

of the abductor pollicis brevis is from the superficial radial ulnar branch of the radial artery. The abductor pollicis brevis can have variation in its anatomy, including additional heads and varying attachments. The main function of the abductor pollicis brevis is abduction and flexion of the thumb metacarpal. This abduction and flexion results in the thumb being pulled away from the palm at a right angle, initiating the act of opposition. The muscle also functions to extend the thumb IP joint through its extensor pollicis longus insertion and ulnarly deviates the MCP joint.[3–6]

The opponens muscle is a short and thick muscle that lies beneath the abductor pollicis brevis. It originates from the carpal metacarpal joint capsule as well as the tubercle of the trapezium and the transverse carpal ligament and inserts onto the volar radial aspect of the thumb metacarpal. Its vascular supply is via the superficial palmar branch of the radial artery. It has innervation from the recurrent branch of the median nerve in most cases but can also have dual innervation or just ulnar innervation.[5–9] The opponens flexes and pronates the thumb metacarpal. The opponens helps magnify the forces of opposition generated by the abductor pollicis brevis.[10]

The flexor pollicis brevis has a superficial (lateral) and a deep (medial) head. The superficial head has its origin from the tubercle of the trapezium and the transverse carpal ligament and inserts onto the radial base of the thumb proximal phalanx. The deep head rises from the trapezoid, capitate, and volar ligament of the distal carpal row and inserts onto the radial sesamoid and the base of the proximal phalanx. It receives its innervation from the recurrent motor branch of the median nerve and its vascular supply from the superficial palmar arch branch of the radial artery. In most cases, the superficial head muscle innervated by the recurrent branch of the median nerve and the deep head is most commonly innervated

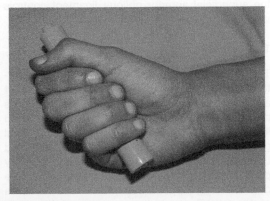

Fig. 6. Power grasp.

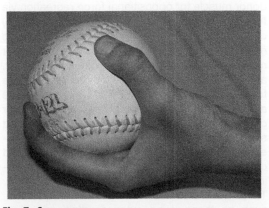

Fig. 7. Span grasp.

by the deep motor branch of the ulnar nerve.[11] The Riche-Cannieu anastomosis is a nerve branch between the deep motor branch of the ulnar nerve and the recurrent motor branch of the median nerve and has been described as occurring in up to 77% of dissections.[12] The primary action of the flexor pollicis brevis is to help flex the MCP joint, as well as extend the distal phalanx, and pronate the thumb metacarpal.[5,6,10,13] It is noted that the thumb does not have a lumbrical, and this is thought (teleologically) to be because the thumb has no PIP joint, thus, no mechanical need for a lumbrical. It also has a highly mobile carpal metacarpal joint that allows for substantial 3-dimensional positioning.

The abductor of the thumb also has 2 heads, an oblique and a transverse. The oblique head has its origin on the capitate and the bases of the second and third metacarpals as well as the volar meta-carpal ligaments and, in some cases, on the sheath of the flexor carpi radialis tendon. Most of its fibers unite to converge with the tendons of the flexor pollicis brevis (deep head), and the transverse head of the adductor inserts on the ulnar base of the thumb proximal phalanx and the dorsal extensor apparatus. This muscle tendon unit does have a sesamoid present. Another group of fibers can coalesce beneath the tendon of the flexor pollicis longus to join the deep head of the flexor pollicis brevis. The first dorsal interosseous muscle lays on the dorsum of the adductor, and the 2 muscles make up the bulk of the first web space. The deep motor branch of the ulnar nerve mainly innervates the adductor, and it gets its blood supply from the princeps pollicis artery. The adductors main action is adduction of the thumb metacarpal. It also helps with the extension of the thumb IP joint.

In considering reconstruction of the oppositional pinch, tendon transfers are an option. Cooney and colleagues[14] studied the muscle cross-sectional area and muscle forces to determine the ideal donor muscle for oppositional force recreation via transfer. The flexor digitorum superficialis (FDS) of the long finger and the extensor carpi ulnaris muscles were closely approximated to thenar muscle strength and potential excursion. However, abduction from the palm was greatest after a transfer of the FDS from the long and ring fingers and after extensor carpi ulnaris and extensor carpi radialis longus transfers. The motion and strength of the transfers were influenced by properly locating them within the hand.[15] Cooney and colleagues[14] emphasized the importance of directing the force of the transfer toward the pisiform. They noted that transfers distal to the pisiform, such as those using extensor digiti minimi or abductor digiti minimi, produced greater amounts of flexion than abduction. Transfers proximal to the pisiform, such as those using FDS and flexor carpi ulnaris, produce more abduction force and less metacarpal flexion.

The trapeziometacarpal joint is very complex because of its inherent instability and the fact that it is on the radial aspect of the wrist with no bony stabilizers. There are 5 major internal liga-mentous stabilizers of the trapeziometacarpal joint:

1. The dorsal radial ligament
2. The posterior oblique ligament
3. The first intermetacarpal ligament
4. Ulnar collateral ligament
5. Anterior oblique ligament

The dorsal radial ligament prevents lateral subluxation. The posterior oblique ligament pro-vides stability in flexion, opposition, and pronation. The first metacarpal is held tightly against the second metacarpal by the first intermetacarpal ligament, which is firm in abduction, opposition, and supination. The ulnar collateral ligament joins the intermetacarpal ligament in preventing lateral subluxation of the first metacarpal on the trape-zium and helps control rotational forces. The fifth ligament, and the most important according to some investigators, is the volar anterior oblique ligament, which has both deep and superficial fibers. The ligament originates from the volar tu-bercle of the trapezium and it attaches on the volar aspect of the thumb metacarpal. This ligament is taut in extension, abduction, and pronation. Its biomechanical purpose is to control pronation forces and mitigate radial translation. The deep aspect of the anterior oblique ligament serves as a pivot point for the trapeziometacarpal joint and guides the metacarpal into pronation while thenar muscles work to produce abduction and flexion. These fibers help control ulnar translocation of the metacarpal during palmar abduction while the superficial anterior oblique ligament controls volar subluxation of the metacarpal.

THE FINGERS

The index finger is probably the next most impor-tant to the hand because of its ability to abduct and adduct, its ability to flex and extend, and its proximity to the thumb. Several studies have noted its importance in precision pinch and directional grip.[16–19] Murray and colleagues[20] have studied the loss of the index finger; they found that key pinch, power grip, and supination strength were diminished by approximately 20% after the loss of the index finger. In the normal hand, the width of the grip extends from the hypothenar region all the way to the index finger. The radial aspect of the palm represents the external fulcrum of movement, and the ulnar aspect represents the internal fulcrum. In this study, those that did not have any dysesthetic pain thought that their overall hand function had improved with removal of the compromised index finger.

The long finger provides the most individual flexion force.[21,22] The central position means that it participates in both power grip and precision movements. The ring finger is noted to have less strength than either the long or the index finger and is uncommonly used for precision grip or pinch maneuvers. Tubiana and colleagues[16] thought that the loss of the ring finger resulted in the least amount of impairment to the hand.

The small finger has the least strength in flexion; however, its loss can result in decreased ability to hold objects in the palm. Part of the small finger's uniqueness is its carpal metacarpal joint, which can move approximately 25° in most people. Also, the hypothenar muscles add stabilization, which augments the flexion of the proximal phalanx of the small finger. The small finger's ability to abduct also helps enhance grasping while spanning an object. Tubiana thought the small finger was of a great impairment value, second only to the thumb.[16]

For finger range of motion, 15% of the intrinsic digital flexion occurs at the DIP joint but the DIP joint only contributes 3% to the overall flexion arc of the finger.[23] The PIP joint contributes 85% of the intrinsic digital flexion and adds 20% to the overall arc of the finger motion.

MCP joints, in many investigators' opinions, represent the most important joint for hand function because they contribute 77% of the total arc of finger flexion.[23–27] The DIP and PIP joints are ginglymoid-type joints that function more like hinges. The MCP joint is diarthrodial, which allows for flexion extension as well as abduction and adduction; they also allow for mild to moderate rotation of the digit.[26,28–30] Most prehension grips require that the digits be able to extend and abduct at the MCP joint. In order to be able to perform a precision pinch, the hand must have functional rotation and ulnar deviation at the MCP joint.[28,29] In order to accomplish a pinch, the radial intrinsic muscles and the collateral ligament to the index finger must hold against the stress applied by the thumb.

LUMBRICALS

Lumbricals are small muscles that are unique in that they arise on their antagonist. Their origin is the flexor digitorum profundus, and their main insertion point is the extensor expansion. The lumbricals contribute to MCP joint flexion, and they assist in IP joint extension. The lumbrical muscle name originates from the Latin word for worm. These 4 cylindrical-shaped muscles are located in the mid palm. Muscles have their origin on the flexor digitorum profundus tendons in the course along the palm in an almost parallel fashion to insert on the radial side of the digits. The most common pattern seen is that the first and second lumbricals originate from the radial side of the index and long finger deep flexors, and the ring and small finger lumbricals originate as bipennate muscle bellies on the adjacent surfaces of the flexor digitorum profundus tendons.[31,32] However, there have been numerous anatomic variants that have been described, and the hand surgeon should be familiar with some of these variants. In general, the muscles tend to follow a pattern of increasing variability as one moves from the radial aspect of the hand to the ulnar aspect.

Lumbricals can also have variable insertions, including the proximal phalanx; the volar plate of the MCP joint; and the extensor apparatus, including the lateral band and transverse oblique fibers of the extensor hood. Even though the lumbricals do insert onto the lateral band, other insertions onto other oblique fibers or transverse fibers have been found in more than 50% of specimens dissected. Furthermore, almost 50% have volar plate and/or bony attachments. Only one-quarter of the muscles went only to the radial lateral band as is classically described.[33]

The lumbrical muscles have very unique biomechanical properties. Their muscle mass and cross-sectional area are lowest in the upper extremity; however, their ratio between fiber and muscle length is largest in the upper extremity. These properties show that the lumbricals are really made for high excursions and that muscle contractile forces are constant over a wide range of fiber lengths.[34] Innervation of the first and second lumbricals is by the median nerve, whereas the third and fourth lumbricals are usually innervated by the ulnar nerve. Of note is that when using lumbricals as a proximally based pedicle flap, the radial-sided lumbricals are a safer option because of the comparatively fewer variations in the origin of the vascular supply and nerve supply.

The lumbrical muscle helps the extensor apparatus. Stimulation of the lumbrical produces IP joint extension followed by metacarpal joint flexion. As classically described, the lumbrical arises from the flexor digitorum profundus tendon; because of this, it is the only muscle that can relax the tendon of its antagonist. When considering lumbrical function, it is best to remember its 2 attachments to the profundus tendon and to the lateral band. Flexion of the proximal phalanx is mainly caused by interossei. However, if the interossei are paralyzed, the lumbrical can initiate flexion at this joint. The lumbrical muscles are richly supplied with muscle spindles. Their passive elongation during contraction of the flexor digitorum profundus is thought to inhibit digit extensor groups and facilitate wrist extensors.[35–38] Because of this, lumbrical muscles have been called tension meters between the flexors and extensors.[39] Leijnse and Kalker[40] thought that the lumbricals provide proprioceptive feedback regarding the PIP and DIP joint motion and positions. Other investigators[41] have thought that their unique properties indicate they are important for fast and sudden changing movements and other fine movements of the hand.

A lumbrical plus finger results when the profundus tendon is lacerated and the normal tone of the muscle belly puts the cut end of the attachment of the lumbrical in a more proximal position. This proximal position causes increased tension on the radial lateral band, and the PIP joint may extend or hyperextend as the finger is actively flexed. This paradoxic extension is known as the lumbrical plus finger[42]; in cases of distal amputation, which severs the profundus tendon, a similar issue can arise. Furthermore, if a flexor tendon graft is placed too loosely, a lumbrical plus finger can result. As patients try to flex IP joints, the profundus pulls first on the lumbrical rather than on the loose tendon graft; this causes paradoxic extension of the PIP joint.

Numerous investigators[43–53] have suggested that carpal tunnel syndrome can be caused by anomalous lumbrical origins as well as hypertrophy of lumbrical muscles. The muscle can be potentially found within the canal resulting in subsequent compression of the median nerve. Carpal tunnel syndrome tends to spare the innervations of the lumbricals because their innervation is in a more dorsal position and better protected from direct compression.[54]

THE INTEROSSEI

The interosseous muscles of the hand are innervated by the ulnar nerve and organized into dorsal and palmar layers. These muscles have a small excursion but a great impact on finger balance, grip, and pinch ability. Their importance is unfortunately only appreciated after denervation and/or contracture, which result in impairment of the hand. The 3 palmar interossei adduct the fingers, and the 4 dorsal interossei abduct the fingers

relative to the midline of the hand. The unique anatomy of the interossei muscles and their insertions and actions allow both sets of muscles to work in synergy. All of the interossei originate from metacarpal shafts. The palmar muscles originate from the ulnar side of the first and second metacarpals and the radial side of the fourth and fifth metacarpals, which positions them nicely for adduction of the fingers. The origin of the dorsal group is from the opposite surfaces of adjacent metacarpal shafts, which allows for finger abduction. The 3 palmar interosseous muscles insert distal to the MCP joint, into the extensor expansion of the finger. The dorsal interossei typically have both a bony insertion to the base of the proximal phalanx and the soft tissue insertion into the extensor aponeurosis. The interossei are key intrinsic balancers of the fingers, acting as flexors of the MCP joints and extensors for the IP joints. The dynamic actions of the interossei help stabilize the hand in the intrinsic plus position. The isometric actions of these muscles help stabilize the fingers throughout their dynamic movements.

It is important to remember that there are fascia boundaries around the interosseous muscles; because of this, compartment syndrome can occur within the interosseous compartments. Because there are both dorsal and palmar muscles, there are fascia layers that enclose both sets of interosseous muscles. These layers need to be released when performing fasciotomies of the hand.

The importance of the interossei on grip and pinch strength has been demonstrated by Kozin and colleagues.[55] They showed decreased grip strength of 38% and a 77% decrease in key pinch strength by measuring them after an ulnar nerve block in otherwise healthy individuals. This article by Kozin and colleagues[55] also showed that each median and ulnar innervated muscle had approximately 40% contribution to overall grip strength. There is a contribution from the interossei and lumbricals to IP extension and MCP flexion.

In high and low ulnar nerve palsies as well as crushing injuries, skin contracture and median nerve injury can all lead to failure and loss of function of the interosseous muscles. Ulnar nerve injury results in disruption of the finger balance with an intrinsic minus deformity: MCP joints hyperextended and the PIP and DIP joints flexed. This injury results because the interossei are mainly flexors of the MCP joints and extensors of the PIP joints. The extrinsic extensors are not strong PIP joint extensors. Ischemic injury as well as prolonged casting can lead to contracture of the interossei with resultant stiff hands and fingers, which may be in either the ulnar plus or ulnar minus position. The optimal positioning of splinting or casting of the hand and wrist keeps the MCP joints flexed approximately 60° and leaves the PIP joints free to move through a flexion and extension arc, which allows for interosseous stretching.

THE HYPOTHENAR MUSCLES

The hypothenar muscles, as a group, originate partially from the transverse carpal ligament, partially from the volar carpal ligament, and partially from the adjacent carpal bones. There has been some concern, theoretically, that a transverse carpal ligament release could result in hypothenar muscle shortening with subsequent grip strength weakness. The abductor digiti minimi muscle originates from the pisiform and the flexor carpi ulnaris tendon as well as the pisohamate ligament. In most cases, it has 2 muscle slips with one inserting onto the ulnar aspect of the small finger proximal phalanx base and the other inserting into the extensor apparatus of the small finger. The main purpose of the abductor digiti minimi is small finger abduction. It also has a small contribution in finger MCP joint flexion and IP joint extension.[56] The flexor digiti minimi muscle has its origin on the hook of the hamate and the ulnar aspect of the flexor retinaculum. It fuses distally with the muscle of the abductor digiti minimi. The flexor digiti minimi muscle has a relatively large moment arm and is responsible for small finger MCP joint flexion. However, it does also have a component of small finger abduction. The biomechanical forces of the flexor digiti minimi and abductor digiti minimi rely on the pisiform. Since Because the pisiform is mobile, the relative position of this bone influences the action of the aforementioned muscles.

The opponens digiti minimi muscle has 2 layers with separate origins. The superficial layer has its origin on the hook of the hamate and inserts onto the distal ulnar aspect of the fifth metacarpal. The deep layer has its origin from the ulnar flexor compartment wall and inserts onto the proximal ulnar aspect of the small finger metacarpal shaft. The opponens digiti minimi muscle is deep to the 2 hypothenar muscles and is separate from them. When the metacarpal is flexed by the hypothenar muscles, the flexor carpi ulnaris contracts to stabilize the pisiform; this results in the ulnar arch becoming further flexed in a position that is otherwise known as *cupping*.

The 3 muscles of the hypothenar eminence also provide a substantial soft tissue envelope over the ulnar aspect of the hand that helps absorb impacts and other trauma that the hand may encounter. In many ways, it can be viewed that these muscles function as shock absorbers.

Almost instinctively people will use the ulnar aspect of the hand with the hypothenar muscles to hammer or apply blunt force to an object, which can be seen in such activities as martial arts. The ulnar artery and its branches provide the vascular supply to these muscles. Specifically, the deep palmar branch of the ulnar artery seems to supply substantial amounts to these muscle groups. The ulnar nerve supplies the innervation specifically through a deep branch of the ulnar nerve, which travels through the canal and around the hook of the hamate where it provides motor innervation to the hypothenar muscles. It is noted that there can be significant variation in the motor nerve distribution in the hypothenar muscles making surgery challenging in this area.

TENDONS

The extensor tendon system has less movement or excursion than the flexor tendon system does.[57] The extensor apparatus also has decreased ability to compensate for shortening because of the connection between the intrinsic and the extrinsic mechanisms of this tendon system. Excursion of the extensor tendon at the level of the PIP joint is only 2 to 5 mm. The profundus flexor tendon provides a terminal pinch. Loss of the flexor profundus tendon may prevent full digital palmar grip.[58,59] Even though the quadralgia effect classically only applies to the long, ring, and small fingers because of the common muscle belly, the quadralgia effect can also involve the index finger because of the copious synovium present at the level of the carpal tunnel. This tissue has been called the *fibromembranous retinaculum*, which can link the index profundus tendon to the long, ring, and small finger tendons. The flexor superficialis tendon helps provide balance to the finger flexion arc. Loss can result in hyperextension at the PIP joint. Even with loss of both flexor tendons, approximately 45° of flexion can be possible at the MCP joints via the intrinsics. The lumbrical plus deformity is caused by the contracted profundus muscle belly placing stretch on the shortened lumbrical while the finger is flexing, this results in a paradoxic extension of the PIP joint. This interesting biomechanical effect can be solved by dividing the lumbrical or by suturing the profundus tendon to the flexor tendon sheath in a relaxed position.[58,60] Of course, during flexor tendon surgery, it is imperative to try and preserve the A2 and A4 pulleys. If these cannot be preserved or have been injured, then repair or reconstruction is needed. The A2 and A4 pulleys are located over the central portions of the proximal and middle phalanges. This location allows them to help prevent bowstringing that would occur with joint flexion if the pulleys were not present. The A1, A3, and A5 pulleys have a variable relationship to the joint axis and are only helpful in restraining some bowstringing. The cruciate pulleys vary in their location and contribute little biomechanical resistance to bowstringing.[61,62]

THE HAND AND WRIST

In order to perform power grip, a stable wrist is needed. Biomechanically, a stable wrist prevents the dissipation of finger flexion and extensor forces as the tendons move over the carpus. The human hand is one of the most complex biomechanical systems. It is a system of bony segments that are arranged in a series of longitudinal and transverse arches.[63] Essentially, there are 2 transverse arches: the proximal transverse arch formed by the carpal bones and the distal transverse arch formed by the metacarpal heads of the fingers. The longitudinal arches are made up of the bones of the 5 digital rays. The proximal aspect of the longitudinal arches and the proximal transverse arches converge at the carpal bones. Therefore, the carpal bones contribute stabilizing components to the longitudinal arches as well as the related structures central to hand function. Biomechanically, the arch resists greater force than other structures, and that is why arches are frequently found throughout ancient and modern architecture and engineering.

Carpal bones help stabilize the motion of the hand and make up part of the joint motion arc. It is well known that the Fibonacci ratio of 1:1.618034 is found in the lengths of the metacarpal, proximal phalanx, middle phalanx, and distal phalanx bones. Other investigators have noted[64,65] that the functional lengths of these bones using the center of rotation about the joints fits the ratio better than absolute bone lengths. This ratio is found in the nautilus shell, sunflowers, eggshells, spiral galaxies of outer space, and the Parthenon in Greece. This geometric design, in this ratio, and the bony structures of the hand make an equiangular spiral of joint motion arcs.

SUMMARY

The biomechanics of the hand are truly amazing. In many ways, the complexity of the hand defies our ability to fully comprehend the marvel of evolutionary engineering that has resulted in its design. Injuries to the bones, tendons, and/or ligaments of the hand can result in permanent loss of function and significant impairment. The goal of the hand

surgeon is to mitigate this functional loss by restoring the anatomy when possible and fooling Mother Nature when needed.

REFERENCES

1. Napier JR. The form and function of the carpometacarpal joint of the thumb. J Anat 1955;89:362.
2. Cooney WP, Lucca MJ, Chao EY, et al. The kinesiology of the thumb trapeziometacarpal joint. J Bone Joint Surg Am 1981;63:1371–81.
3. Botte MJ. Muscle anatomy. In: Doyle JR, Botte MJ, editors. Surgical anatomy of the hand and upper extremity. Philadelphia: Lippincott Williams & Wilkins; 2003. p. 149–55.
4. Standring S, editor. Gray's anatomy. 40th edition. Elsevier limited; 2008.
5. Leversedge FJ. Anatomy and pathomechanics of the thumb. Hand Clin 2008;28(4):681–4.
6. Leversedge F, Goldfarb C, Boyer M. Chapter 1, hand; Chapter 5, neuroanatomy. In: Leversedge F, Goldfarb C, Boyer M, editors. A pocket manual of hand and upper extremity primus manus. Philadelphia: Wolters Kluwer Lippincott Williams &Wilkins; 2010. p. 24–9.
7. Rowntree T. Anomalous innervation of the hand muscles. J Bone Joint Surg Br 1949;31(4):505–10.
8. Day MH, Napier JR. The two heads of flexor pollicis brevis. J Anat 1961;95:123–30.
9. Ajmani ML. Variations in the motor nerve supply of the thenar and hypothenar muscles of the hand. J Anat 1996;189(Pt 1):145–50.
10. Kaplan EB, Smith RJ. Kinesiology of the hand and wrist and muscular variations of the hand and forearm. In: Spinner M, editor. Kaplan's functional and surgical anatomy of the hand. 3rd edition. Philadelphia: J.B. Lippincott; 1984. p. 283–349.
11. Beasley RW. Surgical anatomy of the hand. In: Beasley RW, editor. Beasley's surgery of the hand. New York: Thieme; 2003. p. 18.
12. Harness D, Sekeles E. The double anastomotic innervation of thenar muscles. J Anat 1971;109(Pt 3):461–6.
13. Morris's human anatomy, part II: a complete systematic treatise by English and American authors. 4th edition. Philadelphia: Blakiston's Son & Co; 1907. p. 395–8 *Book digitized by Google from the library of Harvard University and uploaded to the Internet Archive.
14. Cooney WP, Linscheid RL, An KN. Opposition of the thumb: an anatomic and biomechanical study of tendon transfers. J Hand Surg Am 1984; 9:777–86.
15. Bunnell S. Opposition of the thumb. J Bone Joint Surg 1938;20:269–84.
16. Tubiana R, Thomine J, Mackin E. Movements of the hand and wrist. In: Tubiana R, Thomine J,

Mackin E, editors. Examination of the hand and wrist. St Louis (MO): Mosby; 1996. p. 40–125.

17. Duparc J, Alnot JY, May P. Single digit amputations. In: Campbell DA, Gosset J, editors. Mutilating injuries of the hand. Edinburgh (United Kingdom): Churchill Livingstone; 1979. p. 37–44.

18. Buck-Gramcko D, Hoffmann R, Neumann R, editors. Hand trauma: a practical guide. New York: Theime; 1986. p. 60–73.

19. Campbell DA, Gosset J, editors. Mutilating injuries of the hand. Edinburgh (United Kingdom): Churchill Livingstone; 1979. p. 37–44.

20. Murray JF, Carman W, MacKenzie JK. Trans- metacarpal amputation of the index finger: actual assessment of hand strength and complications. J Hand Surg 1977;2:471–81.

21. Ejeskar A, Ortengren R. Isolated finger flexion force: a methodological study. Hand 1981;13:223–30.

22. Hazelton FT, Smidt GL, Flatt AE, et al. The influence of wrist position on the force produced by the finger flexors. J Biomech 1975;8:301–6.

23. Littler JW, Herndon JH, Thompson JS. Examination of the hand. In: Converse JM, Littler JW, editors. Reconstructive plastic surgery, vol. 6. Philadelphia: WB Saunders; 1977. p. 2973.

24. Littler JW, Thompson JS. Surgical and functional anatomy. In: Bowers WH, editor. The interphalangeal joints. New York: Churchill Livingstone; 1987. p. 142.

25. Foucher G, Hoang P, Citron N, et al. Joint reconstruction following trauma: comparison of microsurgical transfer and conventional methods: a report of 61 cases. J Hand Surg Br 1986;11:388–93.

26. Ellis PR, Tsai T. Management of the traumatized joint of the finger. Clin Plast Surg 1989;16:457–73.

27. Swanson AB. Flexible implant arthroplasty for arthritic finger joints: rationale, technique, and results of treatment. J Bone Joint Surg Am 1972;54: 435–55.

28. Beckenbaugh RD, Dobyns JH, Linscheid RL, et al. Review and analysis of silicone-rubber metacarpophalangeal implants. J Bone Joint Surg Am 1976; 58:483–7.

29. Flatt AE. Care of the rheumatoid hand. 4th edition. St Louis (MO): Mosby; 1983.

30. Krishnan J, Chipchase L. Passive and axial rotation of the metacarpophalangeal joint. J Hand Surg Br 1997;22:270–3.

31. Shin YA, Amadio PC. Stiff finger joints. In: Green DP, Hotchkiss RN, Pederson WC, et al, editors. Green's operative hand surgery. 5th edition. Philadelphia: Elsevier; 2005. p. 422–3.

32. Goldberg S. The origin of the lumbrical muscles in the hand of the South African native. Hand 1970;2: 168–71.

33. Eladoumikdachi F, Valkov PL, Thomas J, et al. Anatomy of the intrinsic hand muscles revisited: part II. Lumbricals. Plast Reconstr Surg 2002; 110(5):1225–31.

34. Jacobson MD, Raab R, Fazeli BM, et al. Architectural design of the human intrinsic hand muscles. J Hand Surg Am 1992;17:804–9.

35. Ranney D, Wells R. Lumbrical muscle function as revealed by a new and physiological approach. Anat Rec 1988;222(1):110–4.

36. Buford WL Jr, Koh S, Andersen CR, et al. Analysis of intrinsic-extrinsic muscle function through interactive 3-dimensional kinematic simulation and cadaver studies. J Hand Surg Am 2005;30(6): 1267–75.

37. Backhouse KM, Catton WT. An experimental study of the function of the lumbrical muscles in the human hand. J Anat 1954;88(5):133–41.

38. Devanadan MS, Ghosh S, John KL. A quantitative study of the muscle spindles and tendon organs in some intrinsic muscles of the hand. Anat Rec 1983;207:263–6.

39. Rabischong P. Basic problems in the restoration of prehension. Ann Chir 1971;25(19):927–33.

40. Leijnse JN, Kalker JJ. A two-dimensional kinematic model of the lumbrical in the human finger. J Biomech 1995;28(3):237–49.

41. Leijnse JN. Why the lumbrical muscle should not be bigger – a force model of the lumbrical in the unloaded human finger. J Biomech 1997;30(11–12): 1107–14.

42. Smith RJ. Intrinsic muscles of the fingers: function, dysfunction and surgical reconstruction. In: AAOS instructional course lectures, vol. 24. St Louis (MO): Mosby; 1975. p. 200–20.

43. Butler B Jr, Bigley EC Jr. Aberrant index lumbrical tendinous origin associated with carpal tunnel syndrome: a case report. J Bone Joint Surg 1971;53: 160–2.

44. Schultz RJ, Endler PM, Huddleston HD. Anomalous median nerve and an anomalous muscle belly of the first lumbrical associated with carpal tunnel syndrome. J Bone Joint Surg 1973;55:1744–6.

45. Still JM Jr, Kleinert HE. Anomalous muscles and nerve entrapment in the wrist and hand. Plast Reconsrt Surg 1973;52:394–400.

46. Jabaley ME. Personal observations on the role of the lumbrical muscles in carpal tunnel syndrome. J Hand Surg 1978;3:82–4.

47. Erikson J. A case of carpal tunnel syndrome on the basis of abnormally long lumbrical muscle. Acta Orthop Scand 1973;44:275–7.

48. Robinson D, Aghasi M, Halperin N. The treatment of carpal tunnel syndrome caused by hypertrophied lumbrical muscles. Scand J Plast Reconstr Surg 1989;23:149–51.

49. Gainer JV, Nugent GR. Carpal tunnel syndrome: report of 430 operations. South Med J 1977;70: 325–8.

50. Rothfleisch S, Sherman D. Carpal tunnel syndrome, biomechanical aspects of occupational occurrence and implications regarding surgical management. Orthop Rev 1978;7:107–9.

51. Smith EM, Sonstegard DA, Anderson WH Jr. Carpal tunnel syndrome: contribution of flexor tendons. Arch Phys Med Rehabil 1977;58:379–85.

52. Gelberman RH, Hergenroeder PT, Hargens AA, et al. The carpal tunnel syndrome: a study of canal pressures. J Bone Joint Surg 1981;63:380–3.

53. Skie M, Zeiss J, Ebraheim NA, et al. Carpal tunnel changes and median nerve compression during wrist flexion and extension seen by magnetic resonance imaging. J Hand Surg 1990;15: 934–9.

54. Yates SK, Yaworski R, Brown WF. Relative preservation of lumbrical versus thenar motor fibres in neurogenic disorders. J Neurol Neurosurg Psychiatr 1981;44(9):768–74.

55. Kozin SH, Porter S, Clark P, et al. The contribution of the intrinsic muscles to grip and pinch strength. J Hand Surg Am 1999;24(1):64–72.

56. Brand PW, Hollister AM. Clinical mechanics of the hand. 3rd edition. St Louis (MO): Mosby Inc; 1999. p. 173–5.

57. Verdan CE. Primary and secondary repair of flexor and extensor tendon injuries. In: Flynn JE, editor. Hand surgery. Baltimore (MD): Williams & Wilkins; 1966. p. 220–75.

58. Smith P. Lister's the hand. London: Churchill Livingstone; 2002.

59. Verdan CE. Syndrome of the quadriga. Surg Clin North Am 1960;40:425–6.

60. Louis DS, Jebson PJL, Graham TJ. Amputations. In: Green DP, Hotchkiss RN, Pederson WC, editors. Green's operative hand surgery. 4th edition. New York: Churchill Livingstone; 1999. p. 48–75.

61. Hume EL. Panel discussion: flexor tendon reconstruction. In: Hunter JM, Schneider LH, Mackin EJ, editors. Tendon surgery in the hand. St Louis (MO): Mosby; 1987. p. 658–62.

62. Lin A, Amadio PC, An K, et al. Functional anatomy of the human digital flexor pulley system. J Hand Surg Am 1989;14:949–56.

63. Flatt AE. Biomechanics of the hand and wrist. In: Evarts CM, editor. Surgery of the musculoskeletal system. 2nd edition. New York: Churchill Livingstone; 1983. p. 311–29.

64. Hamilton R, Dunsmuir RA. Radiographic assessment of the relative lengths of the bones of the fingers of the human hand. J Hand Surg 2002;27:546–8.

65. Park AE, Fernandez JJ, Schmedders K, et al. The Fibonacci sequence: relationship to the human hand. J Hand Surg 2003;28:157–60.

The Biomechanics of Fixation Techniques for Hand Fractures

Julie E. Adams, MD[a], Thomas Miller, BS[a],
Marco Rizzo, MD[b],*

KEYWORDS

• Biomechanics • Hand fractures • Fixation devices • Metacarpal fractures • Phalangeal fractures

KEY POINTS

- Although many hand fractures are treated adequately by nonoperative means, operative intervention is indicated in the setting of excessive shortening, angular deformities, rotational malalignment, or intra-articular step-off.
- An understanding of the biomechanics of fracture fixation can aid the clinician in choosing the appropriate fixation options for fractures about the hand.
- Options for fixation, in general, include smooth pin fixation with Kirschner wires, plate and screw constructs (locking and nonlocking), screw fixation, and interosseous wiring.

INTRODUCTION

Most hand fractures are stable either before or after closed reduction and can be effectively treated by closed means. Although many metacarpal and phalangeal fractures may be treated nonoperatively, operative treatment may be indicated in the setting of multiple fractures, excessive shortening, rotational deformity, or excessive angular deformity. Fixation choices depend on the fracture pattern, surgeon preference, and associated injuries. An understanding of the biomechanics associated with fixation techniques can facilitate the choice of appropriate devices. Furthermore, an appreciation of the strength of various constructs can enable an appropriate level of mobilization and the right amount of protection during rehabilitation.

Consideration of the fracture geometry and characteristics is essential, as is an understanding of the deforming forces exerted on the bone. Because of the intrinsic and extrinsic muscle forces on the metacarpus, fractures of the metacarpals tend to have an apex dorsal angulation

deformity. Transverse fractures of the proximal phalanx, in contrast, typically have an apex volar deformity caused by the flexion of the interossei on the base of the proximal phalanx and the extension moment imparted by the central slip. Middle phalanx fractures have more variable deformities depending on the location of the fracture fragments and the actions of the flexor digitorum superficialis and the central slip. In contrast to transverse fractures, spiral or long oblique fractures may be subject to a rotational deformity more so than short oblique fractures, which can both rotate and/or have an angular deformity.[1]

In general, fractures of the diaphyseal region may be considered as one of 4 types. Transverse fractures represent a fracture line that is mostly perpendicular to the long axis of the shaft; oblique fractures may be characterized as short oblique fractures in which the fracture length is equal or less than the diameter of the bone and typically require treatment similar to transverse fractures. Long oblique fractures are those in which the fracture length is less than the diameter of the bone. A

a Department of Orthopaedic Surgery, The University of Minnesota, 2450 Riverside Avenue R200, Minneapolis, MN 55454, USA; b Department of Orthopedic Surgery, The Mayo Clinic, 200 First Street Southwest, Rochester, MN 55905, USA
* Corresponding author.
E-mail address: Rizzo.Marco@mayo.edu

Hand Clin 29 (2013) 493–500
http://dx.doi.org/10.1016/j.hcl.2013.08.004
0749-0712/13/$ – see front matter © 2013 Elsevier Inc. All rights reserved.

fourth fracture type might be considered as a comminuted or combination type.

FIXATION METHODS

Options for fixation of metacarpal and phalangeal fractures, in general, include plating, lag screw fixation, percutaneous or intramedullary fixation, and interosseous wiring.

Kirschner wires (K wires) are commonly used fixation devices for fractures of the hand. The advantages include the ability to remove pins easily once healing is adequate; the low cost; and they are typically easy to apply in a percutaneous fashion, limiting soft tissue damage. The application requires minimal soft tissue disruption, thus preserving soft tissue and periosteal stability. The disadvantages include the need for additional immobilization during the early healing process, pin tract infections, or pin migration; they do not provide compression across the fracture site, and they can occasionally distract the fracture site. Although they do not provide rigid fixation, K wires may provide adequate fixation sufficient for limited mobilization.[2]

Various configurations may be used and have differing stabilities. The options include crossed K wires, parallel K wires across the fracture site, intramedullary wire fixation, transarticular pin fixation or in conjunction with wiring to create a tension band construct, and in combinations.

Several principles apply to the K-wire application, regardless of the orientation. K wires with a trocar tip inserted under slow speeds have more improved fixation ability than do self-cut tips or diamond-cut tips.[3] When crossed K wires are used, they should optimally engage 2 cortices; care should be taken to avoid having the K wires cross at the fracture site.[4,5]

The biomechanics of the orientation of the K-wire application has been investigated. In oblique phalanx fracture models, K wires oriented perpendicular to the fracture line provided more rigid fixation than did crossed K wires.[6] However, compressive loads are better resisted by wires perpendicular to the bone; thus, oblique fractures treated with K wires are often most soundly fixed by multiple K wires in variable orientations.[7]

In models of transverse phalangeal fractures, crossed K wires provided more rigid fixation than other fixation techniques, providing more resistance to torsion or distraction, whereas longitudinal and crossed fixation provide similar bending resistance.[6]

In the setting of border metacarpals, the use of K wires to fix the metacarpal above and below the fracture line to an adjacent digit is a biomechanically sound technique.[8,9]

Augmentation of K wires with tension band wiring is a way to increase the strength of the construct. It requires open exposure but may be useful in transverse or oblique fracture patterns. Typically, 0.035-in K wires are used in a crossed pattern for transverse fractures and in a pattern perpendicular to the fracture for oblique fracture patterns.[10]

Intramedullary placement of K wires or other purpose-made rod devices has been described for use in both phalangeal and metacarpal fractures (**Fig. 1**).[11] This technique involves the placement of one or more bent intramedullary devices. This technique is most appropriately applied in the setting of transverse fractures of the diaphysis but can also be used in the setting of neck fractures.[12–15] In one series of simulated metacarpal fracture, there was no statistically significant difference between fixation with the intramedullary K-wire fixation groups (2 vs 5 pins).[16]

Another series investigated the fixation of transverse osteotomies of the metacarpus with intramedullary K wire, crossed K wires, and plate and screw constructs. When subjected to 3-point bending loads, the intramedullary K-wire fixation was statistically significantly weaker in withstanding torsional loads compared with the other methods of fixation; but the bending moment and rigidity were comparable with plate and screw fixation. These results suggest that a single intramedullary pin fixation may be adequate but should be protected from torsional loads during healing.[17]

LAG SCREW FIXATION

Long oblique fractures (ie, the fracture length is more than the diameter of the bone) or isolated corner articular fractures may be especially amenable to lag screw fixation (**Fig. 2**). For fixation to be effective, the width of the fracture fragment should be at least 3 times as wide as the thread diameter of the screw.

Important considerations regarding screws include outer diameter, inner diameter, and pitch. The pitch of the screw is the distance between the screw threads, which affects the compression.[7,18]

The outer diameter, which is represented by the maximal diameter of the shaft of the screw with the flutes, has a direct affect on the pullout strength, whereas the inner diameter directly affects the bending strength and tensile strength.[7,18]

Lag screw fixation involves drilling a hole in the near fragment that is the same diameter as the outer diameter of the screw. This practice causes the screw to engage only the far fragment and

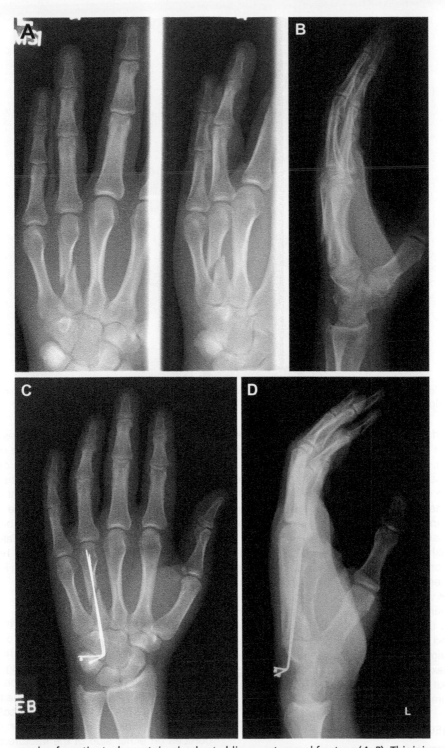

Fig. 1. Case example of a patient who sustained a short oblique metacarpal fracture (*A, B*). This injury was treated with intramedullary K wires (*C, D*), with the wires removed at 6 weeks (copyright Marco Rizzo).

not the near fragment, increasing compression across the construct. The most effective compression across the fracture site occurs with the placement of the screw perpendicular to the fracture line. However, because limited axial stability is provided by this construct alone, it is best to apply multiple lag screws at right angles to both the fracture line and the shaft of the bone.[7,18,19]

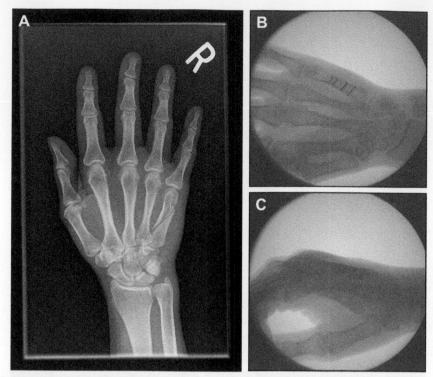

Fig. 2. A patient sustained a spiral metacarpal shaft fracture (*A*). This fracture was amenable to lag screw fixation (*B, C*) (copyright Julie Adams).

Two interfragmentary lag screws were significantly more rigid than crossed K wires, tension band wiring, or dorsal plate fixation in an oblique proximal phalanx apex volar bending model. The most stable construct included plate fixation with 2 interfragmentary lag screws, although no fixation technique approached the strength and rigidity of intact normal phalanges.[20]

Firoozbakhsh and colleagues[16] compared fixation with dorsal plating, 2 lag screws, crossed K wires with tension banding, multiple 0.028-in intramedullary K wires with a bouquet technique versus intramedullary paired 0.045-in K wires; fixation was tested under conditions with an oblique osteotomy and cyclic loading to failure. The plate fixation was significantly more rigid under axial loads than the next strongest method of fixation (2 lag screws), but fixation was not statistically significantly different in bending or torsion.[16]

INTEROSSEOUS WIRING

One series suggests that appropriate interosseous configurations for the fixation of simulated transverse metacarpal fractures (90° loop positioning of two 26-gauge loops) are comparable in strength with nonlocked plating.[21]

Although it can be technically demanding and requires additional soft tissue exposure, the fixation is generally low profile and applies adequate compression at the fracture site. The use is often in transverse fractures, particularly of the phalanges and avulsion-type fractures, such as bony skier's thumb injuries. The placement of the wire dorsal to the central axis of the bone allows it to function as tension banding and can be facilitated by a figure-of-8 configuration.[2,22–24] Failures occur with wire breakage, pullout through holes in the bone, and unraveling of the twist with loading.[2]

PLATE AND SCREW CONSTRUCTS

Plate and screw constructs provide highly stable fixation of fractures; concern exists over the potential bulkiness of the plate in the hand, where there is little room for the many gliding structures. The plate length and thickness may be sacrificed, but the bending resistance of the plate is inversely related to the length cubed and directly proportional to the thickness cubed. Four nonlocking cortices on either side of the fracture are usually adequate for the fixation of metacarpal or phalangeal fractures.[7,18,19]

In metacarpal shaft fractures, plating (**Fig. 3**) has significantly greater stability than internal fixation with K wires.[16,20,25]

The application of the plate on the dorsal side for metacarpal fractures is biomechanically favorable

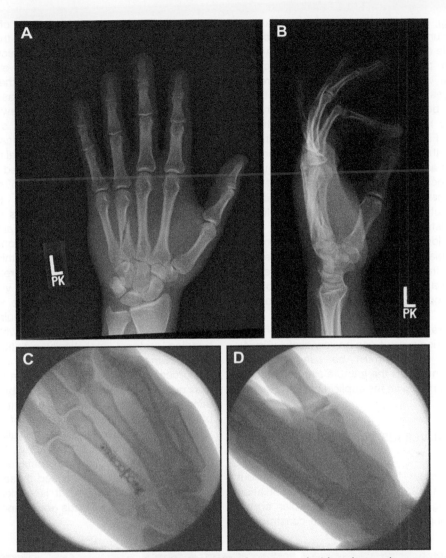

Fig. 3. The injury shown is of the metacarpal shaft (*A, B*) and was treated with a plate and screw construct (*C, D*) (copyright Julie Adams).

because it resists the bending forces on the fracture in vivo. The volar cortex is realigned in contact and, thus, resists compressive forces; the dorsal surface is supported by a plate that resists the tension forces. It is less biomechanically favorable when placed on the dorsal side for phalanx fractures because these fractures are subjected to apex volar bending forces, and a dorsal plate is placed on the compression (rather than tension side) of the bone.[2,16,26]

The challenges associated with plate fixation can relate to location and biology; the application requires relatively more soft tissue dissection and soft tissue stripping of bone than percutaneous techniques. Plate positioning may cause irritation of the extensor tendons; excessive screw length

volarly may cause irritation of the flexor tendons; and in thin individuals, the subcutaneous position of the plate may be bothersome. The advantages of this fixation technique relate to the extremely strong constructs possible.

Black and colleagues[25] investigated the fixation of simulated transverse metacarpal fractures with dorsal plating (with and without lag screw fixation); crossed K wires and interosseous wiring (with and without a single K wire). The plating constructs were significantly more stable than the other constructs, with more resistance to bending and torsional loads.

The factors to be considered when choosing plate and screw construction include the type of device and screws (fixed-angle locking vs nonlocking), unicortical versus bicortical fixation, and the number and configuration of screws. Fixed-angle devices may include locked plates or blade-type plates. Locked plates function as fixed-angle devices and convert shear stresses to compression forces at the interface between screw and bone; because bone resists compressive forces better than shear forces, fixation is enhanced. Fixation strength in locked plating results from the sum of all screw-bone interfaces rather than a single screw's resistance to pullout, as in nonlocking plates.[27,28] The failure of nonlocked constructs, thus, occurs by toggle and loosening of the screws individually while the locked construct fails as a unit.[28]

Notably, locking plates do not rely on friction between the plate and bone to achieve compression across the fracture site, as nonlocking plates do, resulting in a potential biologic advantage of preserved blood supply to the bone with locking plates.[28]

Hybrid fixation using a combination of nonlocking and locking screws can be very useful (**Fig. 4**). Nonlocking screws must be used to apply compression across the fracture site before locking the construct with the application of the locked screws.[28]

BICORTICAL VERSUS UNICORTICAL SCREW FIXATION

Bicortical screw fixation improves the pullout strength of the construct and enhances fixation by engaging the relatively thicker volar cortex and providing a longer stabilization construct. In addition, the mechanism of failure of bicortical screws tends to be the failure of the material (bending of the plate) rather than the screw cutout as in unicortical fixation.[29–31] However, some complications relative to overdrilling the volar cortex or too prominent volar screws has prompted interest in the use of unicortical screw fixation.[32] There have been some series that suggest no biomechanical advantages of bicortical nonlocking screw fixation relative to unicortical nonlocking screw fixation constructs subjected to static 4-point bending protocols, with no statistically significant differences in strength (unicortical 569 N; bicortical 541 N) or stiffness (unicortical 333 N/mm; bicortical 458 N/mm). Failure in this series was by fracture at the screw-bone interface without screw pullout.[33] However, this protocol was a static one, which does not replicate the cyclic bending forces experienced in vivo.

When cyclic loading (which more aptly replicates in vivo forces) is applied to simulated transverse midshaft metacarpal fractures with a 3-point bending protocol, statistically significant differences in mean load to failure were noted (370 N unicortical vs 450 N bicortical).[29] In addition, failures occur in different modes; in the bicortical fixation group, failure occurs primarily with the failure of the implant material (bending of the plate), whereas in the unicortical group, failure occurs because of the cutout of the screw. In addition, estimated forces on the index metacarpus during the simulated grasp can exceed those withstood by the unicortical fixation; it is unclear if these studies replicate the loads experienced during rehabilitation.[29,34]

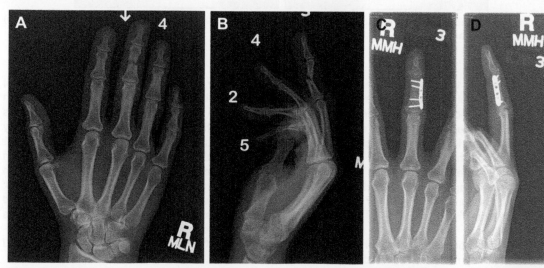

Fig. 4. A case of a patient who sustained a high-energy fracture of the middle phalanx (*arrow*) (*A, B*). Because of the high risk of nonunion, a combination locking and nonlocking screw/plate construct was used (*C, D*) (copyright Marco Rizzo).

LOCKING VERSUS NONLOCKING PLATES/SCREWS

One series compared the strength of locking versus nonlocking plates and demonstrated that nonlocking plates with 4 bicortical screws withstood higher 3-point bending forces (359 ± 90 N) than did locking plates (250 ± 56 N).[35] The strength and stiffness of locking versus nonlocking plates with bicortical versus monocortical screw fixation for the fixation of simulated short oblique midshaft fractures was investigated in a pig metacarpal model using a cantilever bending mode.[36]

Notably, there was no significant difference in stiffness between the nonlocking monocortical and nonlocking bicortical fixation groups or the locking monocortical and locking bicortical fixation groups; however, the stiffness was significantly greater for the locking than nonlocking plates. The maximal load to failure was significantly greater in the bicortical nonlocking versus the monocortical nonlocking fixation but was not significantly different between the locking bicortical or monocortical fixation. The stiffness and load to failure was greater in the monocortical locking than bicortical nonlocking fixation, although not statistically significant.[36]

The configuration of screw fixation with newer double-row plates can enhance stability. In a sawbone study with physiologic loads, Gajendran and colleagues[37] found linear nonlocking (LNL) plates were inferior to double-row nonlocking 3-dimensional (DRNL3D) plates in both bending (LNL 198 ± 18 N; DRNL3D 223 ± 29 N) and torsional resistance (LNL 2033 ± 155 N/mm; DRNL3D3190 ± 235 N/mm). Moreover, double-row locking plates with 8 monocortical screws had the greatest strength and similar stiffness compared with other plating techniques and are theorized to potentially interfere less with the flexor tendons.[36]

SUMMARY

Multiple options are available for the fixation of metacarpal and phalangeal fractures; the treatment options depend largely on the fracture characteristics, concomitant injuries, and surgeon preference. With an understanding of the options available and the biomechanics involved, the appropriate treatment options may be chosen. Although plate and screw constructs provide the strongest fixation for these fractures, many other techniques provide adequate fixation and may be favored for reasons other than biomechanics.

REFERENCES

1. Flatt AE. Closed and open fractures of the hand: fundamentals of management. Postgrad Med 1996;39:17–26.
2. Jones WW. Biomechanics of small bone fixation. Clin Orthop Rel Res 1987;214:11–8.
3. Namba RS, Kabo M, Meals RA. Biomechanical effects of point configuration in Kirschner wire fixation. Clin Orthop Rel Res 1987;214:19–22.
4. Edward GS, O'Brien ET, Hechman MM. Retrograde cross pinning of transverse metacarpal and phalangeal fractures. Hand 1982;14:141–8.
5. Jupiter JB, Koniuch M, Smith RJ. The management of delayed unions and nonunions of the metacarpals and phalanges. J Hand Surg Am 1985;4:457–66.
6. Viegas SF, Ferren EL, Self J, et al. Comparative mechanical properties of various Kirschner wire configurations in transverse and oblique phalangeal fractures. J Hand Surg Am 1988;13:246–53.
7. Tencer AF, Johnson KD, Kyle RF, et al. Biomechanics of fractures and fracture fixation. Instr Course Lect 1993;42:19–34.
8. Lamb DW, Abernathy PA, Raine PA. Unstable fractures of the metacarpal (a method of treatment by transverse wire fixation to intact metacarpals). Hand 1973;5:43–8.
9. Massengill JB, Alexander H, Langrana N, et al. A phalangeal fracture model—quantitative analysis of rigidity and failure. J Hand Surg Am 1982;7:264–70.
10. Tan V, Beredjiklian PK, Weiland AJ. Intraarticular fractures of the hand: treatment by open reduction and internal fixation. J Orthop Trauma 2005;19:518–23.
11. Hall RF. Treatment of metacarpal and phalangeal fractures in noncompliant patients. Clin Orthop Rel Res 1987;214:31–6.
12. Agashe MV, Phadke S, Agashe VM, et al. A new technique of locked, flexible intramedullary nailing of spiral and comminuted fractures of the metacarpals: a series of 21 cases. Hand 2011;6:408–15.
13. Foucher G. "Bouquet" osteosynthesis in metacarpal neck fractures: a series of 66 patients. J Hand Surg 1995;20(3 Pt 2):S86–90.
14. Han SH, Rhee SY, Lee SC, et al. Percutaneous retrograde intramedullary single wire fixation for metacarpal shaft fracture of the little finger. Eur J Orthop Surg Traumatol 2012. [Epub ahead of print].
15. Orbay J. Intramedullary nailing of metacarpal shaft fractures. Tech Hand Up Extrem Surg 2005;9:69–73.
16. Firoozbakhsh KK, Moneim MS, Howey T, et al. Comparative fatigue strengths and stabilities of metacarpal internal fixation techniques. J Hand Surg 1993;18:1059–68.

17. Zhang LS, Pan YW, Tian GL, et al. Biomechanical research of antegrade intramedullary fixation for the metacarpal fractures. Zhonghua Wai Ke Za Zhi 2010;48:606–9 [in Chinese].

18. Kozin SH, Thoder JJ, Lieberman G. Operative treatment of metacarpal and phalangeal shaft fractures. J Am Acad Orthop Surg 2000;8:111–21.

19. Schatzker J. Screws and plates and their application. In: Muller ME, Allguwer M, Schneider R, et al, editors. Manual of internal fixation: techniques recommended by the AO-ASIF Group. New York: Springer-Verlag; 1991. p. 179–290.

20. Black DM, Mann RJ, Constine RM, et al. The stability of internal fixation in the proximal phalanx. J Hand Surg Am 1986;11:672–7.

21. Vanik RK, Weber RC, Matloub HS, et al. The comparative strengths of internal fixation techniques. J Hand Surg Am 1984;9:216–21.

22. Gingrass RP, Fehring BH, Matloub H. Intraosseous wiring of complex hand fractures. Plast Reconstr Surg 1980;66:383–94.

23. Lister G. Intraosseous wiring of the digital skeleton. J Hand Surg 1978;3:427–35.

24. Zimmerman NB, Weiland AJ. Ninety-ninety intraosseous wiring for internal fixation of the digital skeleton. Orthopedics 1989;12:99–104.

25. Black D, Mann RJ, Constine R, et al. Comparison of internal fixation techniques in metacarpal fractures. J Hand Surg Am 1985;10:466–72.

26. Prevel CD, Eppley BL, Jackson JR, et al. Mini and micro plating of phalangeal and metacarpal fractures: a biomechanical study. J Hand Surg 1995; 20:44–9.

27. Cordey J, Borgeaud M, Perren SM. Force transfer between the plate and the bone: relative importance of the bending stiffness of the screws friction between plate and bone. Injury 2000;31(Suppl 3): C21–8.

28. Egol KA, Kubiak EN, Fulkerson E, et al. Biomechanics of locked plates and screws. J Orthop Trauma 2004;18:488–93.

29. Afshar R, Fong TS, Latifi MH, et al. A biomechanical study comparing plate fixation using unicortical and bicortical screws in transverse metacarpal fracture models subjected to cyclic loading. J Hand Surg Br 2012;37:396–401.

30. Khalid M, Theivendran K, Cheema M, et al. Biomechanical comparison of pull-out force of unicortical versus bicortical screws in proximal phalanges of the hand: a human cadaveric study. Clin Biomech 2008;23:1136–40.

31. Lazenby RA. Circumferential variation in human second metacarpal cortical thickness: sex, age, and mechanical factors. Anat Rec 2001;267:154–8.

32. Fambrough R, Green D. Tendon rupture as a complication of screw fixation in fractures in the hand. A case report. J Bone Joint Surg Am 1979;61:781–2.

33. Dona E, Gillies RM, Gianoutsos MP, et al. Plating of metacarpal fractures: unicortical or bicortical screws. J Hand Surg Br 2004;29:218–21.

34. An KN, Chao EY, Cooney WP, et al. Forces in the normal and abnormal hand. J Orthop Res 1985;3: 202–11.

35. Doht S, Jansen H, Meffert R, et al. Higher stability with locking plates in hand surgery? Biomechanical investigation of the trilock system in a fracture model. Int Orthop 2012;36:1641–6.

36. Ochman S, Doht S, Paletta J, et al. Comparison between locking and non-locking plates for fixation of metacarpal fractures in an animal model. J Hand Surg 2010;35:597–603.

37. Gajendran VK, Szabo RM, Myo GK, et al. Biomechanical comparison of double-row locking plates versus single- and double-row non-locking plates in a comminuted metacarpal fracture model. J Hand Surg 2009;34:1851–8.

Selection of Appropriate Treatment Options for Hand Fractures

Douglas M. Sammer, MD*, Tarik Husain, MD,
Rey Ramirez, MD

KEYWORDS

- Hand fractures • Metacarpal fractures • Phalangeal fractures • Principles

KEY POINTS

- The scientific evidence available to guide hand fracture management is poor, so adherence to simple principles can guide decision-making.
- Although anatomic reduction of articular fractures is important, with extra-articular fractures the goal is to restore anatomic relationships.
- Stable fixation should be achieved with minimal soft-tissue injury, and motion should be instituted as early as possible.
- The ultimate goal is to achieve good hand function: treat the patient, not the x-ray.

EVIDENCE-BASED MEDICINE FOR HAND FRACTURES

The decision of how to manage a hand fracture is often made without the support of scientific evidence, and is usually based primarily on the hand surgeon's training and experience. This is in spite of a rapidly expanding body of knowledge. For example, a recent search of PubMed using the term "metacarpal fracture" resulted in 1392 hits, and 66 articles on the topic were published last year alone. When faced with a clinical problem, the individual hand surgeon cannot coherently synthesize all of the relevant information to guide his or her treatment. The sheer volume of information has become an impediment rather than an aid to evidence-based decision making.

Another problem is the poor quality of evidence in the hand surgery literature. The vast majority of studies that address the management of hand fractures are retrospective case series, often without a control cohort.[1,2] There is a paucity of high-quality randomized controlled trials, and those that exist usually compare 2 nonoperative treatments. A recent editorial in the *Journal of Hand Surgery* underlines the need for better evidence in the form of randomized controlled trials that will increase the quality of care provided by the hand surgeon.[3] Unfortunately, there are many hurdles to conducting randomized trials that compare surgical treatment options for hand fractures, not the least of which are the wide spectrum of fracture variations that are seen in the hand, and the difficulty in recruiting patients to undergo randomization.

Due to an increased recognition of these problems, a number of hand surgery–related journals have instituted practices that make it easier to evaluate the quality of evidence, and that help to summarize the existing evidence related to specific topics. Journals have recently begun to display the level of evidence for every article published (**Table 1**),[4,5] and regularly feature articles that focus on applying evidence-based medicine to common hand problems. These and other efforts have greatly helped make the available evidence of more practical use to the hand surgeon.

Department of Plastic Surgery, University of Texas Southwestern Medical School, 1801 Inwood Road, Dallas, TX 75390, USA
* Corresponding author.
E-mail address: Douglas.Sammer@UTSouthwestern.edu

Hand Clin 29 (2013) 501–505
http://dx.doi.org/10.1016/j.hcl.2013.08.005
0749-0712/13/$ – see front matter © 2013 Elsevier Inc. All rights reserved.

Table 1
Levels of evidence for therapeutic studies

Level of Evidence	Therapeutic Studies
I	High-quality randomized controlled trial
II	Prospective comparative, or lesser quality randomized controlled trial
III	Case-control, retrospective comparative
IV	Case series
V	Expert opinion

PRINCIPLES OF HAND FRACTURE MANAGEMENT

Because high-quality scientific evidence cannot be applied to the treatment of most hand fractures, it is critical to have an understanding of the core principles of hand fracture management. These principles should always be kept in mind when treating hand fractures, and should be relied on particularly when scientific evidence is limited or contradictory. These principles include the following:

- Anatomic reduction of articular fractures
- Restoration of anatomic relationships in extra-articular fractures
- Stable fixation that minimizes soft tissue injury
- Institution of early motion

Anatomic Reduction of Articular Fractures

Articular fractures should be reduced to anatomic or near-anatomic alignment to prevent joint pain, loss of motion, and accelerated degenerative changes. Because of the precise reduction required, and because of the deforming forces that ligaments and tendons exert on articular fragments, open reduction with percutaneous or internal fixation is often required. Although it is not known exactly how much articular incongruity can be tolerated in the small joints of the hand, many investigators recommend correction of step-offs of 1 mm or larger. This is supported by the findings of Seno and colleagues,[6] in which the outcomes of 140 intra-articular middle phalanx base fractures were reported. In patients who underwent surgical treatment, the presence of a residual articular step-off of 1 mm or more was associated with poor clinical outcomes. The amount of articular involvement should be considered as well. A displaced fragment that involves 5% of an articular surface is likely to be less

problematic than a fragment that involves 45% of the articular surface. Again, there is little evidence to support a specific threshold for surgical intervention based on the amount of the articular surface involved. Recommendations vary by investigator and by the specific joint or fracture, but displaced articular fractures in the hand that involve more than 15% to 25% of the articular surface benefit from articular reduction.[7,8] Finally, articular fractures that result in persistent subluxation after reduction usually require operative management to maintain a congruous and concentric joint, if not an anatomic articular surface.

Restoration of Anatomic Relationships in Extra-Articular Fractures

For much of the last half of the twentieth century there was an emphasis on achieving anatomic fracture reduction, including in extra-articular fractures. Over the past 2 decades, however, there has been an increased recognition that, for extra-articular fractures in the hand, the restoration of critical anatomic relationships is more important than the anatomic reduction of fracture fragments. This means that the goal of reduction for extra-articular fractures should be the correction of clinically significant shortening, angulation, and rotation so as to avoid problems such as tendon imbalance, weakness, or scissoring. It is not necessary to achieve anatomic fracture reduction to have an excellent clinical outcome.

The amount of shortening, angulation, and rotation that can be tolerated varies by location and fracture pattern. In general, angulation within the primary plane of motion (flexion/extension) is more readily tolerated than angulation in the coronal plane. In the proximal phalanges, biomechanical and clinical studies suggest that a clinically significant proximal interphalangeal extension lag occurs, with more than 20 to 25° of apex volar angulation of the proximal phalanx.[9,10] More than 10° of angulation in the coronal plane, however, may interfere with function. In metacarpal fractures, the degree of angulation that can be tolerated varies depending on the metacarpal and on the location of the fracture within the metacarpal. Because there is very little compensatory motion at the index and long finger carpometacarpal (CMC) joints, index and long finger metacarpal neck fractures only tolerate up to 10° of apex dorsal angulation respectively.[11] In the ring metacarpal neck, 20° to 30° of apex dorsal angulation is acceptable. And because of the highly mobile small finger CMC joint, excellent hand function is observed in small finger metacarpal neck fractures that heal with up to 70° of apex dorsal angulation.[12]

In addition, the more proximal the fracture is within the metacarpal, the greater the clinical impact of angulation. For example, although 70° of apex dorsal angulation can be tolerated at the small finger metacarpal neck, the same amount of angulation at the proximal diaphysis of the small finger metacarpal would markedly impair hand function. Some degree of shortening is also well tolerated in the metacarpals, particularly in the small finger metacarpal. Although biomechanical studies suggest that as little as 3 mm of metacarpal shortening can affect tendon function,[13] there is clinical evidence that shortening of up to 5 mm is well tolerated.[14] Unlike angulation or shortening, rotational deformity is poorly tolerated in the hand. The amount of rotation that can be accepted depends on fracture location. For example, 10° of rotation at the midshaft of the distal phalanx does not result in a clinical deficit; however, the very same amount of rotation in the midshaft of a metacarpal will result in as much as 2 cm of digit overlap with full flexion.[15] For every 1° of metacarpal rotation, as much as 5° of rotation occurs at the fingertips.[15]

Although these radiographic guidelines can help with decision making, it cannot be overemphasized that the most effective way to determine whether residual fracture displacement will be tolerated is by a clinical examination of hand function. If the patient can fully flex and extend the fingers without extension lag or pseudo-clawing, and without scissoring or abutment of adjacent fingers, then surgical intervention to achieve anatomic reduction is unlikely to improve outcomes.

Stable Fixation that Minimizes Soft Tissue Injury

The evidence regarding clinical outcomes after open reduction internal fixation (ORIF) in the hand is limited (level III or IV evidence) and variable. Multiple studies demonstrate poor motion and high complication rates when ORIF is used to treat metacarpal and phalangeal fractures.[16–18] In contrast, other studies show very good clinical outcomes after plate fixation in the hand.[19–21] Furthermore, closed reduction percutaneous pinning is not without complications, such as contractures, loss of motion, and infection.[22] It is likely that the nature of the injury (phalangeal vs metacarpal, articular vs diaphyseal, and open vs closed) has an equal or greater influence on outcomes than the method of fixation. Currently, there is insufficient scientific evidence to guide the selection of fixation in most types of hand fractures.

Because of the need to maintain precise reduction and begin early motion, articular fractures often benefit from ORIF. In contrast, most extra-articular

fractures can be managed successfully with closed reduction and splinting, or percutaneous pin fixation. Although ORIF with plate and screws allows the institution of early aggressive motion,[23,24] extensive soft tissue dissection and periosteal stripping are often required. This can result in increased edema, delayed healing, tendon adhesions, and stiffness, in many cases negating the advantages of plate fixation.[17] Furthermore, complications, such as tendon rupture or delayed union, can result in poor outcomes.[17] Although percutaneous pinning does not provide rigid fixation, it provides sufficient stabilization to maintain the reduction of most extra-articular hand fractures, and, if performed properly, is stable enough to allow early gentle motion at adjacent joints.[11,25]

In summary, there is little evidence to guide the selection of fixation for most hand fractures. The method that achieves the required degree of stabilization and allows early motion, and results in the least damage to soft tissues should be used. For many articular fractures, this is best achieved by ORIF, but most extra-articular fractures can be treated successfully without inflicting significant soft tissue injury.

Institution of Early Motion

The ultimate goal when treating hand fractures is to achieve a mobile, functional hand. To achieve this goal, the surgeon must carefully balance the need to protect the fracture with the absolute imperative to begin motion. In adults, finger immobilization for more than 3 to 4 weeks can result in permanent loss of motion.[26,27] Hand fractures do not need to be solidly united to start joint mobilization, and most hand fractures treated closed have healed sufficiently by 3 weeks to begin gentle protected motion.[11] At this time point, there is often some mild residual tenderness at the site of the fracture, and limited radiographic evidence of healing. However, it is preferable to err on the side of starting motion, and accept the risk of a rare nonunion. As Bob Beasley is quoted as saying,[28] "For every nonunion, the hand surgeon sees a thousand stiff joints." In cases of open reduction with stable internal fixation, it is even more important to start motion early, as soon as edema has subsided and pain is under control, usually within a few days of surgery. The act of opening and plating a fracture leads to increased edema, scarring, and adhesions, and failure to begin early motion will invariably result in stiffness and loss of function.

SUMMARY

The overall quality of evidence that can be used to help guide decision making when treating hand fractures is relatively low. This does not mean that the evidence that exists is not useful, but rather that it should be interpreted and applied cautiously. Fortunately, there are a few straightforward principles that can be used to help guide decision making in cases in which the evidence is limited or contradictory. Articular fractures require a precise, near-anatomic reduction. On the other hand, extra-articular fractures require a reduction that restores anatomic relationships, and restores normal hand function. In many cases, residual displacement is well tolerated. If the hand functions well, surgical intervention to correct the radiographic appearance of a fracture is unlikely to improve function. Rigid internal fixation is not a requirement in most hand fractures, and the less soft tissue injury that occurs as a result of fracture fixation, the better. Extensive dissection and periosteal injury slow fracture healing, and contribute to stiffness and contractures. Finally, the surgeon must balance the need to immobilize the fracture to promote healing, with the need to mobilize the finger joints to prevent stiffness. In general, the surgeon should err on the side of early motion, keeping in mind that the ultimate goal is a mobile, functional hand.

REFERENCES

1. Friedrich JB, Vedder NB. An evidence-based approach to metacarpal fractures. Plast Reconstr Surg 2010;126(6):2205–9.
2. Schadel-Hopfner M, Windolf J, Antes G, et al. Evidence-based hand surgery: the role of Cochrane reviews. J Hand Surg Eur Vol 2008;33(2):110–7.
3. Hammert WC, Ring D, Kozin S. Evidence-based hand and upper extremity surgery: editorial. J Hand Surg Am 2013;38(1):1.
4. Hentz RV, Meals RA, Stern P, et al. Levels of evidence and the *Journal of Hand Surgery*. J Hand Surg Am 2005;30(5):891–2.
5. Sullivan D, Chung KC, Eaves FF 3rd, et al. The level of evidence pyramid: indicating levels of evidence in plastic and reconstructive surgery articles. Plast Reconstr Surg 2011;128(1):311–4.
6. Seno N, Hashizume H, Inoue H, et al. Fractures of the base of the middle phalanx of the finger. Classification, management and long-term results. J Bone Joint Surg Br 1997;79(5):758–63.
7. Green DP, Pederson WC, Hotchkiss RN, et al. Green's operative hand surgery. 5th edition. London: Churchill Livingstone; 2005.
8. Haughton D, Jordan D, Malahias M, et al. Principles of hand fracture management. Open Orthop J 2012; 6:43–53.
9. Vahey JW, Wegner DA, Hastings H 3rd. Effect of proximal phalangeal fracture deformity on extensor tendon function. J Hand Surg Am 1998;23(4): 673–81.
10. Meals RA, Meuli HC. Carpenter's nails, phonograph needles, piano wires, and safety pins: the history of operative fixation of metacarpal and phalangeal fractures. J Hand Surg Am 1985;10(1):144–50.
11. Henry MH. Fractures of the proximal phalanx and metacarpals in the hand: preferred methods of stabilization. J Am Acad Orthop Surg 2008;16(10):586–95.
12. Statius Muller MG, Poolman RW, van Hoogstraten MJ, et al. Immediate mobilization gives good results in boxer's fractures with volar angulation up to 70 degrees: a prospective randomized trial comparing immediate mobilization with cast immobilization. Arch Orthop Trauma Surg 2003; 123(10):534–7.
13. Low CK, Wong HC, Low YP, et al. A cadaver study of the effects of dorsal angulation and shortening of the metacarpal shaft on the extension and flexion force ratios of the index and little fingers. J Hand Surg Br 1995;20(5):609–13.
14. Prokop A, Kulus S, Helling HJ, et al. Are there guidelines for treatment of metacarpal fractures? Personal results and literature analysis of the last 12 years. Unfallchirurg 1999;102(1):50–8 [in German].
15. Freeland AE, Lindley SG. Malunions of the finger metacarpals and phalanges. Hand Clin 2006;22(3): 341–55.
16. Stern PJ, Wieser MJ, Reilly DG. Complications of plate fixation in the hand skeleton. Clin Orthop Relat Res 1987;(214):59–65.
17. Page SM, Stern PJ. Complications and range of motion following plate fixation of metacarpal and phalangeal fractures. J Hand Surg Am 1998;23(5):827–32.
18. Pun WK, Chow SP, So YC, et al. Unstable phalangeal fractures: treatment by A.O. screw and plate fixation. J Hand Surg Am 1991;16(1):113–7.
19. Ford DJ, el-Hadidi S, Lunn PG, et al. Fractures of the metacarpals: treatment by A. O. screw and plate fixation. J Hand Surg Br 1987;12(1):34–7.
20. Dabezies EJ, Schutte JP. Fixation of metacarpal and phalangeal fractures with miniature plates and screws. J Hand Surg Am 1986;11(2):283–8.
21. Takigami H, Sakano H, Saito T. Internal fixation with the low profile plate system compared with Kirschner wire fixation: clinical results of treatment for metacarpal and phalangeal fractures. Hand Surg 2010;15(1):1–6.
22. Faruqui S, Stern PJ, Kiefhaber TR. Percutaneous pinning of fractures in the proximal third of the proximal phalanx: complications and outcomes. J Hand Surg Am 2012;37(7):1342–8.
23. Fyfe IS, Mason S. The mechanical stability of internal fixation of fractured phalanges. Hand 1979;11(1): 50–4.
24. Massengill JB, Alexander H, Langrana N, et al. A phalangeal fracture model—quantitative analysis

of rigidity and failure. J Hand Surg Am 1982;7(3): 264–70.

25. Jones NF, Jupiter JB, Lalonde DH. Common fractures and dislocations of the hand. Plast Reconstr Surg 2012;130(5):722e–36e.

26. Green DP. Complications of phalangeal and metacarpal fractures. Hand Clin 1986;2(2):307–28.

27. Agee J. Treatment principles for proximal and middle phalangeal fractures. Orthop Clin North Am 1992;23(1):35–40.

28. Jabaley ME, Wegener EE. Principles of internal fixation as applied to the hand and wrist. In: Mathes SJ, Hentz VR, editors. Plastic surgery, vol. VII, 2nd edition. Philadelphia: Saunders; 2006. p. 139–50.

Current Management of Metacarpal Fractures

Rafael Diaz-Garcia, MD, Jennifer F. Waljee, MD, MS*

KEYWORDS

- Metacarpal fractures • Hand injury • Bony fixation • Hand fractures

KEY POINTS

- Metacarpal fractures are common, and many can be managed nonoperatively with appropriate reduction and immobilization.
- As with any hand fracture, the primary goals are to achieve anatomic and stable reduction, bony union, and early mobilization to minimize disability.
- Functional outcomes depend on appropriate treatment and early range of motion whenever possible.

OVERVIEW

Metacarpal fractures represent one of the most common orthopedic injuries, and are frequently encountered in emergency departments and ambulatory care clinics. Although most of these injuries can be successfully managed without operative intervention, to achieve optimal outcomes it is important to review the anatomy, principles, and techniques of operative intervention as well as the goals of therapy.

EPIDEMIOLOGY

Metacarpal fractures are among the most prevalent injuries evaluated in the emergency setting, comprising approximately 30% of all hand fractures and 18% of all below-elbow fractures in the United States.[1–3] The majority (70%) occur within the second and third decades of life.[4] Most fractures are due to either accidental falls or direct blows to another object or individual, with small-finger neck fractures and ring-finger shaft fractures among the most common metacarpal fractures.[5] Despite their prevalence, the evidence supporting any single treatment strategy is largely limited to single-center studies, and randomized controlled trials are difficult to implement given the wide spectrum of fracture patterns and mechanisms of injury.[6] Nonetheless, the literature is rich with large, retrospective series with long follow-up that provide insight into the most effective treatments for these common injuries.

ANATOMY

The metacarpals represent the most proximal long bones of the hand, and provide a stable platform for the phalanges and palmar neurovascular structures.[7] The metacarpals form a volar concave arc along their length, with flares at the bases and the necks (Fig. 1). The metacarpal base articulates with the distal carpal row. The metacarpal head is cam-shaped, and articulates with the base of the proximal phalanx as a condylar joint that permits flexion, extension, and radial and ulnar motion.[8] The fibrocartilaginous volar plate lies along the palmar aspect of the metacarpophalangeal (MCP) joint, providing support and resistance to hyperextension. The deep intermetacarpal ligaments connect the volar plates between adjacent digits, and offer further stability by preventing

None of the authors has a financial interest to declare in relation to the content of this article.
Section of Plastic Surgery, Department of Surgery, The University of Michigan Health System, 2130 Taubman Center, SPC 5340, 1500 East Medical Center Drive, Ann Arbor, MI 48109-5340, USA
* Corresponding author.
E-mail address: filip@med.umich.edu

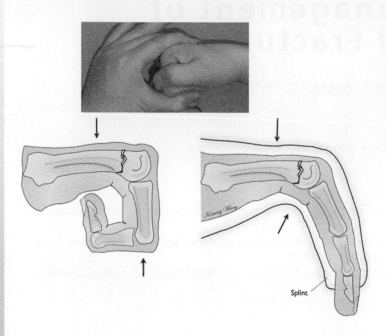

Fig. 1. The Jahss maneuver for reduction of metacarpal neck fractures. *Arrows* indicate direction of force applied across the digit.

shortening from metacarpal shaft fractures. The collateral ligaments arise from the dorsal aspect of the metacarpal head and insert on the volar aspect of the base of the proximal phalanx. The accessory collateral ligaments lie volar to the proper collateral ligaments, and attach at the proximal phalanx and volar plate. When the MCP joint is flexed the collateral ligaments lengthen and tighten, thereby stabilizing the MCP joint.

Unlike phalangeal fractures, the flexor and extensor tendons are less intimately connected with the bony surface, and thus may yield superior outcomes following injury. However, an understanding of the extensor tendon apparatus should be appreciated, as a dorsal approach is typically undertaken to treat these fractures. The interossei originate along the metacarpal shaft, which then insert along the base of the proximal phalanx, the extensor hood, and contribute to the lateral bands of the extensor tendon apparatus.[9] The sagittal bands stabilize the extensor tendon over the head of the metacarpal, and unite the volar plate, collateral ligaments, and deep transverse intermetacarpal ligaments. More proximally, the wrist extensors and flexors insert on the metacarpal bases. Specifically, the extensor carpi radialis longus (ECRL) inserts at the base of the index metacarpal, the extensor carpi radialis brevis (ECRB) inserts at the base of the long-finger metacarpal, and the extensor carpi ulnaris (ECU) inserts at the base of the small-finger metacarpal. Similarly, the flexor carpi radialis (FCR) tendon inserts on the base of the index metacarpal, and the flexor carpi ulnaris inserts at the base of the small finger.

PRINCIPLES OF TREATMENT

The primary goals of treatment are to achieve acceptable alignment, stable reduction, strong bony union, and unrestricted motion. A complete history should be elicited from the patient with a specific focus on hand dominance, occupation, mechanism of injury, time of injury, and previous hand trauma or upper extremity surgical procedures. A thorough physical examination is essential in assessing the presence of rotational deformity, which will not be captured by plain radiographs. The patient is asked to flex and extend the fingers, and the alignment of the nail plates is noted. Rotational deformity may be subtle, and examination of the other hand is often useful. Even a small (5°) degree of rotation will yield a 1.5-cm digital overlap with both aesthetic and functional deformity. For patients who are unable to perform active flexion, the digital cascade can be observed through the tenodesis effect by flexing and extending the wrist. In addition, the neurovascular status of the hand, active and passive range of motion, bony deformity, digit shortening, loss of knuckle contour, and soft-tissue injury should be noted. Standard posterior-anterior, oblique, and lateral radiographs are usually sufficient to evaluate hand fractures, specifically fracture geometry, comminution, angulation, and shortening. Bony apposition should approximate 50% or more, and approximately 5 mm of bony shortening is usually tolerated.

The initial evaluation is focused on assessing stability to determine the need for operative intervention and the potential success of nonoperative management. The general indications for the operative management of metacarpal fractures are listed in **Box 1**. Inherently unstable fractures include those with involvement of 25% or more of the articular surface of the joint or 1 mm of step-off, displaced oblique fractures with rotational deformity, displaced fractures of the metacarpal base with carpometacarpal (CMC) joint subluxation, and displaced Bennett or Rolando fractures. Rotational deformity of a digit is not tolerated in the hand, and is an indication for reduction and fixation (**Table 1**). Finally, metacarpal shortening greater than 5 mm decreases the efficiency of intrinsic muscle contraction, and extensor lag is associated with a significant loss of power.[10,11]

Metacarpal Head Fractures

Although metacarpal head fractures are rare, these injuries are challenging to treat given the presence of hyaline cartilage and the risk of osteonecrosis. Fracture fragments are typically small and comminuted, and reduction and fixation demands a meticulous technique to avoid stripping the collateral ligaments and devascularizing the bony fragments.[12] In addition to plain radiographs, computed tomography scans may be helpful for fractures to better characterize the fracture pattern. For fractures that involve less than 20% of the joint surface, nonoperative management

Table 1	
Degree of acceptable angulation for fractures of metacarpal shaft and neck	
Finger	**Angulation (degrees)**
Neck	
Index	10
Middle	15
Ring	30
Small	40
Shaft	
Index	0
Middle	0
Ring	20
Small	30

can be undertaken with immobilization in the intrinsic plus position.[13] For those fractures with a greater disruption of the articular surface, the goal of treatment is to restore the contour of the metacarpal head in a stable fashion to allow for early range of motion. If possible, these fractures are best treated with lag screws that are countersunk into the cartilage.[14] However, more commonly these fractures present with significant joint disruption and comminution. External fixation that incorporates distraction and early motion may improve long-term function following these injuries, and some investigators have described the use of arthroplasty in the acute setting for treatment of these complex injuries.[15,16] However, despite aggressive treatment, late arthritis is not uncommon.[13,17]

Metacarpal Neck Fractures

Metacarpal neck fractures are most commonly seen in the small finger and are often referred to as "boxer's fractures," given their prevalence in the amateur pugilist. At the time of injury the volar cortex fractures, resulting in an apex-dorsal angulation fracture pattern with flexion of the metacarpal head. The intrinsic muscles of the hand cross the MCP joint and maintain flexion of the metacarpal head, and a pseudoclaw deformity may develop from the imbalance of the extrinsic and intrinsic musculature caused by metacarpal shortening. When the patient attempts to extend the fingers, the proximal interphalangeal (PIP) joint flexes and the MCP joint hyperextends.

In general, metacarpal fractures with angulation of less than 10° for the index finger, less than 15° for the long finger, less than 30° for the ring finger, and less than 40° for the small finger that have no associated rotational deformity may be managed conservatively with immobilization and serial

---

Box 1
Characteristics of unstable fractures requiring operative intervention

Irreducible fractures

Open fractures

Fractures with segmental bony loss

Multiple fractures

Fractures associated with significant soft-tissue injury

Rotational deformity

Angulation

Examples:

>25% Involvement of the articular surface of the metacarpal head or 1-mm step-off

Displaced fractures of oblique shaft with rotational deformity on examination

Displaced fractures of metacarpal base with dislocation or subluxation of the carpometacarpal joint

Displaced fractures of thumb metacarpal base

radiographs. Greater mobility in the ulnar CMC joints of the hand alleviates angulated ring-finger and small-finger neck fractures. By contrast, the index-finger and long-finger CMC joints are relatively fixed, and greater degrees of angulation are poorly tolerated. However, these guidelines are relative, and multiple studies have documented excellent patient-reported outcomes and function with greater degrees of angulation, particularly for small-finger metacarpal neck fractures.[18–22] For example, McKerrell and colleagues[21] followed 40 patients treated nonoperatively and with reduction and pinning for angulated small-finger metacarpal neck fractures, and identified no difference in hand function following treatment. Patients should be counseled regarding the long-term possibility of the loss of dorsal joint/knuckle prominence with a more prominent dorsal deformity more proximally and a palpable metacarpal head in the palm. However, for patients with no rotational deformity or absent pseudoclawing on examination, conservative management is appropriate. Immobilization may consist of cast or splint placement, and should immobilize the wrist, MCP, and PIP joints for 3 weeks in the intrinsic plus position, followed by early active range of motion.

For fractures in which rotational deformity or pseudoclawing is present, reduction can be accomplished using the Jahss maneuver (**Fig. 2**).

Under adequate anesthesia, the MCP and PIP joints are fully flexed, and dorsal force is applied along the proximal phalanx and volarly along the metacarpal shaft, to reduce the metacarpal head from a flexed position. For rotational deformity, additional manipulation can be performed along the flexed proximal phalanx to restore the anatomic position. Percutaneous Kirschner (K) wires can be placed in a variety of configurations to hold the reduction in place and to act as an internal splint. Pins may be placed in a crossed fashion down the metacarpal shaft (**Fig. 3**), or transversely into the head of the adjacent, noninjured ring-finger metacarpal head. K-wires are advantageous because they can easily be placed percutaneously without the need for an extensive dissection. However, they do not provide rigid fixation, and pin-site infections are not uncommon.[23,24] External pins may be difficult for patients to manage, and poor follow-up is common in this patient population.[25] Other investigators have advocated the use of antegrade intramedullary pins inserted percutaneously at the base of the metacarpal (**Fig. 4**).[26,27] Intramedullary fixation offers excellent stability with minimal soft-tissue dissection and protection of the extensor tendon mechanism from adhesions, although joint penetration, loss of reduction, and the need for secondary surgeries has been described.[28,29] Finally, plate fixation using a

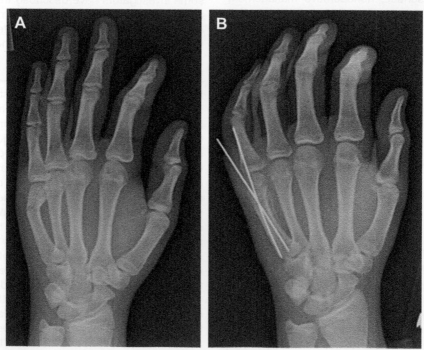

Fig. 2. Percutaneous Kirschner (K)-wire fixation of a closed metacarpal neck fracture in a patient with a pseudoclaw deformity. (*A*) Preoperative. (*B*) Postoperative.

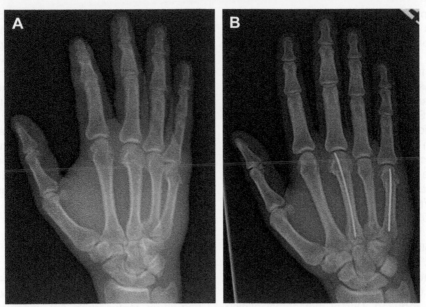

Fig. 3. Intramedullary nailing of a closed metacarpal neck fracture in a polytrauma patient. (*A*) Preoperative. (*B*) Postoperative.

mini-condylar plate can be undertaken for neck fractures. However, this technique requires an open approach with greater dissection, which may increase the risk of adhesions and long-term stiffness.

Metacarpal Shaft Fractures

Metacarpal shaft fractures can result from axial loading, torsion, or a direct blow, and typically present as transverse fractures, oblique fractures, or comminuted fractures. As with metacarpal neck fractures, injuries that are nondisplaced or minimally displaced, without significant angulation,

rotational deformity, or shortening, can be managed conservatively with immobilization. Angulation is better tolerated among the ulnar digits than in the index or middle finger. However, the presence of pseudoclawing, rotational deformity, or significant metacarpal shortening or prominent dorsal deformity should prompt consideration of operative intervention. Although closed reduction may be attempted for displaced transverse metacarpal shaft fractures, the many of these injuries will require operative fixation.

A variety of techniques are available for fracture fixation, including pins, wiring techniques, intramedullary fixation, plate fixation, and interfragmentary

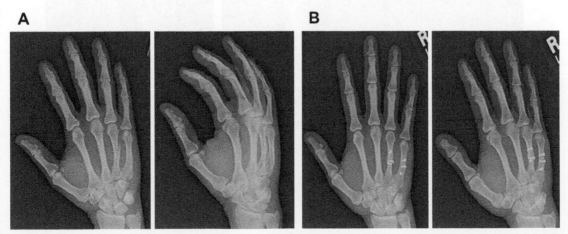

Fig. 4. Lag-screw fixation of an oblique metacarpal shaft fracture in a polytrauma patient. (*A*) Preoperative. (*B*) Postoperative.

compression screws.[30] Although some fracture patterns are ideally suited to specific techniques, the choice for fixation is largely directed by fracture pattern and surgeon preference. As with metacarpal neck fractures, pin fixation is advantageous because pins are readily available, require minimal dissection, and can be applied in a variety of configurations. Similar disadvantages include a lack of rigid fixation, fracture distraction, pin-site infection, and pin migration. Composite wiring or cerclage wiring can be used in conjunction with pins to provide a more stable construct, and can be used for a variety of fracture patterns.[31] Interfragmentary screws can provide compression, and are ideally suited for long oblique fractures in which the fracture length is twice the diameter of the bone, enabling accommodation of at least 2 screws (**Fig. 5**). Achieving compression is technically demanding with little margin for error, and soft-tissue dissection with anatomic fracture reduction is required. Dorsal metacarpal plating using stainless-steel or titanium plates is more straightforward to perform, and may provide more stable fixation compared with pin or wire techniques when 2 or 3 bicortical screws are placed on either side of the fracture (see **Fig. 5**).[32] Despite these advantages, plates are associated with hardware failure, infection, and poor fracture healing, with complication rates of up to 35% in some series.[33,34] Intramedullary fixation can be used with relatively little dissection, and is especially advantageous for multiple transverse shaft fractures.[35] Finally, some investigators have advocated the use of external fixators for shaft

fractures, citing the minimal need for dissection that may potentially devascularize the bone, and formation of a stable construct that permits early motion.[36–38] However, complications may include pin-site infection, nonunion of extensor tendon, and nonunion caused by overdistraction.[39] Bioabsorbable plates have gained popularity for fracture fixation for craniofacial surgery, but as yet have not gained widespread acceptance in hand surgery. Studies in cadaveric and animal models are encouraging, and bioabsorbable plates demonstrate stability similar to that achieved with titanium constructs.[40] Future studies examining the application of these approaches in hand surgery may provide insight into their appropriate use for metacarpal fractures.

Metacarpal Base Fractures

Intra-articular base fractures of the index- through ring-finger metacarpals are uncommon injuries, although some have argued that this likely represents an underreported and underdiagnosed injury.[41–43] These fractures are usually a result of a fall on a flexed wrist with the arm in extension and axial loading of the metacarpal.[44] Because of their low incidence, their presence in the literature is limited to a handful of case series. Their management is somewhat controversial. While some have endorsed conservative management, there is a growing trend toward operative intervention.[43–46] The argument for nonsurgical management is based on the limited motion of the second and third CMC joints, such as to diminish

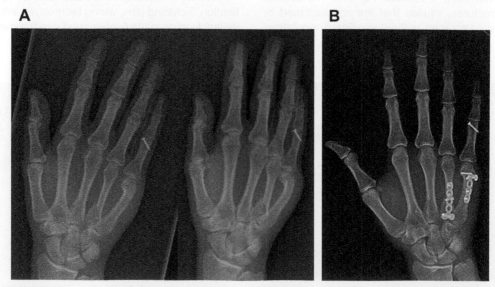

Fig. 5. Multiple metacarpal shaft fractures necessitate open reduction and internal fixation. (*A*) Preoperative. (*B*) Postoperative.

the importance of articular congruity. The counter-argument is that the failure to achieve anatomic reduction is believed to affect the dorsal insertions of the wrist extensors and potentially result in osteoarthritis, which can result in decreased range of motion and diminished wrist extension, in turn causing weakness of grip.

Fractures of the base of the small-finger metacarpal are the most common of these injuries, and can be thought of as mechanically similar to fractures of the thumb, explaining the eponyms "reverse Bennett" and "baby Bennett" fractures. The ECU serves as the deforming force, pulling the metacarpal dorsally, ulnarly, and proximally. The volar-radial segment of the base articular surface remains in situ, owing to the firm attachment to the intermetacarpal ligament and reinforcing insertion of the volar flexor carpi ulnaris.[47] There is no consensus regarding the optimal management of reverse Bennett fractures. Nondisplaced fractures are generally treated nonoperatively. Conservative management with reduction and immobilization of minimally displaced fractures is also possible, with a 100% union rate and return of grip strength, but 41% of patients show radiographic evidence of arthrosis.[48] Most investigators recommend operative management of displaced reverse Bennett fractures, but the clinical outcomes are mixed and do not necessarily support such a recommendation. Regardless of surgical or nonsurgical management, results are similar with regard to return of function, development of posttraumatic arthritis, and long-term pain.[43,49,50]

Thumb Metacarpal Fractures

Fractures of the thumb metacarpal are unique and warrant a distinct discussion, because of both the digit's importance and the compensatory motion of the adjacent joints. Malrotation and angulatory deformity are rarely a functional problem as a result of the motion of the CMC joint, although they may raise cosmetic concerns. Extra-articular fractures can often be managed nonoperatively. Up to 30° of lateral angulation can be tolerated without compromising bony union or overall hand function.[51] However, intra-articular fractures of the thumb metacarpal are almost always treated with surgical intervention for fear of resulting posttraumatic arthritis.

Bennett fractures

Bennett fractures refer to simple intra-articular fractures of the thumb metacarpal base that extend into the CMC joint. There is a single fracture fragment which, held by the anterior oblique ligament, resides volar and ulnar to the rest of the metacarpal base (**Fig. 6**). The metacarpal is

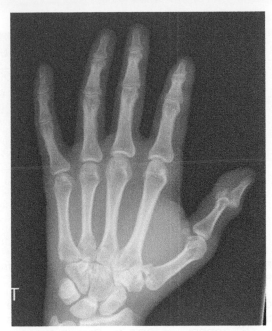

Fig. 6. Fracture at the base of the thumb metacarpal (Bennett fracture).

subluxed by the destabilizing forces of the abductor pollicis longus, which pulls the metacarpal radially and proximally, and the adductor pollicis, which distracts the MCP joint ulnarly.

The fracture is reduced by countering the deforming forces, namely longitudinal traction, thumb pronation, and adduction of the metacarpal base. Closed reduction and percutaneous pinning can be attempted after assuring anatomic reduction under fluoroscopy, with the pin being driven into either the trapezium or the adjacent metacarpal (**Fig. 7**).[52] If anatomic reduction cannot be achieved, open reduction and internal fixation (ORIF) is done through a Wagner incision that is lined up over the subcutaneous border of the metacarpal, between the abductor pollicis longus and the thenar musculature. Anatomic reduction is obtained, and fixation can be with either 1.5-mm screws or K-wires, although the former is obviously more rigid and allows early motion. Some advocate ORIF regardless of reduction if greater than 20% of the articular surface is involved.[53]

Though once commonplace, nonoperative management of Bennett fractures has fallen out of favor because of concern for posttraumatic arthritis. Persistent articular incongruity has been found to lead to degenerative arthritis and subluxation of the joint, leading investigators to conclude that this fracture should not be treated conservatively.[54,55] The best available evidence regarding operative management shows no significant

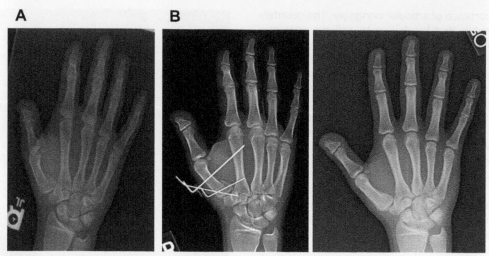

Fig. 7. Closed reduction and K-wire fixation of a fracture of thumb metacarpal base. (*A*) Preoperative. (*B*) Postoperative.

differences in clinical outcome between those treated with closed reduction and percutaneous pinning (CRPP) and ORIF for Bennett fractures with a mean follow-up of 7 years.[56] Pain, range of motion, and strength were similar between the two groups, although the CRPP group tended to have greater adduction deformity and arthrosis on radiographs. However, the arthrosis did not have a clinical impact on outcome.

Rolando fractures

Though initially described as a T-shaped or Y-shaped fracture pattern, the term Rolando fracture is used for any comminuted intra-articular thumb metacarpal base fracture. CRPP is difficult to achieve because of all the individual articular fragments that need to be aligned. Radiographs can appear deceptively benign, but the surgeon must be prepared for more fragments than expected. A classic 3-piece fracture pattern is best treated with an ORIF, using a Wagner incision for exposure and a 2.0- to2.5-mm T-plate for fixation. Fractures with significant articular comminution are often treated with some variation of external fixation, with good clinical results and 100% union rates being reported.[57–59] Buchler and colleagues[51] described a technique with placement of a quadrilateral mini–external fixator between the thumb and index metacarpals, limited internal fixation, and cancellous bone grafting of any voids. This case series represents the longest follow-up at 3 years, with 90% having a good result.

COMPLICATIONS OF METACARPAL FRACTURES

Although most patients with metacarpal fractures do well, complications associated with these injuries are also prevalent, and can arise from either surgical or nonsurgical management of the initial injury. Surgical management can result in hardware-related issues such as adhesions, infection, and tendon rupture, while a more conservative approach can result in malunion or stiffness arising from immobilization. The incidence of complications is highly correlated with the severity of the initial injury, with open fractures and crush injuries decreasing the potential for uneventful union.[60,61]

Malunion

Malunion is the most common complication encountered in the management of metacarpal fractures, particularly after nonoperative management of unstable fracture patterns. The actual prevalence of malunion is difficult to assess given the large number of closed metacarpal fractures that never seek medical care. The eventual malunion appearance can often be predicted from initial radiography, as specific fracture patterns result in specific deformities. Spiral and oblique shaft fractures can result in shortening because of the force of the intrinsic musculature. Shortening of the digit not only can be unaesthetic with blunting of the dorsal prominence of the metacarpal head, it can also alter the balance between the intrinsic and extrinsic muscle forces. Strauch and colleagues[11] demonstrated that each 2 mm of metacarpal shortening resulted in 7° of secondary extensor lag. The MCP joint can hyperextend to compensate for this deformity, but this is normally limited to about 20°. Thus, more than 6 mm of metacarpal shortening requires revision ORIF to reduce the deformity.

Angular malunion in the metacarpal is generally in the sagittal plane with an apex-dorsal deformity. Such malunion is usually seen with transverse shaft fractures, as the combination of the long flexors and intrinsics are stronger than the extrinsic extensors. Some sagittal angulation is acceptable, although the angles vary from 10° to 30° as one transitions from the index-finger to the small-finger metacarpal, owing to the greater mobility of the ulnar CMC joints. If a significant amount of angular malunion is present, it can be addressed with either an opening or closing wedge osteotomy. A closing wedge osteotomy is technically simpler and does not result in significant shortening, because effective length is gained with correction of the angulation.[62]

Rotational malunion is most likely to result in functional impairment as the deformity is magnified distally, and usually results from an unstable spiral or oblique fracture. Five degrees of malrotation in the metacarpal shaft can result in 1.5 cm of digital overlap, resulting in an unacceptable result.[63] Examination requires noting the alignment of the nail plates, as well as looking for "scissoring" or overlap as the patient slowly makes a fist. Correction of any rotational deformity can be achieved with an osteotomy at the previous fracture site or at the metaphysis. Weckesser[64] first described a corrective osteotomy near the base of the metacarpal to address rotational malunion in the 1960s. Gross and Gelberman[65] later described the limits of these osteotomies in cadavers, noting that the transverse metacarpal ligament was the main limiting factor in further rotation, and that 20° to 30° was the upper limit.

Nonunion

Nonunion after a closed metacarpal fracture is rare, and is more often found in the setting of a complex open injury with bony loss. Jupiter and colleagues[66] defined a delayed union or nonunion as fractures without clinical or radiographic evidence of healing at 4 months. The incidence of delayed union or nonunion may be as high as 6% after ORIF.[34,67] Bony nonunions can be classified as either hypertrophic or atrophic, and their management varies somewhat. The former is usually a result of inadequate stabilization, be it from failed fixation or poor compliance with immobilization. The management requires more stable fixation, usually with ORIF. Atrophic nonunions are more common in open fractures and are associated with bony infection. Any fibrous tissues or infected bone must be aggressively debrided, and bone grafts should be used to bridge any osseous defects.[68]

Decreased Range of Motion

Limitations in range of motion can occur after both conservative and operative management, albeit for different reasons. While ORIF predisposes the patient to tendinous adhesions, prolonged immobilization leads to tightening of the joint capsules and collateral ligaments, emphasizing the importance of splinting in a functional or safe position. Predisposing factors to postinjury stiffness include crush injuries, open fractures, multiple digit involvement, segmental injury and immobilization for longer than 4 weeks.[34,69] Overall, most patients undergoing ORIF for metacarpal fractures do well, with more than 75% having 220° of total active motion.[70–72]

Infection

Acute infections, including osteomyelitis, are much more common in open fractures of the hand. The deep-infection rate of open injuries is as high as 11%, compared with less than 0.5% in closed fractures undergoing operative intervention.[69,73] The rate of infection is correlated with contamination and soft-tissue injury, including periosteal stripping and devascularization. The stakes are high, as once osteomyelitis has set in the risk of eventual amputation is greater than 50%.[74] Traditional inflammatory markers such as erythrocyte sedimentation rate and C-reactive protein are of little value in the hand, and the diagnosis must be made with operative bone biopsy and pathologic examination. The management requires external fixation, aggressive debridement, systemic intravenous antibiotics, and secondary reconstruction with bone grafts and internal fixation.

REHABILITATION AFTER METACARPAL FRACTURE

Postinjury rehabilitation after metacarpal fracture is based on multiple variables including, but not limited to, the reliability of the patient, the location of the fracture, the stability of the fracture pattern, and the stability of fixation (if any). Early motion is generally considered appropriate when there are inherently stable fracture patterns or rigid fixation, the assumption being that early motion has the potential for improved outcomes.[75,76] It remains unclear as to whether early mobilization with conservative management offers a clinically relevant functional benefit, as most of the literature is based on limited case series and retrospective reviews.[77]

Protocols for postoperative hand therapy are largely predicated on operative technique and the confidence in the stability of the construct. After CRPP, gentle active range-of-motion exercises without resistance are usually commenced 2 to 3 weeks after surgery in adjacent or uninvolved joints, and this activity is advanced with Kirschner wire removal at 4 to 6 weeks. ORIF provides a more stable construct, so it is usually safe to begin active range of motion at the first postoperative period. The additional stability does come at a cost, with an increase in the incidence of tendinous adhesions, thus making early therapy not only possible but necessary.

SUMMARY

Metacarpal fractures are a common entity in both the emergency room and ambulatory care setting, making up one-third of the fractures seen in the hand. Fortunately, with proper management most patients do well after these injuries. Appropriate treatment requires a keen understanding of the types of fractures, their inherent stability, and the available treatment options. Further research with prospective cohorts and randomized controlled trials are needed to determine the ideal management strategies.

ACKNOWLEDGMENTS

The authors would like to thank Dr Keming Wang for the artwork contributed to this article.

REFERENCES

1. Aitken S, Court-Brown CM. The epidemiology of sports-related fractures of the hand. Injury 2008; 39(12):1377–83.
2. Chung KC, Spilson SV. The frequency and epidemiology of hand and forearm fractures in the United States. J Hand Surg Am 2001;26(5):908–15.
3. van Onselen EB, Karim RB, Hage JJ, et al. Prevalence and distribution of hand fractures. J Hand Surg Br 2003;28(5):491–5.
4. Stanton JS, Dias JJ, Burke FD. Fractures of the tubular bones of the hand. J Hand Surg Eur Vol 2007;32(6):626–36.
5. Soong M, Got C, Katarincic J. Ring and little finger metacarpal fractures: mechanisms, locations, and radiographic parameters. J Hand Surg Am 2010; 35(8):1256–9.
6. Poolman RW, Goslings JC, Lee JB, et al. Conservative treatment for closed fifth (small finger) metacarpal neck fractures. Cochrane Database Syst Rev 2005;(3):CD003210.
7. Chin SH, Vedder NB. MOC-PSSM CME article: metacarpal fractures. Plast Reconstr Surg 2008; 121(Suppl 1):1–13.

8. Minami A, An KN, Cooney WP 3rd, et al. Ligamentous structures of the metacarpophalangeal joint: a quantitative anatomic study. J Orthop Res 1984; 1(4):361–8.
9. Rayan GM, Murray D, Chung KW, et al. The extensor retinacular system at the metacarpophalangeal joint. Anatomical and histological study. J Hand Surg Br 1997;22(5):585–90.
10. Meunier MJ, Hentzen E, Ryan M, et al. Predicted effects of metacarpal shortening on interosseous muscle function. J Hand Surg Am 2004;29(4): 689–93.
11. Strauch RJ, Rosenwasser MP, Lunt JG. Metacarpal shaft fractures: the effect of shortening on the extensor tendon mechanism. J Hand Surg Am 1998;23(3):519–23.
12. Kumar VP, Satku K. Surgical management of osteochondral fractures of the phalanges and metacarpals: a surgical technique. J Hand Surg Am 1995; 20(6):1028–31.
13. McNemar TB, Howell JW, Chang E. Management of metacarpal fractures. J Hand Ther 2003;16(2): 143–51.
14. Tan JS, Foo AT, Chew WC, et al. Articularly placed interfragmentary screw fixation of difficult condylar fractures of the hand. J Hand Surg Am 2011;36(4): 604–9.
15. Stassen LP, Logghe R, van Riet YE, et al. Dynamic circle traction for severely comminuted intra-articular finger fractures. Injury 1994;25(3): 159–63.
16. Nagle DJ, af Ekenstam FW, Lister GD. Immediate silastic arthroplasty for non-salvageable intraarticular phalangeal fractures. Scand J Plast Reconstr Surg Hand Surg 1989;23(1):47–50.
17. Houshian S, Jing SS. A new technique for closed management of displaced intra-articular fractures of metacarpal and phalangeal head delayed on presentation: report of eight cases. J Hand Surg Eur Vol 2013. [Epub ahead of print].
18. Hunter JM, Cowen NJ. Fifth metacarpal fractures in a compensation clinic population. A report on one hundred and thirty-three cases. J Bone Joint Surg Am 1970;52(6):1159–65.
19. Kuokkanen HO, Mulari-Keranen SK, Niskanen RO, et al. Treatment of subcapital fractures of the fifth metacarpal bone: a prospective randomised comparison between functional treatment and reposition and splinting. Scand J Plast Reconstr Surg Hand Surg 1999;33(3):315–7.
20. Statius Muller MG, Poolman RW, van Hoogstraten MJ, et al. Immediate mobilization gives good results in boxer's fractures with volar angulation up to 70 degrees: a prospective randomized trial comparing immediate mobilization with cast immobilization. Arch Orthop Trauma Surg 2003;123(10):534–7.

21. McKerrell J, Bowen V, Johnston G, et al. Boxer's fractures—conservative or operative management? J Trauma 1987;27(5):486–90.

22. Lowdon IM. Fractures of the metacarpal neck of the little finger. Injury 1986;17(3):189–92.

23. Hargreaves DG, Drew SJ, Eckersley R. Kirschner wire pin tract infection rates: a randomized controlled trial between percutaneous and buried wires. J Hand Surg Br 2004;29(4):374–6.

24. Botte MJ, Davis JL, Rose BA, et al. Complications of smooth pin fixation of fractures and dislocations in the hand and wrist. Clin Orthop Relat Res 1992;(276):194–201.

25. ten Berg PW, Ring D. Patients lost to follow-up after metacarpal fractures. J Hand Surg Am 2012;37(1):42–6.

26. Kelsch G, Ulrich C. Intramedullary k-wire fixation of metacarpal fractures. Arch Orthop Trauma Surg 2004;124(8):523–6.

27. Wong TC, Ip FK, Yeung SH. Comparison between percutaneous transverse fixation and intramedullary K-wires in treating closed fractures of the metacarpal neck of the little finger. J Hand Surg Br 2006;31(1):61–5.

28. Ozer K, Gillani S, Williams A, et al. Comparison of intramedullary nailing versus plate-screw fixation of extra-articular metacarpal fractures. J Hand Surg Am 2008;33(10):1724–31.

29. Rhee SH, Lee SK, Lee SL, et al. Prospective multicenter trial of modified retrograde percutaneous intramedullary Kirschner wire fixation for displaced metacarpal neck and shaft fractures. Plast Reconstr Surg 2012;129(3):694–703.

30. Henry MH. Fractures of the proximal phalanx and metacarpals in the hand: preferred methods of stabilization. J Am Acad Orthop Surg 2008;16(10):586–95.

31. Teoh LC, Tan PL, Tan SH, et al. Cerclage-wiring-assisted fixation of difficult hand fractures. J Hand Surg Br 2006;31(6):637–42.

32. Yaffe MA, Saucedo JM, Kalainov DM. Non-locked and locked plating technology for hand fractures. J Hand Surg Am 2011;36(12):2052–5.

33. Fusetti C, Meyer H, Borisch N, et al. Complications of plate fixation in metacarpal fractures. J Trauma 2002;52(3):535–9.

34. Page SM, Stern PJ. Complications and range of motion following plate fixation of metacarpal and phalangeal fractures. J Hand Surg Am 1998;23(5):827–32.

35. Blazar PE, Leven D. Intramedullary nail fixation for metacarpal fractures. Hand Clin 2010;26(3):321–5, v.

36. Parsons SW, Fitzgerald JA, Shearer JR. External fixation of unstable metacarpal and phalangeal fractures. J Hand Surg Br 1992;17(2):151–5.

37. Schuind F, Cooney WP 3rd, Burny F, et al. Small external fixation devices for the hand and wrist. Clin Orthop Relat Res 1993;(293):77–82.

38. Margic K. External fixation of closed metacarpal and phalangeal fractures of digits. A prospective study of one hundred consecutive patients. J Hand Surg Br 2006;31(1):30–40.

39. Dailiana Z, Agorastakis D, Varitimidis S, et al. Use of a mini-external fixator for the treatment of hand fractures. J Hand Surg Am 2009;34(4):630–6.

40. Waris E, Ashammakhi N, Raatikainen T, et al. Self-reinforced bioabsorbable versus metallic fixation systems for metacarpal and phalangeal fractures: a biomechanical study. J Hand Surg Am 2002;27(5):902–9.

41. Cobbs KF, Owens WS, Berg EE. Extensor carpi radialis brevis avulsion fracture of the long finger metacarpal: a case report. J Hand Surg Am 1996;21(4):684–6.

42. Rotman MB, Pruitt DL. Avulsion fracture of the extensor carpi radialis brevis insertion. J Hand Surg Am 1993;18(3):511–3.

43. Bushnell BD, Draeger RW, Crosby CG, et al. Management of intra-articular metacarpal base fractures of the second through fifth metacarpals. J Hand Surg Am 2008;33(4):573–83.

44. Crichlow TP, Hoskinson J. Avulsion fracture of the index metacarpal base: three case reports. J Hand Surg Br 1988;13(2):212–4.

45. DeLee JC. Avulsion fracture of the base of the second metacarpal by the extensor carpi radialis longus. A case report. J Bone Joint Surg Am 1979;61(3):445–6.

46. Tsiridis E, Kohls-Gatzoulis J, Schizas C. Avulsion fracture of the extensor carpi radialis brevis insertion. J Hand Surg Br 2001;26(6):596–8.

47. Lilling M, Weinberg H. The mechanism of dorsal fracture dislocation of the fifth carpometacarpal joint. J Hand Surg Am 1979;4(4):340–2.

48. Lundeen JM, Shin AY. Clinical results of intraarticular fractures of the base of the fifth metacarpal treated by closed reduction and cast immobilization. J Hand Surg Br 2000;25(3):258–61.

49. Kjaer-Petersen K, Jurik AG, Petersen LK. Intra-articular fractures at the base of the fifth metacarpal. A clinical and radiographical study of 64 cases. J Hand Surg Br 1992;17(2):144–7.

50. Niechajev I. Dislocated intra-articular fracture of the base of the fifth metacarpal: a clinical study of 23 patients. Plast Reconstr Surg 1985;75(3):406–10.

51. Buchler U, McCollam SM, Oppikofer C. Comminuted fractures of the basilar joint of the thumb: combined treatment by external fixation, limited internal fixation, and bone grafting. J Hand Surg Am 1991;16(3):556–60.

52. van Niekerk JL, Ouwens R. Fractures of the base of the first metacarpal bone: results of surgical treatment. Injury 1989;20(6):359–62.

53. Foster RJ, Hastings H 2nd. Treatment of Bennett, Rolando, and vertical intraarticular trapezial fractures. Clin Orthop Relat Res 1987;(214):121–9.

54. Livesley PJ. The conservative management of Bennett's fracture-dislocation: a 26-year follow-up. J Hand Surg Br 1990;15(3):291–4.

55. Kjaer-Petersen K, Langhoff O, Andersen K. Bennett's fracture. J Hand Surg Br 1990;15(1):58–61.

56. Lutz M, Sailer R, Zimmermann R, et al. Closed reduction transarticular Kirschner wire fixation versus open reduction internal fixation in the treatment of Bennett's fracture dislocation. J Hand Surg Br 2003;28(2):142–7.

57. Gelberman RH, Vance RM, Zakaib GS. Fractures at the base of the thumb: treatment with oblique traction. J Bone Joint Surg Am 1979; 61(2):260–2.

58. El-Sharkawy AA, El-Mofty AO, Moharram AN, et al. Management of Rolando fracture by modified dynamic external fixation: a new technique. Tech Hand Up Extrem Surg 2009;13(1):11–5.

59. Niempoog S, Waitayawinyu T. Comminuted Rolando's fractures: treatment with modified wrist external fixator and transmetacarpal pinning. J Med Assoc Thai 2007;90(1):182–7.

60. Bannasch H, Heermann AK, Iblher N, et al. Ten years stable internal fixation of metacarpal and phalangeal hand fractures-risk factor and outcome analysis show no increase of complications in the treatment of open compared with closed fractures. J Trauma 2010;68(3):624–8.

61. Duncan RW, Freeland AE, Jabaley ME, et al. Open hand fractures: an analysis of the recovery of active motion and of complications. J Hand Surg Am 1993;18(3):387–94.

62. Green DP. Complications of phalangeal and metacarpal fractures. Hand Clin 1986;2(2):307–28.

63. Jupiter J, Axelrod T, Belsky M. Fractures and dislocations of the hand. In: Browner B, editor. Skeletal trauma. 3rd edition. Philadelphia: W.B. Saunders; 2003. p. 1153.

64. Weckesser EC. Rotational osteotomy of the metacarpal for overlapping fingers. J Bone Joint Surg Am 1965;47:751–6.

65. Gross MS, Gelberman RH. Metacarpal rotational osteotomy. J Hand Surg Am 1985;10(1):105–8.

66. Jupiter JB, Koniuch MP, Smith RJ. The management of delayed union and nonunion of the metacarpals and phalanges. J Hand Surg Am 1985; 10(4):457–66.

67. Yan YM, Zhang WP, Liao Y, et al. Analysis and prevention of the complications after treatment of metacarpal and phalangeal fractures with internal fixation. Zhongguo Gu Shang 2011;24(3):199–201 [in Chinese].

68. Ring D. Malunion and nonunion of the metacarpals and phalanges. Instr Course Lect 2006;55:121–8.

69. Balaram AK, Bednar MS. Complications after fractures of metacarpal and phalanges. Hand Clin 2010;26(2):169–77.

70. Stern PJ, Wieser MJ, Reilly DG. Complications of plate fixation in the hand skeleton. Clin Orthop Relat Res 1987;(214):59–65.

71. Dabezies EJ, Schutte JP. Fixation of metacarpal and phalangeal fractures with miniature plates and screws. J Hand Surg Am 1986;11(2):283–8.

72. Ford DJ, el-Hadidi S, Lunn PG, et al. Fractures of the metacarpals: treatment by A. O. screw and plate fixation. J Hand Surg Br 1987;12(1):34–7.

73. McLain RF, Steyers C, Stoddard M. Infections in open fractures of the hand. J Hand Surg Am 1991;16(1):108–12.

74. Reilly KE, Linz JC, Stern PJ, et al. Osteomyelitis of the tubular bones of the hand. J Hand Surg Am 1997;22(4):644–9.

75. Stern PJ. Fractures of the metacarpals and phalanges. In: Green D, editor. Operative hand surgery, vol. 1. New York: Churchill Livingstone; 1993. p. 695–758.

76. Feehan LM. Early controlled mobilization of potentially unstable extra-articular hand fractures. J Hand Ther 2003;16(2):161–70.

77. Feehan LM, Bassett K. Is there evidence for early mobilization following an extraarticular hand fracture? J Hand Ther 2004;17(2):300–8.

Treatment of Phalangeal Fractures

Shannon Carpenter, MD, Rachel S. Rohde, MD*

KEYWORDS

- Phalanx • Phalangeal fracture • Treatment • Hand fracture

KEY POINTS

- Fractures involving the tubular bones of the hand are the most common skeletal injuries.
- The primary goals of phalangeal fracture treatment are to restore anatomy and preserve function. Lost productivity attributed to these fractures exceeds $2 billion every year, making early return to activities a key goal as well.
- The preferred method of treatment is one that offers limited soft tissue damage and enables mobilization of the injured digit(s) as soon as fracture stability permits.
- Technical treatment of phalangeal fractures depends on characteristics of the fracture, requirements of the patient, and judgment of the treating physician. In general, operative treatment is reserved for unstable fractures or those creating unacceptable articular incongruity.
- Optimal outcome from surgical treatment demands appropriate surgical plan, atraumatic soft tissue handling, and stable fixation to facilitate early motion; however, complications such as nonunion, malunion, infection, and stiffness can occur even in the setting of appropriate treatment.

INTRODUCTION

Philosophies regarding phalangeal fracture treatment have evolved over time. The principle of complete immobilization espoused by Sir Reginald Watson-Jones in 1943 remained uniformly accepted for many years.[1] It was not until 1962 that James proposed what is now known as the "safe position" for immobilization,[2] also posing the question of whether complete immobilization of every hand fracture was necessary.[3,4]

Contemporaneously, Swanson[5] asserted that fractures of the hand can be complicated by deformity from no treatment, stiffness from overtreatment, and both deformity and stiffness from poor treatment. Ultimately, the primary objectives of phalangeal fracture treatment are to restore anatomy and preserve function. Given that the lost productivity associated with phalangeal fractures

exceeds $2 billion per year,[6] a third goal is to minimize recovery time and expedite return to activity. The preferred treatment restores anatomy, minimizes soft tissue injury, and enables mobilization of the injured digit as soon as fracture stability permits.

TREATMENT CONSIDERATIONS

Thorough clinical evaluation is required to determine the appropriate treatment course for each patient. The patient's age, hand dominance, occupation, avocations, medical comorbidities (including tobacco use), goals, limitations, and tolerances are important factors for the treating physician to consider. The mechanism of injury and associated injuries also may dictate course of treatment. A careful examination, including clinical and radiographic evaluation is needed, and sometimes is

The authors have nothing to disclose with relation to this publication.
Department of Orthopaedic Surgery, Oakland University William Beaumont School of Medicine, Beaumont Health System, 3535 West Thirteen Mile Road #742, Royal Oak, MI 48073, USA
* Corresponding author. Michigan Orthopaedic Institute, P.C., 26025 Lahser Road, Second Floor, Southfield, MI 48033.
E-mail address: rohders@gmail.com

supplemented with advanced medical imaging (eg, computed tomography).[7,8]

Acceptable alignment limitations vary based on the anatomic location of the fracture as well as the age of the patient, which suggests remodeling potential. However, one of the key general determinants of whether a fracture will require operative treatment is its inherent stability (**Table 1**).[9]

TREATMENT OPTIONS

A phalanx fracture can be addressed using one (or more) of several treatments based on clinical and radiographic assessment of the fracture and any associated injuries.

Nonoperative Treatment

A vast majority of phalangeal fractures can be managed nonoperatively.[10–13] These include fractures that are incomplete, nondisplaced, or able to be reduced so that acceptable alignment and stability are maintained without operative fixation. Nonoperative treatments include the following:

- Closed reduction (if needed) and casting or functional bracing (**Fig. 1**)
- Closed reduction and dorsal block splinting (**Fig. 2**)
- Buddy strapping or taping (**Fig. 3**)

It is important to emphasize that "nonoperative" treatment is not without its pitfalls, and using the appropriate nonsurgical technique is as critical as using the appropriate operative one. The "safe" or "intrinsic plus" position of James[3] is used to prevent collateral ligament and volar plate contractures. The metacarpophalangeal joints

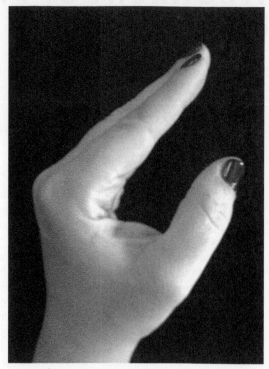

Fig. 1. Unless there is a specific rationale, casting of the digits should be performed in intrinsic plus position: 70° of flexion at the MCPJs and full extension at the IPJs.

(MPJs) are maintained at 70° of flexion and the proximal interphalangeal joints (PIPJs) in full extension (see **Fig. 1**). Exceptions to this are made when the position must be altered for

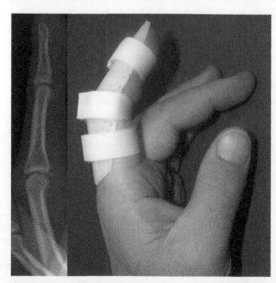

Fig. 2. Dorsal block splinting of the PIPJ allows active flexion exercises while maintaining reduction of potentially unstable volar plate avulsion injuries.

Table 1 Characteristics predictive of phalangeal fracture stability		
	Stable	**Unstable**
Anatomic location	Distal phalanx	Subcondylar proximal phalanx
Fracture characteristics	Simple, transverse Impacted	Short oblique, spiral Comminuted
Displacement	None or minimal	Displaced, malrotated
Articular incongruity	None or minimal	Incongruous surface
Soft tissue injury	Minimal	Severe

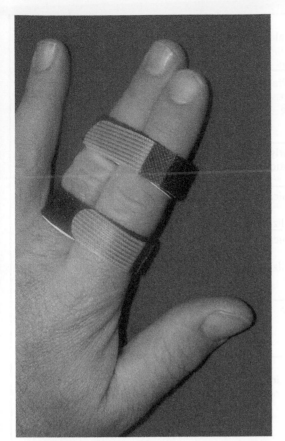

Fig. 3. Buddy straps or buddy tape allows the neighboring digit to act as a splint that provides support but allows early motion.

treatment purposes (eg, dorsal block splinting of PIPJ fracture-dislocations).

Operative Treatment

Surgical treatment is necessary if the fracture pattern is unstable or if the fracture is intra-articular and creates an unacceptable articular incongruity (see **Table 1**).[9] Operative options and their potential uses are introduced in **Table 2**.[7,14,15]

TREATMENT OF DISTAL PHALANX FRACTURES

Fractures of the distal phalanx constitute almost half of all hand fractures.[7,9,16] Caused by crushing or axially loading mechanisms, these have been classified by the following:

- Type of fracture (transverse, longitudinal split, or comminuted)[9]
- Anatomically/soft tissue injury[16]

The authors prefer to consider these as extra-articular fractures of the tuft, shaft, or base, and intra-articular fractures.

Distal Phalangeal Tuft Fractures

Tuft fractures usually occur secondary to a crushing injury and are often associated with a laceration of the nail matrix, pulp, or both. "Closed" fractures, therefore, result in the formation of a subungual hematoma, which often is more painful than the fracture itself. In this case, decompression of the hematoma using a trephine or electrocautery will provide pain relief. This perforation of the nail bed converts a closed fracture into an open one and a short course of oral antibiotics should be considered as a result.[14,17–19]

Open tuft fractures are less stable than closed fractures because the supporting pulp and nail plate are disrupted. Nevertheless, these rarely require internal fixation. Careful approximation of the associated lacerations of the pulp and nail matrix (following removal of the nail plate, if necessary) will restore alignment of the associated bony injury. Replacement of the nail plate or appropriate substitute beneath the eponychial fold prevents adherence of the fold to the matrix and serves as a splint for the fracture (**Fig. 4**). Rarely, a 0.028-inch Kirschner wire (K-wire) is used to support a fracture that remains unstable or displaced despite restoration of the soft tissue envelope.

A short (10–14-day) period of immobilization of the middle and distal phalanges will provide symptomatic relief and support of the fracture. Unrestricted PIPJ movement should be allowed to minimize subsequent motion loss. Radiographic delayed or nonunion frequently occurs, but symptom resolution is suggestive of fibrous union.

Potential complications following distal phalangeal tuft injuries include persistent pain, infection, cold intolerance, altered sensibility, nail bed and nail deformity, malunion, and nonunion.[20]

Distal Phalangeal Shaft Fractures

The distal phalangeal diaphysis generally fractures either longitudinally or transversely. Because of the inherent stability and minimal displacement of these fractures (**Fig. 5**), most require limited immobilization. Support is maintained until the patient's comfort resolves or until radiographic union is evident.

Open distal phalangeal shaft fractures are associated with disruption of the overlying nail matrix. As in treatment of an open tuft fracture, the nail

Table 2
Operative techniques available for treatment of phalangeal fractures

Technique	Primary Uses	Advantages	Disadvantages	Complications
K-wires	Unstable fractures amenable to a closed reduction	Minimal effect on soft tissue envelope	Need for additional immobilization (cast/brace) Often delays mobilization	Infection Loosening Pin migration Symptomatic hardware
Intraosseous wires	Transverse fractures or articular avulsion fractures	Possible early mobilization	Soft tissue irritation	Symptomatic hardware
Tension band wires	Avulsion fractures	Biomechanically stable Early mobilization	Increased operative exposure Technical difficulty	Symptomatic hardware
Compression screws	Large intra-articular fragments Long oblique diaphyseal fractures	Biomechanically stable Early mobilization	Increased operative exposure Technical difficulty	Fragmentation of fracture intraoperatively
Open reduction internal fixation plate and screws	Complex periarticular or intra-articular fractures	Most stable fixation	Most operative exposure Technical difficulty	Prominent hardware Adhesion formation
External fixation	Open fractures with extensive soft tissue injury Extensive bone loss or severe comminution	Limits soft tissue injury Preserves length	Potential interference with other digits Nonanatomic reduction	Pin site infections Hardware failure

should be removed, the fracture reduced, and the nail bed repaired with absorbable suture under loupe magnification. Although most of these fractures are supported adequately by the overlying (or replaced) nail plate, fractures that remain unstable can be supported by a 0.028-inch or 0.035-inch K-wire (**Fig. 6**). The distal phalanx and middle phalanx are splinted for 10 to 14 days.[9]

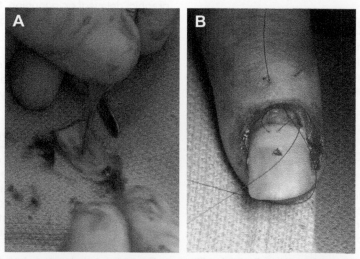

Fig. 4. An avulsed or extruded nail plate can be debrided and used as a biologic splint for distal phalanx and nail bed injuries. (*A*) The nail plate is prepared for reinsertion. (*B*) The nail plate is inserted beneath the eponychial fold and loosely sutured to prevent migration during the early postoperative period.

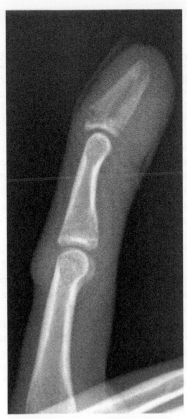

Fig. 5. Alignment of this longitudinal distal phalanx fracture resulting from crush injury is maintained by surrounding soft tissues and the nail plate.

Distal Phalangeal Base Fractures

Deforming forces of the flexor and extensor tendons and lack of intrinsic nail plate support render fractures at the base of the distal phalanx unstable. Because of these forces, the fracture tends to angulate with the apex pointing volarly (**Fig. 7**).

Fractures in the skeletally immature

Although most pediatric fractures are beyond the scope of this text, 2 distinct physeal injury patterns occur in children and bear mentioning:

- The Seymour fracture is a complete physeal separation that occurs from a hyperflexion injury.[21] Typically seen in toddlers, this often is mistaken for a distal interphalangeal joint (DIPJ) dislocation or a mallet injury. The extensor tendon remains attached to the proximal ephiphyseal fragment while the unopposed flexor digitorum profundus (FDP) tendon pulls the remainder of the distal phalanx into flexion. A transverse laceration of the nail bed occurs, and the avulsed nail plate lies superficial to the proximal nail fold. Interposition of the germinal matrix within the

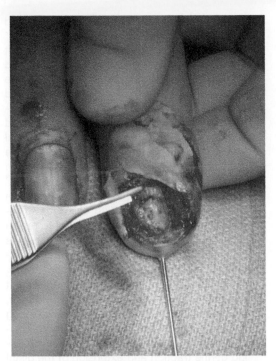

Fig. 6. A small K-wire can be inserted percutaneously just below the hyponychium if fixation of distal phalanx fragments is needed.

distracted dorsal physis can prevent reduction.[19] High suspicion and immediate recognition of this fracture pattern is imperative to prevent recurrent deformity, infection,

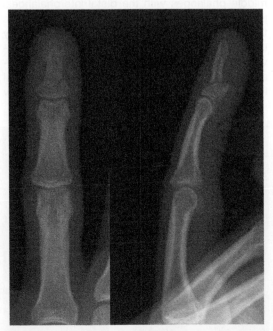

Fig. 7. Flexion of the proximal fragment of a distal phalangeal base fracture is noted due to the deforming force of the FDP tendon.

residual nail deformity, DIPJ stiffness, and premature physeal closure.[22]

- Simple reduction without treatment of the soft tissue injury can result in loss of reduction and infection. After irrigation and debridement, the fracture is reduced using slight traction and manipulation of the distal fragment into extension. The nail matrix laceration is repaired and the nail plate replaced beneath the proximal nail fold. The use of K-wires should be avoided because these are associated with a higher risk of infection in these injuries.[23] Although 30° of dorsal or volar angulation can be tolerated in a young child due to remodeling, it is preferable to attempt to regain anatomic reduction.[9] A splint or cast is applied to hold the distal fragment in extension for approximately 4 weeks.
- Older children incur physeal injuries that resemble closed mallet injuries; the deformity, however, is due to dorsal physeal opening rather than extensor tendon disruption. Typically, closed reduction is easily achieved using gentle traction and extension of the distal fragment. Subsequent immobilization in a splint incorporated into a cast or a cast alone should be maintained for 4 weeks.[22]

Fractures in adults

In adults, a closed fracture at the base of the distal phalanx is best treated by splinting the distal and middle phalanges with the distal interphalangeal joint extended for a minimum of 4 weeks. If the fracture is open, it is more likely to be rotationally unstable and may require K-wire insertion to provide internal stability. Penetration of the DIPJ usually can be avoided, however, if the proximal fragment is too small or too comminuted to allow

adequate fixation, a transarticular K-wire can be used.

Intra-articular Fractures of the Distal Phalanx

Intra-articular fractures of the distal phalanx most commonly are encountered as avulsion fractures.

- Mallet fractures occur when the dorsal base of the distal phalanx is avulsed by the attached extensor tendon (**Fig. 8**). In past years, several operative techniques have been used to restore the articular congruity of these fractures. However, closed treatment for 6 to 8 weeks in a DIPJ hyperextension splint results in excellent outcomes with fewer complications than operative treatment.[24,25]
- FDP avulsion injuries (Jersey finger) can be associated with fracture when the FDP tendon avulses a fragment of the volar distal phalanx. This fracture fragment serendipitously can prevent proximal migration of the tendon through the pulley system. Open reduction and internal fixation (ORIF) of a large fragment might be considered (**Fig. 9**). Most fragments, however, are small, and are inconsequential when planning reinsertion of the FDP tendon into the distal phalanx.

TREATMENT OF PROXIMAL AND MIDDLE PHALANX FRACTURES

Treatment decisions regarding proximal and middle phalanx fractures merit consideration of the following:

- Anatomic location within the phalanx (head [condylar], neck, shaft, base)
- Articular involvement
- Stability of the fracture

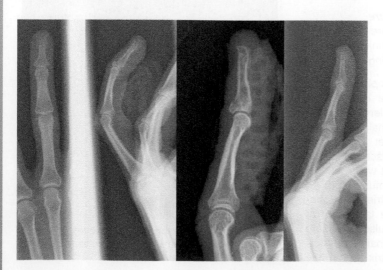

Fig. 8. Mallet fractures are treated as soft tissue injuries. Splinting of the DIPJ in extension or slight hyperextension allows restoration of DIPJ extension. These radiographs show reduction of the fracture fragment in the splinted position and subsequent healing without extensor lag. Radiographs are not necessary to confirm healing, which generally is assessed clinically.

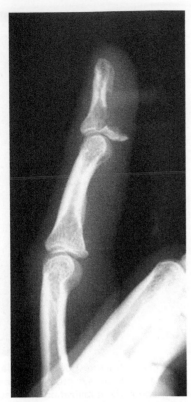

Fig. 9. Avulsion of a large fragment of the distal phalanx by the FDP tendon (bony Jersey finger) was treated by ORIF of the fragment to its distal phalanx insertion.

Inherently stable fractures generally are amenable to nonoperative treatment and protected early mobilization. Unstable fractures or those associated with articular incongruity are candidates for operative intervention.

Proximal and Middle Phalangeal Condylar (Intra-Articular) Fractures

Because of their articular involvement and tendency for rotational displacement, fractures of the condylar architecture of the phalangeal head can result in pain, deformity, and loss of motion. Any displacement of a condylar fracture is an indication for operative management.[14,26,27] Condylar fractures can be classified into the following 3 categories depending on their severity and stability[9,15]:

- Type I Condylar Fractures
  o Stable and nondisplaced
  o Can be treated nonoperatively in a digital splint for 7 to 10 days followed by buddy taping and protected mobilization
  o Weekly radiographs are useful to monitor for displacement

- Type II Condylar Fractures
  o Unicondylar fractures are inherently unstable fractures that result from shearing forces
  o Closed reduction with or without assistance of a manipulative K-wire, compression using a pointed reduction clamp, and percutaneous K-wire fixation or percutaneous screw fixation is preferable if possible to avoid disruption of the tenuous vascular supply
  o Multiple screws or K-wires are necessary to prevent rotation and loosening
  o Superimposition of the condyles on a true lateral radiograph confirms restoration of alignment
  o ORIF is reserved for displaced fractures not amenable to closed reduction (see later in this article)
  o Stable fixation allows early motion, and the PIPJ is splinted in extension, when not in motion, to prevent extensor lag
- Type III Condylar Fractures
  o Bicondylar or comminuted
  o Require ORIF, first of the condyles to each other using K-wires or screw, followed by fixation of the reassembled head to the diaphysis
  o A minicondylar plate can be used if needed
  o In the case of significant comminution of the condyles and/or the adjacent metaphysis, external fixation can be considered

Technical Pearls Specific to Open Treatment of Phalangeal Condyle Fracture:

- The condyle is approached dorsally by using a Chamay approach[28] or the interval between the extensor tendon/central slip and lateral band
- Before reduction, the condylar fragment dimensions are evaluated to determine appropriate screw size and the insertion of the collateral ligament is identified
- The fragment is reduced under direct visualization and fixed provisionally using a 0.028-inch K-wire
- A 1.5-mm headless compression screw is placed just dorsal and proximal to the origin of the collateral ligament to preserve the vascular supply
- A mincondylar blade plate can be used as a neutralization or buttress plate if there is metaphyseal or diaphyseal extension of the fracture

Proximal and Middle Phalangeal Neck Fractures

These fractures are far more common in children than in adults.[29] Adult fractures usually are amenable to closed reduction and splinting or crossed K-wire fixation.[30,31] Phalangeal neck fractures in children are divided into the following:

- Type I: Nondisplaced fractures are treated nonoperatively in a splint for 4 weeks. Bony union and full range of motion without residual deformity is common.
- Type II: Displaced fractures with persistent bone-to-bone contact account for about 70% of these fractures. Treatment and outcome depend greatly on initial presentation and management. These fractures are unstable and maintaining reduction often requires K-wire fixation. However, the authors note that these frequently present late (as "finger jams") with radiographic evidence of some healing. It is controversial whether these should be manipulated or left to remodel at that point, but the authors observationally have found that these fractures remodel quite well in young children (**Fig. 10**).
- Type III: Completely displaced fractures often demonstrate rotation of the distal fragment up to 180°; these are treated with ORIF using K-wire fixation.

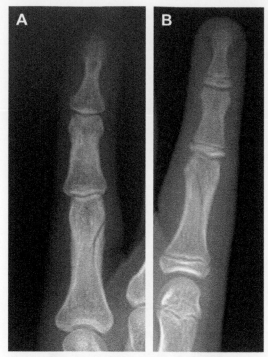

Fig. 11. Incomplete fractures of the phalanx are treated successfully with symptomatic protection, buddy taping, and early mobilization in an adult (*A*) and in a child (*B*).

Proximal and Middle Phalangeal Shaft Fractures

Nondisplaced fractures of the phalangeal diaphysis, particularly those that are incomplete, are stable (**Fig. 11**).[7,10] Fractures that are displaced initially can be classified following closed reduction as stable, unstable because of fracture obliquity (spiral, oblique, or transverse), or unstable because of significant bone loss.

The initial degree of displacement is more predictive of stability than the direction or number of fracture planes.[8] Even crush injuries without

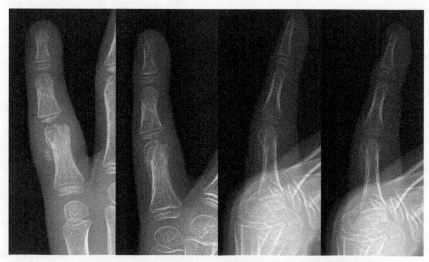

Fig. 10. Phalangeal neck fractures often present late, as in the case of this 6-year-old, whose fracture was partially healed 3 weeks following injury (*left*). Operative treatment was not chosen because of the likelihood of devascularization of the phalangeal head. Closed treatment in a cast resulted in some remodeling even 3 weeks later (*right*).

significant displacement are relatively more stable than less comminuted fractures if the periosteal sleeve is maintained.[27] In terms of obliquity, a transverse fracture is inherently more stable than spiral or long oblique fractures, which tend to angulate, rotate, or shorten with the deforming forces affecting the phalanx.

Stable fractures can be treated with buddy taping and early mobilization. Fractures that are unstable after reduction or have great potential to displace must be treated operatively or at minimum followed closely to prevent malunion and subsequent malfunction.

Unstable transverse fractures can be treated with percutaneous fixation or ORIF with plates and screws. The nature of the phalangeal shaft is such that crossed K-wire fixation can be difficult, depending on the configuration of the fracture. The authors prefer to use a retrograde intramedullary K-wire for unstable transverse middle phalanx fractures or a transarticular intramedullary K-wire across the MPJ for unstable transverse proximal phalanx fractures. This prevents translation, while buddy strapping of the digit to its neighbor helps maintain rotational stability.[7]

Unstable spiral or long oblique fractures can be stabilized by placing K-wires or compression screws across the fracture site (see Technique: Compression Screws). The screw diameter should be less than one-third of the length of the fracture line, and multiple screws are placed to maintain stability. Percutaneous screw fixation is an option, but requires perfect closed reduction; if this cannot be achieved or confirmed, then open reduction before screw fixation is preferred.[15,32]

If stable fixation is achieved, digital motion can be initiated immediately as comfort allows. Protective splinting is suggested to prevent extensor lag and accidental reinjury.[14,33,34]

Proximal and Middle Phalangeal Base Fractures

Fractures of the proximal and middle phalangeal bases can be either extra-articular or intra-articular:

- Proximal Phalangeal Base: Intra-articular result from ligamentous avulsions, crush, or rotation. Operative treatment is considered if the fragment interferes with joint motion or if joint stability is compromised.[35] Most ligament avulsions can be treated successfully with buddy taping or functional bracing of the affected digit to its neighboring digit (**Fig. 12**A). Joint instability at the ulnar aspect of the thumb metacarpophalangeal joint (MCPJ) ("boney gamekeeper") or the radial aspect of the index MCPJ is poorly tolerated and fixation of the fracture fragment versus debridement and ligament repair should be considered. Intra-articular injuries that involve significant joint incongruity and/or are unstable should be treated operatively (see **Fig. 12**B).
- Proximal Phalangeal Base: Extra-articular are relatively common.[36,37] They result in an apex volar angulation seen on a lateral radiograph; unfortunately, this might remain unrecognized following attempted closed reduction because the fracture site is obscured by

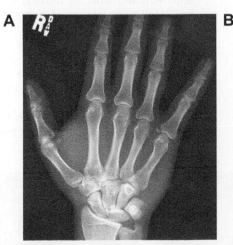
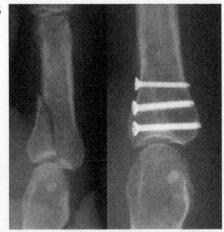

Fig. 12. (A) This intra-articular avulsion fracture at the base of the proximal phalanx was treated by functional bracing and buddy taping, rendering stability of the joint without pain despite the apparent incongruity. (B) This intra-articular fracture at the base of the proximal phalanx created significant articular incongruity and is considered unstable due to obliquity. This was treated with ORIF using compression screw technique.

plaster or fiberglass. Although stability some-times can be achieved following closed reduction, the chance of loss of reduction is high.[38] If acceptable reduction cannot be maintained, crossed K-wires inserted through the dorsal proximal phalangeal base, crossing the fracture site, and purchasing the cortex of the distal fragment are helpful (**Fig. 13**). The hand is splinted in the position of function with unobstructed interphalangeal joint (IPJ) motion until radiographic healing is noted (4 to 6 weeks), at which time the K-wires are removed and range of motion exercises instituted.

- Middle Phalangeal Base: Intra-articular
  - Partial articular
    - Dorsal: Avulsion fractures of middle pha-lanx by the central slip (**Fig. 14**) can be treated with closed reduction and dy-namic extension splinting of the PIPJ. If closed reduction fails, operative fixation of the fracture fragment or tendon rein-sertion is considered.
    - Volar: Volar plate avulsion fractures most often involve only a small fragment of the middle phalangeal base avulsed by the detached volar plate. Resulting from hyperextension injuries or dorsal dislocations, nonoperative treatment consists of buddy taping or, if there is a potential for redislocation, dorsal block splinting. Active range-of-motion exercises are initiated early to minimize stiffness and edema. Instability of the joint results when the fracture fragment involves more than 40% of the articular surface.[39] In this case, volar plate ar-throplasty, ORIF (**Fig. 15**), or hemiha-mate autograft procedures are indicated to restore joint congruity and stability.
    - Lateral middle phalanx fractures usually are ligamentous avulsion fractures; un-less there is unacceptable joint congru-ity, these are treated with buddy taping and early range of motion.
  - Complete articular, pilon, impaction, and lateral plateau fractures can occur at the base of the middle phalanx. These create unacceptable articular congruity and are treated with ORIF, external fixation, or reconstruction arthroplasty.[15,27,40–47]

Surgical Approaches for ORIF of Proximal and Middle Phalangeal Fractures

When necessary, open approach to the proximal or middle phalanx can be accomplished via dorsal, midaxial, or dorsolateral longitudinal skin inci-sions.[48] Rarely, a volar approach is necessary to address intra-articular fractures at the volar base of the middle phalanx. Gentle dissection and thoughtful technique is recommended to minimize soft tissue disruption. Preserving vascular supply will promote union, and minimizing tendon manip-ulation is thought to decrease adhesion forma-tion.[34] Stable fixation will allow early mobilization, which also can help prevent tendon adhesions.[49] Repair of periosteum to protect gliding surfaces and repair of the extensor tendon mechanism are critical to ensure a reasonable functional outcome.[9]

Dorsal Approach to the Phalanx

- A midline dorsal incision is made, and the dor-sal veins are preserved.[50]
- The extensor mechanism is divided longitudi-nally. Alternatively, in the dorsolateral approach, an interval is created between the extensor tendon/central slip and the lateral band. The extensor tendon can be elevated and retracted ulnar or radially; this can be facilitated by an incision of the transverse ret-inacular ligament at the PIPJ.
- PIPJ exposure may require additional approach:
  - Tendon splitting, in which the central slip insertion is reflected but remains attached to the periosteum
  - Chamay[28] approach, in which the central tendon is divided at the level of the proximal

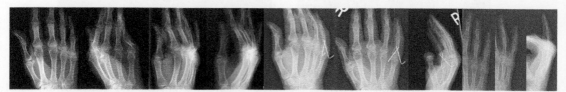

Fig. 13. Fractures at the base of the proximal phalanx are most easily noted on the lateral and oblique radio-graphic views. Closed reduction can be maintained using crossed K-wires. These are removed in the office setting at 4 to 6 weeks postoperatively and range-of-motion activities are instituted.

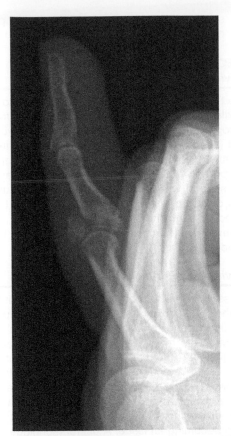

Fig. 14. The central slip attachment to the dorsal base of the middle phalanx can result in avulsion of part of the articular surface, as seen in this lateral radiograph.

phalanx and the tendon flap with intact central slip insertion is reflected distally

Midaxial Approach to the Phalanx

The midaxial approach allows exposure of the lateral phalanges, IPJs, and collateral ligaments for fracture fixation and PIPJ arthroplasty.[48,51,52] It is indicated for oblique, spiral, comminuted, or transverse fractures of the diaphysis and metaphysis. It provides visualization of phalangeal fractures for placement of internal fixation (either screws or plates) on the radial or ulnar aspect of the bone. Hardware is less likely to interfere with tendon gliding in the midaxial than in a dorsal or palmar position.

- The digit is flexed and the dorsal aspect of each flexion crease is marked with a dot. The digit is extended and these markings are connected to create the incisional marking. The digital artery and nerve will lie palmar to this line.
- The skin is incised, the soft tissues dissected, and Clelands ligaments are divided to expose the neurovascular bundle. The neurovascular bundle is maintained in the palmar flap and the periosteum of the phalanx can be visualized. Palmarly, the flexor tendon sheath can be identified.
- Two structures limit the proximal dissection of this approach: the dorsal branch of the digital nerve and the lateral band. The nerve should

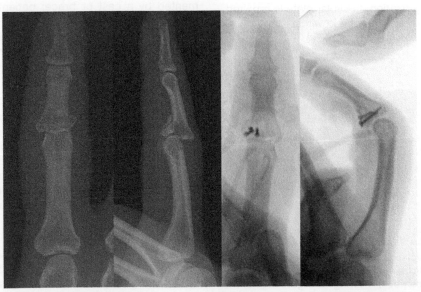

Fig. 15. This unstable articular fracture of the middle phalangeal base was treated via ORIF using three 1.0-mm screws.

be identified and protected as it travels palmar to dorsal over the proximal phalanx. The lateral band may be incised longitudinally or even excised for better exposure of the proximal phalanx. Repair is optional if the contralateral lateral band is intact.

Volar Approach to the Middle Phalangeal Base

The volar approach to the middle phalangeal base (or the PIPJ) is reserved primarily to address PIPJ fracture-dislocations (also discussed in the article "Intra-Articular Fractures" by Lawton elsewhere in this issue)[27,48]:

- A modified Brunner incision is made centered over the PIPJ.
- A thick flap of soft tissue is elevated and retracted to reveal the flexor tendon within the pulley system.
- The A3 pulley is incised and reflected, allowing retraction of the FDS and FDP tendons radially and/or ulnarly.
- The volar plate may already be avulsed (as in an acute PIPJ fracture dislocation pending volar plate arthroplasty or acute fracture) or remain healed to the middle phalanx (as in chronic or pilon injuries). If necessary, reflection of the volar plate from the base of the middle phalanx allows visualization of the base of the middle phalanx.
- Further middle phalangeal base exposure is facilitated by release of the collateral ligaments in anticipation of "shotgunning" the joint in preparation for ORIF or hemihamate autograft placement (**Fig. 16**).
- Following fixation, the volar plate is repaired, the tendons realigned within the pulley

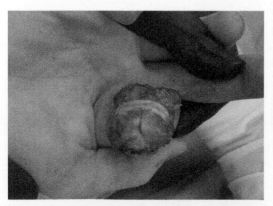

Fig. 16. The volar approach usually is used to treat volar intra-articular injuries. Here, the volar approach was used as described, allowing "shotgunning" of the joint in preparation for hemi-hamate autograft reconstruction.

system, and the skin is closed with interrupted nylon sutures.

SPECIFIC SURGICAL TECHNIQUES
K-wire Insertion into Distal Phalanx

The tuft of the distal phalanx lies just volar to the sterile matrix. Hence, the starting point for a retrograde K-wire is just volar to the hyponychial fold (see **Fig. 6**). If the initial pass of the wire is unsatisfactory, leaving the errant wire in place temporarily while passing the next can prevent the second wire from taking that initial course. The distal tip of the exposed wire can be truncated beneath the skin or bent, truncated, and covered with a protective cap until later removal.

K-wire Cross-Pinning

Crossed K-wire fixation is one of the most useful methods of fixation of phalangeal fractures. Confirmation of anticipated insertion point and direction are made with the use of fluoroscopic imaging. The fracture is crossed by multiple K-wires to promote rotational and translational stability (**Fig. 17**). Although K-wires have the potential for migration, careful bending, truncating, and protecting the end will help prevent this from becoming an issue. A useful technique also is to drive the sharp end of the K-wire through the far cortex, through the skin, truncate the sharp tip, and draw it back to the appropriate length. This can minimize symptomatic irritation of soft tissues by the sharp point should the K-wire move. This fixation generally is supplemented by a cast or brace; patients wearing a removable brace are able to shower with running water over the pins but should be cautioned against soaking in standing water to prevent infection.

Intraosseous Wiring

Intraosseous wiring involves passing a 26-gauge wire transversely across the fracture line dorsal to the midaxis and looping it around oblique K-wires to help neutralize the rotational forces. Although excellent success has been reported using this technique for transverse fractures and replants,[53] it has become less popular in recent years.

Tension Band Wiring

Tension band wiring entails inserting K-wires across the fracture site and using supplemental 26-gauge wire looped around the protruding K-wire ends to create a compressive force at the

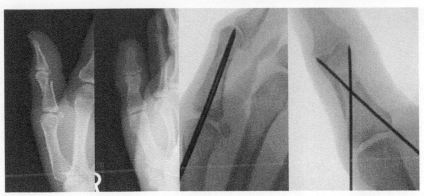

Fig. 17. K-wires are inserted in a crossed fashion, aiming to achieve multidirectional stability and maintain reduction.

fracture site. Useful for avulsion fractures, its popularity also has decreased, possibly supplanted by the availability of suture anchors.

Compression Screws

Despite widespread familiarity of surgeons who treat fractures with compression screw fixation, the unique anatomic considerations in the phalanges (gliding structures, thin cortices, and small fracture fragments with tenuous vascular supplies) render compression screw fixation one of the more technically difficult methods of phalanx fracture surgery. However, the stability achieved affords the option of immediate mobilization, a distinct advantage over some other methods. The following general principles of compression screw placement apply:

- The screw diameter should not exceed one-third of the length of the fracture.
- In the diaphysis, the fracture line itself should be at least twice the diameter of the bone.
- At least 2 and preferably 3 screws should cross the fracture site to provide multiplanar stability (see **Fig. 13B**).
- The fracture reduction should be held by either K-wires or a clamp. The tap drill, equal to the core diameter for the chosen screw size, is used to drill both the near and far cortices along a line halfway between a perpendicular to the phalangeal shaft and a perpendicular to the fracture line. The near cortex is then overdrilled with a drill bit that is the same size as the screw's outer diameter to create a gliding hole. The screw is placed in a lag fashion to provide compression of the fracture site.[15,27,54]
- It is not recommended to countersink the screw head in the metaphysis because of the thin cortex.[15]

ORIF Plate and Screws

As in compression screw fixation, ORIF using a small plate and screws is technically difficult but can provide unparalleled restoration of anatomy with stability to allow immediate motion (**Fig. 18**). T plates are typically used for phalanx fractures.[15] The plate is aligned perpendicular to the joint line and secured with a single screw. The distal portion of the fracture is then brought into alignment and secured with an additional screw. The length, angulation, and rotation are all assessed radiographically and clinically before filling the plate with the remaining screws. Plate placement is relevant to outcome in the phalanx. Lateral plate placement effectively resists compressive forces and has less disruption to the extensor mechanism and potentially less risk of adhesions[55] than dorsal plating. If a plate is applied to the dorsal surface, care must be taken to avoid damaging the flexor tendons with screws that are overdrilled.

External Fixation

External fixation of phalangeal fractures is useful if there is extensive comminution requiring distraction or if there is significant soft tissue disruption precluding internal fixation.[42,45] Although rarely needed, the authors prefer using the dynamic external fixator described by Ruland and colleagues.[56]

Complications

Complications can arise with either nonoperative or operative management of phalangeal fractures. Potential complications include delayed union, nonunion, malunion, soft tissue adhesions, joint contractures, infection, posttraumatic arthritis, hardware issues, and tendon rupture.[27,34,49,57]

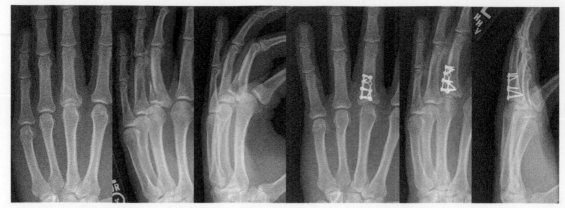

Fig. 18. This unstable intra-articular fracture at the base of the proximal phalanx required early motion and was too comminuted for simple screw fixation. Therefore, a buttress plate and screws were used. (*Courtesy of* Jennifer M. Wolf, MD Farmington, CT)

Authors' Preferred Method of Treatment

The authors treat phalangeal fractures guided by the principles of restoring anatomy to maximize function. In general, this entails minimizing joint stiffness and pain by restoring articular congruity, minimizing digit deformity and malrotation by addressing phalangeal shortening and angulation, and preventing functional loss by achieving early mobilization without compromising fracture stability. In most cases, this can be accomplished without surgery. However, in the case of an unstable fracture or one that unacceptably disrupts the articular surface, operative fixation balancing the goals of fracture healing, soft tissue preservation, and early return to function is preferred.

REFERENCES

1. Watson-Jones R, Wilson JN. Fractures and joint injuries, 6th edition. Edinburgh (United Kingdom), New York: Churchill Livingstone; 1982.
2. James JI. Fractures of the proximal and middle phalanges of the fingers. Acta Orthop Scand 1962;32:401–12.
3. James JI. The assessment and management of the injured hand. Hand 1970;2(2):97–105.
4. Barton B. Fractures of the hand. J Bone Joint Surg Br 1984;66(2):159–67.
5. Swanson AB. Fractures involving the digits of the hand. Orthop Clin North Am 1970;1(2):261–74.
6. Van Onselen EB, Karim RB, Hage JJ, et al. Prevalence and distribution of hand fractures. J Hand Surg Br 2003;28(5):491–5.
7. Gaston RG, Chadderdon C. Phalangeal fractures: displaced/nondisplaced. Hand Clin 2012;28(3):395–401.
8. Kozin SH, Thoder JJ, Lieberman G. Operative treatment of metacarpal and phalangeal shaft fractures. J Am Acad Orthop Surg 2000;8(2):111–21.
9. Jupiter J, Axelrod TS, Belsky MR. Fractures and dislocations of the hand. In: Browner BD, Green NE, editors. Skeletal trauma. 4th edition. Edinburgh (United Kingdom): Saunders; 2008. p. 1221–341.
10. Reyes FA, Latta LL. Conservative management of difficult phalangeal fractures. Clin Orthop Relat Res 1987;(214):23–30.
11. Maitra A, Burdett-Smith P. The conservative management of proximal phalangeal fractures of the hand in an accident and emergency department. J Hand Surg Br 1992;17(3):332–6.
12. Barton NJ. Fractures of the shafts of the phalanges of the hand. Hand 1979;11(2):119–33.
13. Moberg E. Fractures and ligamentous injuries of the thumb and fingers. Surg Clin North Am 1960;40:297–309.
14. Day C, Stern P. Fractures of the metacarpals and phalanges. In: Green DP, editor. Green's operative hand surgery. 5th edition. Philadelphia: Elsevier/Churchill Livingstone; 2005. p. 239–90.
15. Harman TW, Graham TJ, Uhl RL. Operative treatment of extra-articular phalangeal fractures. In: Wiesel SW, editor. Operative techniques in orthopaedic surgery. 1st edition. Philadelphia: Lippincott Williams & Wilkins; 2012. Chapter 32 p. 2378–91.
16. Schneider LH. Fractures of the distal phalanx. Hand Clin 1988;4(3):537–47.
17. Sloan J, Dove A, Maheson M, et al. Antibiotics in open fractures of the distal phalanx? J Hand Surg Br 1987;12(1):123–4.
18. Roser SE, Gellman H. Comparison of nail bed repair versus nail trephination for subungual hematomas in children. J Hand Surg Am 1999;24(6):1166–70.
19. Krusche-Mandl I, Köttstorfer J, Thalhammer G, et al. Seymour fractures: retrospective analysis

and therapeutic considerations. J Hand Surg Am 2013;38(2):258–64.

20. Schneider LH. Fractures of the distal interphalangeal joint. Hand Clin 1994;10(2):277–85.

21. Seymour N. Juxta-epiphysial fracture of the terminal phalanx of the finger. J Bone Joint Surg Br 1966;48(2):347–9.

22. Dolan M, Water P. Fractures and Dislocations of the forearm, wrist, and hand. In: Green NE, Swiontkowski MF, editors. Skeletal trauma in children. 4th edition. Philadelphia: Saunders/Elsevier; 2009. p. 159–205.

23. Rider DL. Fractures of the metacarpals, metatarsals, and phalanges. Am J Surg 1937;38(3): 549–59.

24. Moss JG, Steingold RF. The long term results of mallet finger injury. A retrospective study of one hundred cases. Hand 1983;15(2):151–4.

25. Handoll HH, Vaghela MV. Interventions for treating mallet finger injuries. Cochrane Database Syst Rev 2004;(3):CD004574.

26. Weiss AP, Hastings H. Distal unicondylar fractures of the proximal phalanx. J Hand Surg Am 1993; 18(4):594–9.

27. Henry M. Hand fractures and dislocations. In: Rockwood CA, Green DP, Bucholz RW, editors. Rockwood and Green's fractures in adults. 7th edition. Philadelphia: Wolters Kluwer Health/Lippincott Williams & Wilkins; 2010. p. 710–829.

28. Chamay A. A distally based dorsal and triangular tendinous flap for direct access to the proximal interphalangeal joint. Ann Chir Main 1988;7(2): 179–83.

29. Al-Qattan MM. Phalangeal neck fractures in children: classification and outcome in 66 cases. J Hand Surg Br 2001;26(2):112–21.

30. Al-Qattan MM. Phalangeal neck fractures in adults. J Hand Surg Br 2006;31(5):484–8.

31. Al-Qattan MM. Phalangeal neck fractures of the proximal phalanx of the fingers in adults. Injury 2010;41(10):1084–9.

32. Horton TC, Hatton M, Davis TR. A prospective randomized controlled study of fixation of long oblique and spiral shaft fractures of the proximal phalanx: closed reduction and percutaneous Kirschner wiring versus open reduction and lag screw fixation. J Hand Surg Br 2003;28(1):5–9.

33. Orbay JL, Touhami A. The treatment of unstable metacarpal and phalangeal shaft fractures with flexible nonlocking and locking intramedullary nails. Hand Clin 2006;22(3):279–86.

34. Balaram AK, Bednar MS. Complications after the fractures of metacarpal and phalanges. Hand Clin 2010;26(2):169–77.

35. Shewring DJ, Thomas RH. Avulsion fractures from the base of the proximal phalanges of the fingers. J Hand Surg Br 2003;28(1):10–4.

36. Chung KC, Spilson SV. The frequency and epidemiology of hand and forearm fractures in the United States. J Hand Surg Am 2001;26(5):908–15.

37. Feehan LM, Sheps SB. Incidence and demographics of hand fractures in British Columbia, Canada: a population-based study. J Hand Surg Am 2006;31(7):1068–74.

38. Coonrad RW, Pohlman MH. Impacted fractures in the proximal portion of the proximal phalanx of the finger. J Bone Joint Surg Am 1969;51(7):1291–6.

39. Schenck RR. Classification of fractures and dislocations of the proximal interphalangeal joint. Hand Clin 1994;10(2):179–85.

40. Calfee RP, Kiefhaber TR, Sommerkamp TG, et al. Hemi-hamate arthroplasty provides functional reconstruction of acute and chronic proximal interphalangeal fracture-dislocations. J Hand Surg Am 2009;34(7):1232–41.

41. Inanami H, Ninomiya S, Okutsu I, et al. Dynamic external finger fixator for fracture dislocation of the proximal interphalangeal joint. J Hand Surg Am 1993;18(1):160–4.

42. Parsons SW, Fitzgerald JA, Shearer JR. External fixation of unstable metacarpal and phalangeal fractures. J Hand Surg Br 1992;17(2):151–5.

43. Geissler WB. Operative fixation of metacarpal and phalangeal fractures in athletes. Hand Clin 2009; 25(3):409–21.

44. Stern PJ. Management of fractures of the hand over the last 25 years. J Hand Surg Am 2000; 25(5):817–23.

45. Slade JF, Baxamusa TH, Wolfe SW. External fixation of proximal interphalangeal joint fracture-dislocations. Atlas of the Hand Clin 2000;5(1):1–29.

46. Kuhn KM, Dao KD, Shin AY. Volar A1 pulley approach for fixation of avulsion fractures of the base of the proximal phalanx. J Hand Surg Am 2001;26(4):762–71.

47. Hastings H, Carroll C. Treatment of closed articular fractures of the metacarpophalangeal and proximal interphalangeal joints. Hand Clin 1988;4(3): 503–27.

48. Catalano LW, Zlotolow DA, Purcelli Lafer M, et al. Surgical exposures of the wrist and hand. J Am Acad Orthop Surg 2012;20(1):48–57.

49. Kurzen P, Fusetti C, Bonaccio M, et al. Complications after plate fixation of phalangeal fractures. J Trauma 2006;60(4):841–3.

50. Bickel KD. The dorsal approach to silicone implant arthroplasty of the proximal interphalangeal joint. J Hand Surg Am 2007;32(6):909–13.

51. Field LD, Freeland AE, Jabaley ME. Midaxial approach to the proximal phalanx for fracture fixation. Contemp Orthop 1992;25:133–7.

52. Carlson MG, Szabo R, Lipscomb P. Principles of hand surgery and surgical approaches to the hand and wrist. In: Chapman MW, editor. Chapman's

orthopaedic surgery. 3rd edition. Philadelphia: Lippincott Williams & Wilkins; 2001. p. 1226–46.

53. Zimmerman NB, Weiland AJ. Ninety-ninety intraosseous wiring for internal fixation of the digital skeleton. Orthopedics 1989;12(1):99–103.

54. Perren SM, Allgöwer M, Osteosynthesefragen AF. Manual of internal fixation: techniques recommended by the AO-ASIF Group. Berlin, New York: Springer-Verlag; 1991.

55. Lins RE, Myers BS, Spinner RJ, et al. A comparative mechanical analysis of plate fixation in a proximal phalangeal fracture model. J Hand Surg Am 1996;21(6):1059–64.

56. Ruland RT, Hogan CJ, Cannon DL, et al. Use of dynamic distraction external fixation for unstable fracture-dislocations of the proximal interphalangeal joint. J Hand Surg Am 2008;33(1): 19–25.

57. Page SM, Stern PJ. Complications and range of motion following plate fixation of metacarpal and phalangeal fractures. J Hand Surg Am 1998; 23(5):827–32.

Intra-Articular Fractures of the Hand

Nikhil Oak, MD, Jeffrey N. Lawton, MD*

KEYWORDS

- Hand • Fractures • Intra-articular • Open reduction and internal fixation (ORIF)

KEY POINTS

- Management of intra-articular fractures depends upon Fracture Location and Pattern of Injury.
- Treatment should seek to allow for Early Motion to prevent long-term stiffness, pain, and arthritis.
- Restoration of Joint Congruity and Early ROM supercedes Anatomic Alignment.
- Maintain respect for Soft Tissue and Tendon Gliding.

INTRODUCTION

Fractures of the hand are a common problem seen by primary care physicians and hand surgeons. In a survey of 36,518 patients,[1] fractures of the hand accounted for 19% of all fractures. In another series,[2] of 2655 patients with fractures, 28% involved the hand. The distribution of fractures also varies within the hand, with the small finger ray the most fractured digit and fractures of the phalanges more common than metacarpal fractures.[1,2] Fractures involving the articular surface such as the interphalangeal, metacarpophalangeal (MCP), or carpometacarpal joints (CMC), can often present challenges to the treating physician. Although the treatment of these fractures needs to be individualized based on fracture pattern and location, the overriding goals for these fractures is to restore the alignment, stability, and congruity and also allow for early motion to prevent stiffness and traumatic arthritis. This article classifies the various types of intra-articular hand fractures as well as the workup and management of these injuries.

CMC JOINT FRACTURES
Anatomy and Classification

Intra-articular fractures occur infrequently through the base of the metacarpals and are more common in the border digits. These fractures have some stability provided by dorsal and palmar CMC and interosseous ligaments[3]; however, stability decreases toward the ulnar aspect of the hand because of the greater degree of motion in the fourth and fifth CMC joints.[4] Isolated intra-articular fractures are rare for the second and third metacarpals because of lack of motion.[5] The second and third metacarpals form the central pillar of the hand and are fixed rigidly by the bony and ligamentous anatomy of the CMC articulations.[3] The irregular structure and articulations of the bases with the trapezium and capitate allow the second and third metacarpals to key together, allowing for stability. The mechanism of intra-articular fracture to these central metacarpal bases has often been postulated as a fall onto the dorsal aspect of a flexed hand.[3,5,6] Fracture fragments could potentially displace or become avulsed from the metacarpal bases from the pull of the extensor carpi radialis longus (ECRL) or extensor carpi radialis brevis (ECRB).[7–9]

The fourth and fifth CMC joints have a greater range of motion than the second and third CMC joints, with motion in all 3 directions necessary for normal hand function.[3,4] Both fourth and fifth CMC allow for flexion extension, with the fifth having close to 44° if the fourth CMC joint is intact.[4] Fourth and fifth CMC joint fractures occur more

Department of Orthopaedic Surgery, University of Michigan, 1500 East Medical Center Drive, 2912 Taubman Center, Ann Arbor, MI 48109, USA
* Corresponding author.
E-mail address: jeflawto@med.umich.edu

Hand Clin 29 (2013) 535–549
http://dx.doi.org/10.1016/j.hcl.2013.08.007
0749-0712/13/$ – see front matter © 2013 Elsevier Inc. All rights reserved.

frequently and are often associated with CMC dislocations.[10] These fractures can occur from a closed fist striking an immobile object, resulting in a combination of axial load and shear stresses.[11,12] The hamate articulates with the fourth and fifth metacarpal bases by 2 concave facets.[5] When a fracture involves more than one-third of the dorsal articular side of the hamate, stability of the MC-hamate joint may be lost.[11] The fifth metacarpal base has an ulnar slope and lacks a supporting buttress on the ulnar side of the hand, which contributes to ulnar instability during axial loading.[3] The extensor carpi ulnaris (ECU), flexor carpi ulnaris, and abductor digiti minimi may further exert deforming forces on fracture fragments,[10] with ulnar and proximal displacement common because of the ECU force vector. Kjaer-Peterson and colleagues[13] discussed a classification system for metacarpal base fractures, which divided fractures into 4 types based on articular involvement and comminution **Fig. 1**.

The articular surface of the hamate can also be involved in fracture/dislocations of the CMC. These fractures are uncommon and can result in a coronal split of the hamate or a die-punch fracture of the articular surface.[14,15] Lee and colleagues[11] described a classification of CMC fracture/dislocations based on amount of hamate articular surface involved as well as involvement of metacarpal base fracture.

Presentation and Workup

Injuries to metacarpal bases can occur from both high-energy and low-energy trauma, so patient presentation is variable. Fractures to the base of the second and third metacarpals may not be easily seen on standard radiographs and can often be missed.[6] For these central intra-articular metacarpal base fractures, a history of fall onto the back of a flexed wrist with examination showing tenderness, bruising, and swelling over the metacarpal bases can raise suspicions of such an injury. Pain or limitations in active wrist extension,

diminished grip strength or range of motion are common physical examination findings.[6,8,9] For fourth and fifth metacarpal base fractures, a history of axial loading injury through the metacarpal head with pain and swelling at the bases of metacarpals and dorsoulnar aspect of the hand are common findings.[3,16,17] Patients should also have a thorough neurovascular examination, because the deep motor branch of the ulnar nerve courses over the bases of the fourth and fifth metacarpals and could be affected.[3]

Initial radiographs should always include standard posterior-anterior, lateral, and oblique views. The lateral view may show dorsal displacement and subluxation of metacarpal bases but may be inconclusive because of overlying the carpal bones.[3] If there is high clinical suspicion, a 30° anterior oblique view and 30° pronated lateral view may aid in visualizing the articular surface.[5,6,18] For difficult visualization and to further assess articular comminution, a computed tomography (CT) scan is occasionally necessary.[5] CT scans can aid in recognizing rotational deformity and help direct treatment options.[3]

Treatment and Outcomes

The treatment of intra-articular fractures to the bases of the metacarpals varies from closed reduction and casting to open reduction and internal fixation (ORIF). There is no consensus for optimal treatment, because these injuries occur infrequently. In a review of reported cases, Bushnell and colleagues[3] describe the integrity of the ECRL and ECRB to protect wrist stability and extension strength as being important by many investigators in deciding for operative treatment. Some investigators report open reduction to visualize the joint surfaces and tendinous insertions followed by stabilization with K-wires and immobilization for 4 weeks followed by wire removal and gradual return to activities.[6–9] Most investigators reported good results after restoration of ECRL

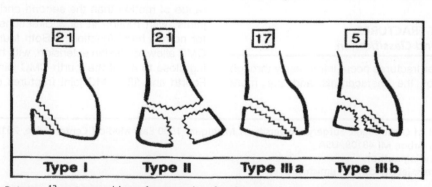

Fig. 1. Kjaer-Peterson[13] metacarpal base fracture classification.

or ECRB and return to normal function and grip/extension strength by 4 months to a year.[3,6–9]

Intra-articular fractures of the fourth and fifth metacarpal bases resemble Bennett and Rolando fractures, because they have a tendency to be unstable.[13] However, treatment remains controversial, because larger studies recommend a variety of treatment options, ranging from closed reduction and casting to ORIF.[13,18] It is recommended that before a definitive plan is made, all patients should be initially immobilized with a dorsal and volar splint with the wrist in 30° of extension and the MCP joints free; this position minimizes the deforming pull of the ECU and can aid in reduction.[3] Closed reduction and casting is a treatment option for minimally displaced intra-articular fractures. Lundeen and Shin[16] studied a series of 37 patients with intra-articular fifth metacarpal base fractures, who all underwent closed reduction using longitudinal traction and digital pressure over the dorsal proximal portion of the displaced fifth metacarpal base followed by a short-arm plaster cast immobilization for an average of 4 to 5 weeks with return to work at 6 weeks and did not have any nonunions/malunions. These investigators reported equivalent grip strength compared with contralateral hand, and 8 of 37 patients had intermitted pain but no disability.[16] Bora and Didizian[18] noted that significantly displaced fractures require closed reduction and percutaneous pinning (CRPP) or ORIF to prevent pain and loss of grip strength.

Kjaer-Petersen and colleagues[13] analyzed a series of 64 intra-articular fractures to the base of the fifth metacarpal, in which minimally displaced fractures were treated conservatively with closed reduction and casting, whereas displaced fractures were either treated with CRPP or ORIF was performed for more comminuted fractures. In that study, 38% of patients had some residual symptoms and 1 went on to have an arthrodesis. These investigators concluded that reduction should be held by internal fixation if casting alone does not improve the positioning.[13] Lee and colleagues[11] reviewed 43 patients with fourth and fifth CMC fracture dislocations and treated fractures that involved less than one-third of the articular surface of the hamate with closed reduction and percutaneous K-wire fixation, whereas fractures that were unstable or coronally split were treated by ORIF. All patients were splinted initially then casted in neutral position for 3 to 4 weeks before graduating to activities as tolerated. With this treatment, average time to union was 45 days with good to excellent results for all cases, except 2 that had fair results. Average loss of grip strength in that study was 8% compared with uninjured side.[11]

Intra-articular fractures of the index and middle finger metacarpals are uncommon; treatment should aim to reestablish integrity of the ECRL and ECRB. Fourth and fifth metacarpals are more common, but treatment of these fractures varies. Undisplaced or stable fractures can be treated nonoperatively, with similar return to work and incidence of pain to surgical management, which can be reserved for unstable and malreduced fractures. Failure to properly diagnose and treat these intra-articular fractures can lead to decreased range of motion, arthritis, and diminished grip strength and wrist extension.[3]

THUMB CARPOMETACARPAL FRACTURES (ROLANDO, BENNETT)
Anatomy and Classification

The thumb ray is involved in 14% of all hand fractures.[1] Intra-articular fractures have been coined either Bennett fractures, which are intra-articular fractures separating the volar-ulnar aspect of the metacarpal base from the remaining metacarpal, or Rolando fractures, which are now used to describe any comminuted intra-articular fracture to the base of the first metacarpal.[19,20] The thumb CMC acts as a biconcavoconvex saddle joint; on a lateral view, the trapezium is convex and thumb metacarpal is concave, whereas in the anteroposterior (AP) plane, the trapezium is concave and thumb metacarpal is convex.[21,22] Its unique geometry allows for thumb movement in multiple planes, allowing power grip, power pinch, and precision pinch.[22] The stability and function of the thumb CMC depends on this articular surface, the anterior oblique, and the dorsal ligament complex.[22,23]

A Bennett fracture results from an axial load on a partially flexed metacarpal. This situation results in the metacarpal shaft subluxating in a dorsal, proximal, and radial direction because of the muscular forces of the adductor pollicus longus, extensor pollicus longus, extensor pollicus brevis, and abductor pollicus longus, whereas the volar-ulnar fragment remains in place held by the anterior oblique, also known as the volar beak ligament, anchoring it to the trapezium.[19] The vertical fracture line exists near the metaphyseal-diaphyseal junction along the ulnar border of the bone, with deformation common at the fracture site.[20] A classification schema by Gedda and colleagues[24] divided Bennett fractures into 3 types. Type 1 includes fractures with a large ulnar fragment and subluxation of the metacarpal base, type 2 are impaction fractures without subluxation, and type 3 are metacarpal dislocations with a small ulnar avulsion fragment.[19,24]

Rolando's fracture was initially described as a T-shaped or Y-shaped intra-articular fracture of the thumb metacarpal base, but is now used to describe other comminuted intra-articular fractures.[25] These fractures include the volar-ulnar Bennett fragment as well as a dorsal radial fragment, but often there is articular comminution.[19] These fractures are also caused by an axial load injury on a flexed metacarpal and are usually higher-velocity injuries, which are more difficult to treat compared with Bennett fractures.[23] These fractures usually show volar angulation of the metacarpal shaft in relation to the joint surface.[25]

Presentation and Workup

Patients with these injuries have pain at the base of the thumb, deformity, ecchymosis, and edema. It is also important to note any previous thumb pain that could indicate preexisting CMC arthritis.[20] Radiographic workup should include standard posteroanterior (PA) and lateral views as well as a true AP of the thumb, or a Roberts view, which requires hyperpronation with the dorsum of the thumb against the radiograph plate.[19,20] A Betts view, or a true lateral of the metacarpotrapezial joint, is also useful to view fracture displacement and joint congruency with the hand pronated 15° to 35° and radiograph beam angled 15° from distal to proximal.[19] A CT scan is usually unnecessary unless there is severe comminution, deformity, or rotation of fracture fragments to help in operative planning **Fig. 2**.

Treatment and Outcomes

For Bennett fractures, initial treatment of these fractures should include attempting closed reduction and splinting, which requires axial traction, palmar abduction, and pronation while downward pressure is applied to the metacarpal base.[5,19] These fractures must be appropriately treated to avoid stiffness and posttraumatic arthritis. Maintaining reduction can be difficult, and most investigators recommend mandatory joint reduction, with an emphasis on anatomic reduction to prevent joint incongruity and degenerative changes. Cannon and colleagues[26] reported on long-term follow-up, mean of 9.6 years after Bennett fractures, for 25 patients, of whom 22 were managed conservatively with plaster casting. In that study, 21 of 25 patients showed loss of CMC motion, with malrotation in 20% of patients. Surgical treatment varies from closed reduction and pinning to open reduction with interfragmentary fixation or pinning. Percutaneous pin fixation can be performed with a reduction maneuver as described earlier with a K-wire passed obliquely from the metacarpal to the trapezium under fluoroscopic guidance.[5,27,28] Alternatively, the fracture can be stabilized with K-wire fixation from the first to second metacarpals, with an additional K-wire through the volar-ulnar fragment and the metacarpal.[19] After pin fixation, the fracture should be immobilized for 4 to 5 weeks in a thumb spica cast before range of motion and return to function are begun.[20] Open reduction is most often performed via a Wagner approach along the subcutaneous border of the first metacarpal between the abductor pollicus longus and thenar musculature.[5] The thenar muscles are elevated subperiosteally off the thumb metacarpal, the joint capsule is incised, and the fracture can be reduced and provisionally fixed with a pin followed by fragment fixation with pins or via lag technique ensuring that 1.5-mm or 2-mm screws have not penetrated the joint.[5,19,29,30] During the open approach, care is taken not to elevate the volar oblique ligament from the metacarpal fracture fragment. Postoperatively, the thumb is immobilized in a thumb spica cast for 4 weeks if pins are used or range of motion can be initiated 5 to 10 days after screw fixation **Fig. 3**.

Lutz[29] described 32 patients with Bennett fractures treated by ORIF versus closed reduction and K-wiring. They concluded that the type of treatment did not influence the prevalence of posttraumatic arthritis and advised CRPP for fractures with a large volar ulnar fragment and ORIF when fractures are irreducible. Leibovic[20] recommended surgical reduction and fixation if articular displacement exceeds 1 mm. Kjaer-Peterson and colleagues[30] studied 41 Bennett fractures treated using closed reduction, CRPP, and ORIF and concluded that better outcomes correlated with

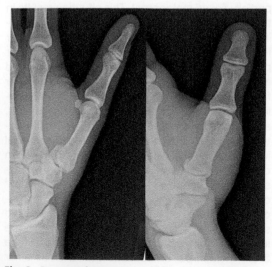

Fig. 2. Bennett fracture.

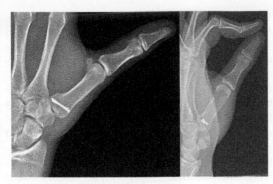

Fig. 3. ORIF of Bennett fracture.

superior anatomic reduction. With a median of 7.3 years of follow-up, these investigators found that 83% of patients whose fractures had healed in excellent position were symptom free as opposed to 46% of those who had residual articular surface displacement.[30] Surgical intervention via either CRPP or ORIF is often necessary to ensure a near-anatomic reduction in treating Bennett fractures to prevent long-term pain and arthrosis.

Rolando fractures are generally more challenging to treat, because there can be articular comminution and difficulty restoring the joint surface. Numerous methods have been described to treat this fracture pattern, including multiple K-wire pinning, ORIF with lag screws or plate, and traction pinning. A Wagner approach can be used for surgical exposure. Day and Stern[5] described longitudinal traction and reduction of articular fragments with a clamp or pins followed by application of a 2.4-mm to 2.7-mm L or T plate for definitive fixation. Leibovic[20] advises reducing the articular components first and when using the T plate, to insert the screws eccentrically to compress across the fracture site. Bone graft may be used if there is a metaphyseal defect. Complications to ORIF include malunions, damage to dorsal sensory branches of the radial nerve or palmar cutaneous branch of median nerve, and stiffness.[20] In cases with severe comminution, distraction and reduction by ligamentotaxis may be achievable.[19] Gelberman and colleagues[31] discussed using oblique traction with an outrigger splint and K-wire through the first metacarpal for 8 patients with comminuted intra-articular fractures. These investigators described using a 0.062 K-wire drilled obliquely through the first metacarpal exiting in the first web-space, crimped at the proximal aspect for traction, and reported satisfactory maintenance of reduction for all patients.[5,31] Langhoff and colleagues[25] reported on 17 cases of Rolando fractures and did not establish a correlation between quality of reduction

and symptoms at follow-up. Of the 14 operative cases, 11 required open reduction, and the occurrence of osteoarthritic changes (55%) at median 5.8-year follow-up was unrelated to the quality of reduction.[25] For comminuted fractures, Buchler and colleagues[32] described external fixation using a quadrilateral frame with pins inserted into the first and second metacarpals and interconnected with rods.

If lag screw or plate fixation seems secure, patients can be started on postoperative protected active motion. However, in fractures needing oblique traction or external fixation, immobilization remains in place for 5 to 6 weeks before removal and initiation of therapy.[5,20] For persistent pain and arthritis, arthrodesis of the trapeziometacarpal joint is always a late option.[5]

MCP JOINT FRACTURES
Anatomy and Classification

MCP joint fractures are less common than fractures of the proximal interphalangeal (PIP) joint but can have a severe impact on hand function and pain.[33] The MCP joint is a multiaxial condyloid joint, with a large articular surface, permitting an arc of motion from 10° to 15° of hyperextension to 110° of flexion.[33] The geometry of the MCP joint shows that the center of rotation is not fixed and moves as a function of flexion, and the eccentric attachment of the collateral ligaments results in a complex sliding and rolling action on the articular surfaces.[34] The metacarpal head is broader and longer volarly than dorsally, and the collateral ligaments tighten when the proximal phalanx is flexed.[33]

McElfresh and Dobyns[35] reviewed 103 intra-articular metacarpal head fractures and found that the most commonly injured was the second metacarpal, with athletic injuries causing the greatest number of fractures, followed by striking objects and fights. These investigators divided intra-articular head fractures into 10 groups based on anatomy: epiphyseal injuries involving the metacarpal head, collateral ligament avulsion fractures, osteochondral fractures, oblique fractures, vertical (coronal) fractures, horizontal (transverse) fractures, comminuted fractures, boxer-type metacarpal neck fractures with intra-articular split, fractures involving loss of substance, and occult fractures leading to avascular necrosis of the metacarpal head.[35] These investigators found that 22 of 103 patients had open injuries; the most common intra-articular type was comminuted (31/103), followed by oblique (22/103).[35] Proximal phalangeal fractures may be caused by an axial load, collateral ligament avulsion, or physeal injury.[33]

Presentation and Workup

Patients commonly present with pain, swelling, tenderness, and loss of motion of their MCP joint. Sometimes with impaction fractures, the widening of the articular base can produce a mechanical block to flexion.[36] Any lacerations over the metacarpal head after a fistfight or striking injury could signify an open injury prone to infection.[37] Intra-articular MCP head fractures can be difficult to appreciate on routine radiographs **Fig. 4**.[33,37] In addition to standard PA, lateral, and oblique radiographs, the Brewerton view, with the MCP joint flexed 60° to 70° and radiograph source angled 15° from an ulnar to radial direction, has been described for identifying collateral injuries.[33,38] Oblique and skyline views may be helpful in showing impaction injuries.[33] CT scans with fine (1-mm) cuts can also help define the injuries and aid in treatment planning.[37]

Treatment and Outcomes

Minimally displaced metacarpal head fractures or collateral ligament avulsion fractures can be treated with closed management and early-protected motion.[33,37] The MCP joint can be immobilized in flexion to prevent contracture of the collateral ligaments. Treatment with internal fixation may be difficult for severely comminuted fractures; therefore, treatment with a traction splint allowing passive motion is acceptable.[33] Traction treatments are further described in the treatment section for comminuted PIP joint fractures. Articular defects may remodel over time, and incongruous MCP joints may still function satisfactorily.[5] Treatment of displaced intra-articular metacarpal head fractures should be individualized. ORIF may be performed for displaced and unstable MCP joint fractures. Commonly, a midline longitudinal extensor tendon splitting incision provides adequate exposure of the metacarpal head while the collateral ligaments are preserved.[33] Internal fixation can be performed with K-wires, minifragment screws, minicondylar plates, and pins.[33,35,39,40] The minicondylar plate can be used for sagittal and coronal patterns with metaphyseal extension.[40] Self-compressing Herbert screws, which are countersunk under the chondral surface, can minimize impedance on soft tissues and articular surface.[37] For avulsion fractures to the base of the proximal phalanx, fragments involving less than 20% of the articular surface can be treated with buddy taping and motion, whereas fragments involving more than 20% should be treated with ORIF.[33] Hastings and Carroll[39] reported an average postoperative range of motion 1° to 83° of MCP flexion. Some of the complications include avascular necrosis[40] and joint stiffness if mobilization is delayed more than 3 weeks.[33] In delayed diagnosis, malunions or nonunion salvage procedures can include osteotomies, resection arthroplasty, silicone arthroplasty, surface replacement arthroplasty, and arthrodesis.

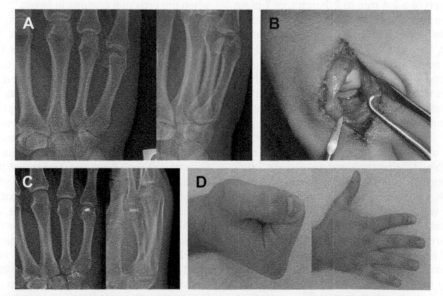

Fig. 4. Intra-articular metacarpal head fracture: injury PA and oblique views of small metacarpal head fracture. (*A*) Injury PA and oblique views of small metacarpal head fracture. (*B*) Articular surface after reduction and internal fixation. (*C*) Follow-up films. (*D*) Final range of motion.

PIP JOINT FRACTURES
Anatomy and Classification

Injuries to the PIP joint are among the most common in the hand.[41] The PIP joint is crucial in our ability to grasp objects, contributing to 85% of the total motion necessary because of its unique anatomy, with 110° arc of motion.[42,43] Inadequate treatment can commonly result in permanent pain, swelling, and stiffness.[44] The head of the proximal phalanx is bicondylar and has almost complete articular congruency with the middle phalanx, allowing for joint stability with axial loading.[45] The cross-sectional shape of the PIP head is trapezoidal, with the anterior surface sloping toward the ring finger, acting as a trochlea in a cone and a hinge joint.[43] Its axis of rotation is not perpendicular to the longitudinal axis of the bone and allows for the fingers to cascade toward the distal pole of the scaphoid in flexion.[42,43] The stability of the PIP joint through a flexion extension arc is provided by the thick volar plate, lateral collateral ligaments, and joint capsule, forming a 3-sided box, with the dorsal aspect relatively devoid of stabilizing structures.[43] Its precise anatomy allows for flexor and extensor moment arms to equally load the articular surface through its arc of motion; any subluxation of the joint can cause abnormal wearing and arthritis.[43,46]

Fractures of the PIP joint can involve the proximal phalanx or the middle phalanx and can be classified based on articular surface involved and displacement. Injuries to the joint can occur with hyperextension, rotation, or lateral stresses; however, it is often difficult to ascertain a single force vector.[43] Proximal phalanx articular fractures can be classified as type 1, stable fractures without displacement, type 2 unicondylar and unstable, and type 3 bicondylar or comminuted fractures.[5] Mechanism of injury for these fractures has been believed to be an axial load through the tip of the finger.[45] Weiss and Hastings[47] reviewed 38 cases of unicondylar fractures and radiographically divided fractures into oblique volar, long sagittal, dorsal coronal, and volar coronal. These investigators concluded that even nondisplaced unicondylar fractures can result in instability and displacement, because the bicondylar surface of the joint normally provides inherent lateral and rotational stability.[45–47]

Middle phalanx fractures can be divided into 3 basic types: palmar lip fractures, dorsal lip fractures, and pilon fractures.[48] Palmar lip fractures with dorsal subluxation are the most common, caused by a hyperextension or axial load injury.[45,48] The severity of this injury can be graded based on percentage of articular surface involved and amount of joint subluxation: I (<10% surface, <25% subluxation), II (11%–20% surface, 25%–50% subluxation), III (21%–40% surface, >50% subluxation), and IV (>40% surface with complete dislocation).[46] Dorsal lip fractures occur with palmar subluxation of the middle phalanx and can be caused by axial loading with hyperextension or an avulsion fracture by hyperflexion.[48] Pilon fractures to the middle phalanx are those in which the volar and dorsal margins are disrupted, with comminution of the central articular surface.[48] These fractures are caused by high-energy axial load with the joint in extension.[48,49]

Presentation and Workup

Initial workup of PIP injuries includes an adequate history and physical examination. The finger should be inspected for localization of swelling, point tenderness, capillary refill, sensation, and malrotation. Range of motion and stability of the joint should be assessed as well; a digital nerve block may be necessary for a thorough examination.[42] Passive testing of joint stability allows for assessment of the volar plate and collateral ligaments, whereas subluxation during active range of motion suggests ligament disruption or significant intra-articular fracture.[41] Treatment of palmar lip fracture/dislocations should be tailored to stability on clinical examination. Radiographic views should include AP, lateral, and oblique views of the entire finger. A true lateral allows superimposition of the condyles of the proximal phalanx, allowing for detection of subluxation.[42] Dorsal subluxation of the joint produces a V sign caused by the separation of the dorsal proximal and middle phalanx articular surfaces, which indicates subtle joint instability.[49] Closed reduction should be followed by radiographic confirmation. Palmar lip fractures can be classified into 3 functional groups: stable (<30% articular surface involvement), tenuous (30%–50% surface involvement), and unstable (>50% surface involvement).[48] After reduction, stable fractures remain congruent with the PIP joint fully extended, and tenuous fractures stay reduced with less than 30° of flexion, whereas unstable fractures require greater than 30° of flexion to maintain joint congruency (**Fig. 5**).[42,45,48,49]

Dorsal lip fractures are not as common as palmar lip fractures. Stability is assessed in full extension (the position of maximum stability) to classify fractures as either stable or unstable on a true lateral radiograph.[48] Articular surface involvement is usually less than 50% when stable, but if there is any palmar subluxation or dislocation in full extension, these fractures are deemed unstable.[42,48] Dorsal lip fractures can also present

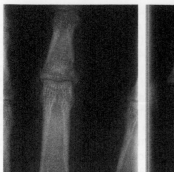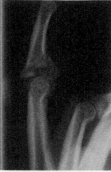

Fig. 5. Intra-articular proximal phalanx fracture.

as an avulsion of the insertion of the central slip of the extensor mechanism.[45] All pilon fractures are grossly unstable and involve up to 100% of the articular surface. These fractures show the greatest amount of joint surface disruption, with areas of central depression and comminution.[45]

Condylar fractures of the proximal phalanx should also undergo the same workup as middle phalangeal base fractures. It is also important to check oblique radiographs along with a true lateral to assess the fracture orientation; an AP radiograph is beneficial to visualize articular step-off.[5]

Treatment and Outcomes

Goals of treatment of PIP joint fractures are to obtain a concentric joint reduction, restore a stable arc of motion, and allow early motion to minimize adhesions and contractures.[49] Anatomic restoration is desirable but not as important as the other goals.[39,48,50]

Treatment of fractures of the proximal phalanx consists of immobilization, with frequent radiographic examination for minimally displaced fractures or closed reduction and pinning versus ORIF for malrotated or displaced fractures.[45] For unicondylar fractures, CRPP with 2 K-wires provides adequate fixation and can be removed in 3 to 4 weeks.[47] If a closed reduction cannot be achieved, then proceeding to open reduction with 1.5-mm to 2-mm lag screws is an alternative.[5] Bicondylar fractures are more difficult to treat. Screw fixation is recommended for triplane fractures; a minicondylar plate can also achieve good results with large condylar fragments.[51] A frequent complication is PIP joint stiffness.[5,51]

The goals of treating middle phalanx dorsal lip fractures are to obtain concentric reduction of the PIP as well as reestablishing the continuity of the central slip of the extensor mechanism.[48] Stable dorsal lip fractures with less than 2 mm of displacement can be treated by splinting the PIP joint in extension or with a transarticular K-wire

for 3 to 4 weeks followed by a return to motion protocol.[44,48] Fractures with greater than 2 mm of displacement can cause an extensor deficit and necessitate ORIF with lag screws, suture, K-wire, or tension banding, which allows for immediate postoperative motion.[44] Unstable dorsal lip fractures are treated by repairing the central tendon and ORIF if possible to restore joint reduction and stability. With high degrees of comminution, ORIF may be difficult and the PIP joint can be pinned in full extension, allowing the dorsal fragments and central slip insertion to consolidate.[44,48] Other options include a dynamic external fixator or suturing the central slip into the dorsal fracture bed to restore stability.[48]

Treatment of middle phalanx volar lip fractures is tailored based on the stability of the fracture. Stable fractures, with less than 30% articular involvement and congruency throughout motion, can be treated with buddy taping, figure-of-8 splint, or extension block splint. Phair and colleagues[52] studied 74 stable volar lip fractures treated with various techniques and concluded that fracture size and displacement are unimportant if the joint remains concentrically reduced. These investigators also concluded that excessive immobilization was the only factor leading to persistent stiffness.[52] For tenuous volar lip fractures, with 30% to 50% articular surface involvement, treatment is aimed at maintaining a concentric joint until the palmar fracture fragments can consolidate to restore the palmar buttress.[48] These fractures can be treated in a variety of ways: extension block splinting, extension block pinning, static splinting, figure-of-8 splint, transarticular K-wire, ORIF, volar plate arthroplasty, and external fixation. Hastings and Carroll[39] advised a trial of dorsal extension block splinting and increasing the limit of extension by 10° weekly, with radiographic confirmation of joint reduction. When the PIP is stable in full extension, by 6 to 8 weeks, the splint can be discontinued and the finger can be buddy taped until comfortable.[39,48] Extension block pinning involves flexing the PIP joint until the joint is concentrically reduced, followed by pinning the proximal phalanx to act as a dorsal block to extension and allowing active/passive flexion of the PIP joint.[53,54]

Other surgical treatment options for unstable PIP fractures include traction, dynamic external fixation, ORIF, volar plate arthroplasty, and a hamate osteochondral autograft arthroplasty. All these strategies seek to obtain a reduction allowing for normal glide around the proximal phalangeal head without hinging on the fracture site.[48,49]

Traction uses the concept of ligamentotaxis to maintain general joint reduction. Agee[55] used a force-couple device with K-wires to lever the base of the middle phalanx palmarly and lift the head of the proximal phalanx dorsally to maintain reduction through the motion arc. Schenck[56] described another method of traction by using a K-wire placed transversely through the middle phalanx attached to an external ring to distract the PIP joint and allowing range of motion. In that series, patients had an average of 63% of articular surface involvement and at 16-month follow-up, patients had an average of –5° to 87° of flexion and all joints were asymptomatic.[56] Another method of traction described by Hastings and Ernst[57] is called traveling traction or dynamic external fixation. In their model, a K-wire is placed through the proximal phalangeal head axis of rotation and also through the middle phalanx. This wire is then bent back to attach to the proximal wire and distract the joint **Fig. 6**. It provides longitudinal traction and permits passive and active motion.[57] When using traction techniques, it is important to have an intact dorsal cortex to keep the joint from subluxating. Salter[58] reviewed effect of motion on articular cartilage and found that cartilage undergoes deterioration if motion is limited and that the articular surface remodels over time. Numerous studies have reported good outcomes by accepting incomplete articular reduction and instituting early motion.[50,56,59] Agee[59] reported good results despite unreduced central fragments in a series of 16 patients treated with a force-couple device and immediate motion. Schenck[56] treated 10 patients with PIP fracture dislocations with traction and

passive motion. He reported that 2 patients had persistent articular surface irregularities but regained a nearly full pain-free arc of motion.[56] Stern and colleagues[50] noted that the middle phalanx base remodels and assumes a widened shape that matches the head of the proximal phalanx after treatment of PIP fractures with traction and motion.

ORIF with lag screws is another option when there is minimal comminution if there is a large fracture fragment. The PIP joint can be approached volarly, mobilizing the neurovascular bundles and flexor tendons to allow for hyperextension of the joint and a shotgun view of the articular surfaces **Fig. 7**. In cases of comminution and instability, cerclage wiring is another method described to treat articular PIP fractures. Weiss[60] described 12 patients treated with 20-gauge or 22-gauge volar cerclage wiring that is used to stabilize the fragments by providing circumferential compression with wire tightening. After an average of 2.1 years' follow-up, 11 of 12 patients reported no degenerative changes, average total arc of motion was 89° without implant failure, and all patients treated had pain-free motion **Fig. 8**.[60]

Volar plate arthroplasty has been described as a treatment option when the articular surface cannot be restored.[61] Some investigators primarily use this technique to salvage late dislocations; others prefer this procedure for many acute fracture dislocations.[48,49] This method advances the volar plate into the middle phalanx fracture defect to restore stability and simultaneously resurfaces

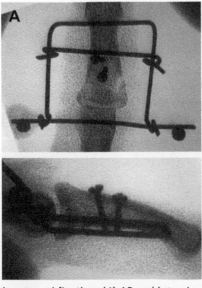
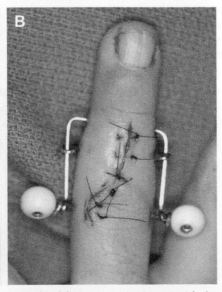

Fig. 6. Dynamic external fixation. (*A*) AP and lateral radiographs. (*B*) Postoperative image with dynamic external fixator in place.

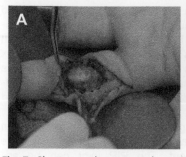
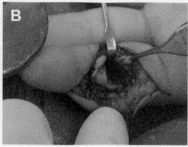
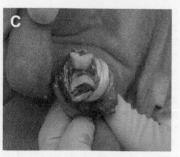

Fig. 7. Shotgun volar approach to PIP joint of a left small finger: (*A*) digital neurovascular bundles shown with dotted lines; (*B*) volar plate elevated and grasped in pickups; (*C*) articular surfaces of proximal phalanx (*above*) and middle phalanx (*below*) showing depressed portion of middle phalangeal base articular surface.

the articular surface.[61] Of the 17 reconstructive cases described,[62] only 3 reported mild pain and an average of 95° of motion was restored. Follow-up radiographs showed marked remodeling of the disrupted surface; however, they reported an average of 6° to 12° of flexion contracture, and redislocation remains a concern if greater than 50% of the base is involved.[62]

Hamate osteochondral autografting is a method for reestablishing the palmar base of the middle phalanx when traction is unable to maintain the joint and when fracture comminution does not allow for restoration of the surface.[48,49] Capo and colleagues[63] proposed this approach by using the anatomically similar contour of the hamate articulation with the fourth and fifth metacarpal bases to reconstruct the contour of the palmar articular surface of the middle phalanx. Calfee and colleagues[64] studied 33 patients treated with hemihamate arthroplasty; all patients healed and maintained joint reduction. These investigators reported an average PIP arc of motion of 71° for acute fractures treated with this method and 69° in chronic injuries. They concluded that it is the treatment of choice for fractures involving 50%

of the volar articular surface that are not amenable to primary internal fixation **Fig. 9**.[64]

Implant resection arthroplasty can be indicated for painful posttraumatic or degenerative joint destruction or subluxation of the joint with stiffness that cannot be corrected.[65] Pyrolytic carbon and silicone implants can be used to resurface the joint and allow for better motion.[66] An intact flexor tendon mechanism, adequate bone stock, soft tissue coverage, and neuromuscular structures are essential for implant arthroplasty.[65] Pyrolytic implants are unlinked and minimally constrained and the stability of these implants in the PIP joint requires intact collateral ligaments.[66]

Joint arthrodesis is another option for unreconstructable bony injury. Arthrodesis is indicated in high-demand patients such as heavy laborers, patients with soft tissue concerns such as burns or contractures, and patients with loss of bone stock.[67] PIP joints of the index and middle fingers are typically functional when fused at 15° to 30° of flexion, because having them slightly extended allows for improved dexterity and allows for posting. Ring and small fingers are functional when fused at 30° to 45°, because they are more

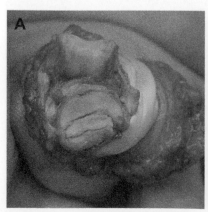
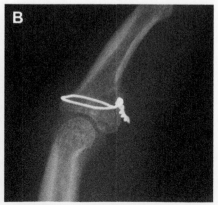

Fig. 8. Cerclage wire ORIF of intra-articular middle phalanx base fracture. (*A*) Intraoperative image showing fracture reduction with cerclage wire. (*B*) AP and lateral postoperative radiographs.

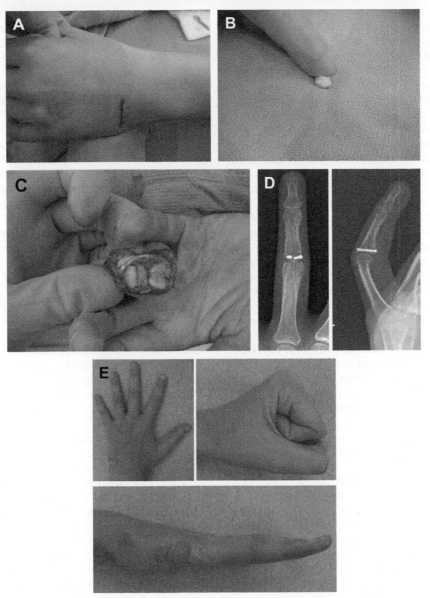

Fig. 9. Hemihamate autograft technique. (*A*) Incision for hamate autograft harvest. (*B*) Hamate autograft. (*C*) Hamate autograft restoring volar aspect of middle phalanx secured with two 1.2-mm screws. (*D*) Postoperative AP and lateral radiographs showing restoration of articular surface–middle phalangeal base to left side of image with proximal phalangeal head to right. (*E*) Clinical images at final follow-up.

involved in gripping. The PIP joint can be fused with a transarticular screw, K-wires, or tension band technique.[67,68]

DORSAL INTERPHALANGEAL JOINT FRACTURES
Anatomy and Classification

The distal interphalangeal joint is an intrinsically stable joint. It has strong collateral ligaments that provide lateral stability, the dorsum is stabilized by the terminal extensor tendon and palmar

aspect stabilized by the flexor digitorum profundus (FDP) tendon.[69,70] Articular fractures can be caused by different mechanisms and can be classified into palmar or dorsal injuries of the distal phalanx[71] and fractures of the head of the middle phalanx.[69]

Articular fractures to the head of the middle phalanx can be caused by torsional or crush injuries of the dorsal interphalangeal (DIP) joint. London[67] classified these in 3 grades: grade 1, unicondylar nondisplaced; grade 2, unicondylar displaced; and grade 3, bicondylar comminuted.

Fractures to the dorsal aspect of the joint, also termed bony mallet fractures, are avulsions to the terminal tendon typically caused by an axial load applied to the finger.[69] Sudden forced flexion can cause an avulsion injury to the extensor mechanism at the DIP joint.[71] Wehbe and Scheider[72] categorized mallet fractures as: type I, with no subluxation of the DIP; type II, with DIP joint subluxation; and type III with epiphyseal/physeal injuries. These types were further subtyped by articular surface involvement with (A) being less than one-third surface involvement, (B) as between one-third and two-thirds involvement, and (C) with greater than two-thirds articular surface involvement.[72] In a biomechanical study of DIP mallet fractures, subluxation was not observed with the fracture fragment measuring less than 43% of the joint surface, with subluxation consistently occurring if the defect measured greater than 52% of the articular surface.[73] Digits with persistent subluxation can progress to having a swan-neck deformity, dorsal joint prominence, and degenerative arthritis.[49]

Palmar-sided articular fractures, or jersey finger, can occur during forced extension during active finger flexion, which causes an avulsion injury of the FDP tendon from the palmar lip. A classic example of this injury is after a football or rugby player grabs an opponent's jersey while attempting a tackle.[37,71] Horiuchi and colleagues[74] described that 75% of cases were caused by injuries during ball sports. A classification system by Leddy and Packer[75] divided fractures based on the FDP tendon: type I, the FDP ruptures and retracts into the palm; type II, the FDP ruptures and retracts to the PIP joint; and type III, a large bony fragment is avulsed with the FDP.[75] Fractures to the distal phalanx are common injuries that can cause significant difficulties in activities of daily living and at work.[70,71]

Presentation and Workup

Clinically, a DIP joint fracture presents with a swelling, ecchymosis, pain, and tenderness at the site of avulsion/fracture.[37] For palmar FDP avulsions, the patient is still able to actively flex the MCP and PIP joints but is unable to actively flex at the DIP joint. Often, with FDP avulsions, radiographs of the finger may appear normal. The injury can be overlooked and considered a jammed finger.[37] Therefore, an appropriate history with examination of active DIP joint flexion is necessary to avoid a delayed or missed diagnosis.[71] There can be a painful nodule in the palm that demarcates the retraction of the FDP tendon (type I). Radiographic views should include AP, lateral, and

oblique views of the DIP joint. Mallet fractures are commonly seen after an axial trauma. Patients are unable to fully extend at the DIP joint, with tenderness over the dorsal surface. Swelling may mask the flexed posture of the joint.[37] AP, lateral, and oblique radiographs show the extent of joint subluxation and fracture fragment size.

Treatment and Outcomes

Fractures of the middle phalangeal head can be guided by the London classification.[76] Grade 1 injuries are stable and treated with closed splinting, whereas grade 2 can be reduced and fixed with K-wires. However, grade 3 injuries are comminuted bicondylar and unstable injuries, which may require arthrodesis or amputation depending on the soft tissue injury.[69]

Although treatment of type I/II FDP avulsion injuries fall outside the scope of this article, with type III fractures with a large fracture fragment, an anatomic reduction of the joint surface is necessary with either pullout suture technique or ORIF with interfragmentary screws or K-wire fixation.[71] DIP joint stiffness is common after such repairs, with an average loss of 10° to 15° of DIP motion.[75] With late presentations or for patients with DIP instability, DIP arthrodesis can yield predictable outcomes.[77]

Many dorsal articular fractures or bony mallet fractures can be treated nonoperatively. Wehbe and Schneider[72] described good results with nonoperative treatment of all mallet fractures and noted the capacity of the articular surface to remodel. Kalainov and colleagues[78] treated mallet fractures with more than one-third articular surface loss nonoperatively with continuous extension splinting of the DIP joint for 5 to 6 weeks. These investigators noted at 2-year follow-up that patients had minimal difficulties with activities of daily living and pain was negligible; however, patients with palmar subluxation may develop an extensor lag, swan-neck deformity, dorsal joint prominence, and degenerative changes.[78] With fractures involving more than 50% of the articular surface and impaction injuries of the distal phalanx base and in patients with persistent volar subluxation, operative treatment can give predictable results.[37,79] A dorsal H-shaped or S-shaped incision centered over the DIP joint is used with full-thickness flaps from the extensor tendon to assess the joint. Fracture can then be reduced and fixed with K-wire or 30-gauge steel pullout wire.[37,70,80] Zhang and colleagues[80] described 65 closed mallet fractures reduced and stabilized with pullout wire fixation of the fragment and K-wire fixation of the DIP joint. These investigators noted an average extensor loss of 7° and flexion loss of 1°, with 52 excellent results.[80] When there is no palmar joint subluxation and less than 30% to 40% of the articular surface is involved, splinting in extension is the treatment of choice.[70,71]

SUMMARY

Fractures of the hand are common injuries and in particular, fractures involving the articular surfaces can present difficulties to the orthopedic surgeon in practice. An overall theme in taking care of these injuries was well encapsulated by Swanson,[81] hand fractures can be complicated by deformity from no treatment, stiffness from over treatment, and both deformity and stiffness from poor treatment.

Treatment of intra-articular fractures of the hand depends on fracture location and pattern of injury. Overall goals must include restoring the alignment and stability and allow for early motion to prevent long-term stiffness, pain, and arthritis.

REFERENCES

1. Van Onselen E, Karim R, Hage J, et al. Prevalence and distribution of hand fractures. J Hand Surg Br 2003;28:491–5.
2. Packer GJ, Shaheen MA. Patterns of hand fractures and dislocations in a district general hospital. J Hand Surg Br 1993;18:511–4.
3. Bushnell BD, Draeger RW, Crosby CG, et al. Management of intra-articular metacarpal base fractures of the second through fifth metacarpals. J Hand Surg Am 2008;33:573–83.
4. El-shennawy M, Nakamura K, Patterson RM, et al. Three-dimensional kinematic analysis of the second through fifth carpometacarpal joints. J Hand Surg Am 2001;26:1030–5.
5. Day CS, Stern PJ. Fractures of the metacarpals and phalanges. In: Wolfe SW, Hotchkiss RN, Pederson WC, et al, editors. Green's operative hand surgery. 6th edition. Philadelphia: Churchill Livingstone; 2011. p. 239–90.
6. Crichlow TP, Hoskinson J. Avulsion fractures of the index metacarpal base: three case report. J Hand Surg Br 1988;13:212–4.
7. Treble N, Arif S. Avulsion fractures of the index metacarpal. J Hand Surg Br 1987;12:1–2.
8. Jena D, Giannikas K, Din R. Avulsion fracture of the extensor carpi radialis longus in a rugby player: a case report. Br J Sports Med 2001;35:133–5.
9. Cobbs KF, Owens WS, Berg EE, et al. Extensor carpi radialis brevis avulsion fracture of the long finger metacarpal: a case report. J Hand Surg Am 1996;21:684–6.
10. Weinstein LP, Hanel DP. Metacarpal fractures. J Am Soc Surg Hand 2002;2:168–80.
11. Lee S, Park I, Kim H, et al. Fourth and fifth carpometacarpal fracture and dislocation of the hand: new classification and treatment. Eur J Orthop Surg Traumatol 2012;22:571–8.
12. Yoshida R, Sha MA, Patterson RM, et al. Anatomy and pathomechanics of ring and small finger carpometacarpal joint injuries. J Hand Surg Am 2003;28:1035–43.
13. Kjaer-Peterson K, Jurik AG, Peterson LK. Intraarticular fractures of the base of the fifth metacarpal. J Hand Surg Br 1992;17:144–7.
14. Jones RS, Kutty S. Intra-articular fractures of the hamate. Injury 1993;24:272–3.
15. Wharton DM, Casaletto JA, Choa R, et al. Outcome following coronal fractures of the hamate. J Hand Surg Eur 2010;35:146–9.
16. Lundeen JM, Shin AY. Clinical results of the intraarticular fractures of the base of the fifth metacarpal treated by closed reduction and cast immobilization. J Hand Surg Br 2000;25:258–61.
17. Liaw Y, Kalnins G, Kirsh G, et al. Combined fourth and fifth metacarpal fracture and fifth carpometacarpal joint dislocation. J Hand Surg Br 1995;20:249–52.
18. Bora FW Jr, Didizian NH. The treatment of injuries to the carpometacarpal joint of the little finger. J Bone Joint Surg Am 1974;56:1459–63.
19. Carlsen BT, Moran SL. Thumb trauma: Bennett fractures, Rolando fractures, and ulnar collateral ligament injuries. J Hand Surg Am 2009;34:945–52.
20. Leibovic SJ. Treatment of Bennett's and Rolando's fractures. Tech Hand Up Extrem Surg 1998;2:36–46.
21. Bosmans B, Verhofstad MH, Gosens T. Traumatic thumb carpometacarpal joint dislocations. J Hand Surg Am 2008;33:438–41.
22. Edmunds JO. Current concepts of the anatomy of the thumb trapeziometacarpal joint. J Hand Surg Am 2011;36:170–82.
23. Leversedge FJ. Anatomy and pathomechanics of the thumb. Hand Clin 2008;24:219–29.
24. Gedda KO. Studies on Bennett's fracture; anatomy, roentgenology, and therapy. Acta Chir Scand Suppl 1954;193:1–114.
25. Langhoff O, Andersen K, Kjaer-Peterson K. Rolando's fracture. J Hand Surg Br 1991;16:454–9.
26. Cannon S, Dowd G, Williams D, et al. A long-term study following Bennett's fracture. J Hand Surg Br 1986;11:426–31.
27. Wagner CJ. Method of treatment of Bennett's fracture dislocation. Am J Hand Surg 1950;80:230–1.
28. Van Niekerk JL, Ouwens R. Fractures of the base of the first metacarpal bone: results of surgical treatment. Injury 1989;20:359–62.
29. Lutz M. Closed reduction transarticular Kirschner wire fixation versus open reduction internal fixation

in the treatment of Bennett's fracture dislocation. J Hand Surg Br 2003;28:142–7.

30. Kjaer-Petersen K, Langhoff O, Andersen K. Bennett's fracture. J Hand Surg Br 1990;16:454–9.

31. Gelberman RH, Vance RM, Zakaib GS. Fractures at the base of the thumb: treatment with oblique traction. J Bone Joint Surg Am 1979;61:260–2.

32. Buchler U, McCollam SM, Oppikofer C. Comminuted fractures of the basilar joint of the thumb: combined treatment by external fixation, limited internal fixation, and bone grafting. J Hand Surg Am 1991;16:556–60.

33. Light TR, Bednar MS. Management of intraarticular fractures of the metacarpophalangeal joint. Hand Clin 1994;10:303–14.

34. Pagowski S, Piekarski K. Biomechanics of metacarpophalangeal joint. J Biomech 1977;10:205–9.

35. McElfresh EC, Dobyns JH. Intra-articular metacarpal head fractures. J Hand Surg 1982;8:383–92.

36. Wolfe SW, Katz LD. Intra-articular impaction fractures of the phalanges. J Hand Surg Am 1995;20:327–33.

37. Jupiter JB, Axelrod TS, Belsky MR. Fractures and dislocations of the hand. In: Browner BD, Jupiter JB, Levine AM, et al, editors. Skeletal trauma. 4th edition. Philadelphia: Saunders Elsevier; 2009. p. 1221–341.

38. Brewerton DA. A tangential radiographic projection for demonstrating involvement of the metacarpal heads in rheumatoid arthritis. Br J Radiol 1967; 40:233–4.

39. Hastings H, Carroll C. Treatment of closed articular fractures of the metacarpophalangeal and proximal interphalangeal joints. Hand Clin 1988;4:503–27.

40. Buechler U, Fischer T. Use of a minicondylar plate for metacarpal and phalangeal periarticular injuries. Clin Orthop 1987;214:53–8.

41. Chinchalkar SJ, Gan BS. Management of proximal interphalangeal joint fractures and dislocations. J Hand Ther 2003;16:117–28.

42. Freiberg A, Pollard BA, Macdonald MR, et al. Management of proximal interphalangeal joint injuries. Hand Clin 2006;22:236–42.

43. Leibovic SJ, Bowers WH. Anatomy of the proximal interphalangeal joint. Hand Clin 1994;10:169–78.

44. Kiefhaber TR, Stern PI. Clinical perspective fracture dislocations of the proximal interphalangeal joint. J Hand Surg Am 1998;23:368–80.

45. Blazar PE, Steinberg DR. Fractures of the proximal interphalangeal joint. J Am Acad Orthop Surg 2000;8:383–90.

46. Schenck RR. Classification of fractures and dislocations of the proximal interphalangeal joint. Hand Clin 1994;10:179–85.

47. Weiss AC, Hastings H. Distal unicondylar fractures of the proximal phalanx. J Hand Surg Am 1993;18:594–9.

48. Kang R, Stern PJ. Fracture dislocations of the proximal interphalangeal joint. J Am Soc Surg Hand 2002;2:47–59.

49. Calfee RP, Sommerkamp TG. Fracture-dislocation about the finger joints. J Hand Surg Am 2009;34:1140–7.

50. Stern PJ, Roman RJ, Kiefhaber TR, et al. Pilon fractures of the proximal interphalangeal joint. J Hand Surg Am 1991;16:844–50.

51. Freeland AE, Sud V. Unicondylar and bicondylar proximal phalangeal fractures. J Am Soc Surg Hand 2001;1:14–24.

52. Phair IC, Quinton DN, Allen MJ. The conservative management of volar avulsion fractures of the P.I.P. joint. J Hand Surg Br 1989;14:168–70.

53. Inoue G, Tamura Y. Treatment of fracture-dislocation of the proximal interphalangeal joint using extension-block Kirschner wire. Ann Hand Surg 1991;10:564–8.

54. Viegas SF. Extension block pinning for proximal interphalangeal joint fracture dislocations: preliminary report of a new technique. J Hand Surg Am 1992;17:896–901.

55. Agee JM. Unstable fracture dislocations of the proximal interphalangeal joint of the fingers: a preliminary report of a new treatment technique. J Hand Surg Am 1978;3:386–9.

56. Schenck RR. Dynamic traction and early passive movement for fractures for the proximal interphalangeal joint. J Hand Surg Am 1986;11:850–8.

57. Hastings H II, Ernst JM. Dynamic external fixation for fractures of the proximal interphalangeal joint. Hand Clin 1993;9:659–74.

58. Salter RB. The physiologic basis of continuous passive motion for articular cartilage healing and regeneration. Hand Clin 1994;10:211–20.

59. Agee JM. Unstable fracture dislocations of the proximal interphalangeal joint treatment with the force couple splint. Clin Orthop 1987;214:101–12.

60. Weiss AP. Cerclage fixation for fracture dislocation of the proximal interphalangeal joint. Clin Orthop Relat Res 1996;327:21–8.

61. Eaton RG, Malerich MM. Volar plate arthroplasty for the proximal interphalangeal joint: a ten year review. J Hand Surg Am 1980;5:260–8.

62. Malerich MM, Eaton RG. The volar plate reconstruction for fracture-dislocation of the proximal interphalangeal joint. Hand Clin 1994;10:251–60.

63. Capo JT, Hastings H, Choung E, et al. Hemicondylar hamate replacement arthroplasty for proximal interphalangeal joint fracture dislocations: an assessment of graft suitability. J Hand Surg Am 2008;33:733–9.

64. Calfee RP, Kiefhaber TR, Sommerkamp TG, et al. Hemi-hamate arthroplasty provides functional reconstruction of acute and chronic proximal interphalangeal fracture-dislocations. J Hand Surg Am 2009;34:1232–41.

65. Swanson AB, Swanson G. Flexible implant resection arthroplasty of the proximal interphalangeal joint. Hand Clin 1994;10:261–6.

66. Branam BR, Tuttle HG, Stern PJ. Resurfacing arthroplasty versus silicone arthroplasty for proximal interphalangeal joint osteoarthritis. J Hand Surg Am 2007;32:775–88.

67. Jones BF, Stern PJ. Interphalangeal joint arthrodesis. Hand Clin 1994;10:267–75.

68. Uhl RL. Proximal interphalangeal joint arthrodesis using the tension band technique. J Hand Surg 2007;32:914–7.

69. Schneider LH. Fractures of the distal interphalangeal joint. Hand Clin 1994;10:277–85.

70. Lubahn JD, Hood JM. Fractures of the distal interphalangeal joint. Clin Orthop Relat Res 1996;327:12–20.

71. Chen F, Schneider LH. Fractures of the distal phalanx. Oper Tech Orthop 1997;7:107–15.

72. Wehbé MA, Schneider LH. Mallet fractures. J Bone Joint Surg Am 1984;66:658–69.

73. Husain SN, Dietz JF, Kalainov DM, et al. A biomechanical study of distal interphalangeal joint subluxation after mallet fracture injury. J Hand Surg Am 2008;33:26–30.

74. Horiuchi Y, Itoh Y, Sasaki T, et al. Dorsal dislocation of the D.I.P. joint with fracture of the volar base of the distal phalanx. J Hand Surg Br 1989;14:177–82.

75. Leddy JP, Packer JW. Avulsion of the profundus tendon insertion in athletes. J Hand Surg Am 1977;2:66–9.

76. London PS. Sprains and fractures of the interphalangeal joints. Hand 1971;3:155–8.

77. Ruchelsman DE, Christoforou D, Wasserman B, et al. Avulsion injuries of the flexor digitorum profundus tendon. J Am Acad Orthop Surg 2011;19:152–62.

78. Kalainov DM, Hoepfner PE, Hartigan BJ, et al. Nonsurgical treatment of closed mallet finger fractures. J Hand Surg Am 2005;30:580–6.

79. Stark HH, Gainor BJ, Ashworth CR, et al. Operative treatment of intra-articular fractures of the dorsal aspect of the distal phalanx of digits. J Bone Joint Surg Am 1987;69:892–6.

80. Zhang X, Meng H, Shao X, et al. Pull-out wire fixation for acute mallet finger fractures with K-wire stabilization of the distal interphalangeal joint. J Hand Surg Am 2010;35:1864–9.

81. Swanson AB. Fractures involving the digits of the hand. Orthop Clin North Am 1970;1:261–74.

Open Fractures of the Hand with Soft Tissue Loss

David Ruta, MD, Kagan Ozer, MD*

KEYWORDS

- Antibiotics • Flap • Fracture • Graft • Open • Primary • Reconstruction • Tissue

KEY POINTS

- Clinical decision-making for open fractures of the hand associated with soft tissue loss is influenced by the mechanism, time and environment of injury, medical and social histories, comorbidities, and patient goals and expectations.
- Guidelines for antibiotic use in open hand fractures remain less definitive than for other anatomic areas, given conflicting literature.
- Segmental bone and soft tissue loss can be reconstructed primarily with improved outcomes as described throughout the literature. This includes thorough irrigation and debridement, corticocancellous bone grafting, and soft tissue coverage.
- There is a wide selection of local, regional, and distant flaps, which vary based on defect location. Options are discussed in the text, including the pros and cons of each.
- Worse outcomes in open hand injuries have been associated with increased grade of soft tissue injury, increased comminution, and concomitant tendon injury, among others.

INTRODUCTION

Open fractures associated with soft tissue loss in the hand may result from high-energy trauma that can put the patient's life at risk. Therefore, care should be taken to ensure that an appropriate primary survey is initially performed, with strict adherence to advanced trauma life support protocols.

This primary survey should be followed by a secondary survey, starting with a detailed history of the time, mechanism, and environment of injury. A medical, social, and medication history must be obtained, because patient comorbidities, habits, and addictions can influence clinical decision making. Physical examination must evaluate the size and condition of any wounds, with note of gross contamination and whether a zone of injury is visible extending beyond the wound edges. Especially in the presence of soft tissue loss,

motor, sensory, and independent tendon function must be determined, as well as an assessment of vascularity and any threat to it. However, the definitive examination typically occurs at the time of surgery.

Having a discussion with the patient regarding clear goals for outcome before any surgical management is of utmost importance, as such information can alter the treatment course.

ANTIMICROBIAL TREATMENT

The benefit of antibiotic treatment of open fractures in other areas of the body has been well documented.[1–5] In 2 prospective studies of open fractures, including wrist or hand injuries, Patzakis and colleagues[2,4] concluded early administration of antibiotics to be the single most important factor in preventing infections following open fractures.

Disclosure: Neither the authors nor any immediate family member has any financial relationship to disclose with any commercial company or institution directly or indirectly related to the subject of this article.
Department of Orthopaedic Surgery, University of Michigan, 2098 South Main Street, Ann Arbor, MI 48103, USA
* Corresponding author.
E-mail address: kozer@umich.edu

Hand Clin 29 (2013) 551–567
http://dx.doi.org/10.1016/j.hcl.2013.08.008
0749-0712/13/$ – see front matter © 2013 Elsevier Inc. All rights reserved.

The literature on antibiotic use specifically in open hand fractures is less definitive, because there are few prospective, randomized controlled trials and they are often confounded by the heterogeneity of these injuries.[6–12] Sloan and colleagues[13] performed a prospective, randomized trial of 85 open distal phalanx fractures of various severities, all treated with irrigation, primary closure, and intravenous or oral cephradine within 6 hours versus no antibiotics. Although only 1 infection occurred in the antimicrobial groups combined (n = 73), 3 infections developed in the 40 patients treated without antibiotics. The investigators recommended a single dose of antibiotics both before and after surgery as appropriate therapy. In contrast, Peacock and colleagues[12] and Suprock and colleagues,[14] in two separate prospective studies, found no difference in infection rates following irrigation, debridement, and primary closure versus the same with the addition of prophylactic antibiotics. In a larger cohort, Stevenson and colleagues[15] performed a prospective, randomized controlled trial comparing flucloxacillin and placebo in 193 distal phalanx fractures with a range of mechanisms and severity. All underwent irrigation and primary closure, and all received oral antimicrobials or placebo within 12 hours of injury with continuation for 5 days. Seven total superficial infections developed, without significant difference between groups. Chow and colleagues[11] reported on their experience treating 245 open digital fractures, 51% associated with significant soft tissue injuries. Although all received antibiotic therapy, their infection rate of 2.04% is consistent with those in placebo groups of other studies. In a prospective, randomized, double-blind, controlled trial, Madsen and colleagues[16] compared a single intravenous penicillin dose, 6 days of oral penicillin, and placebo as treatment of 599 patients with traumatic wounds to the hands or feet, with exposed fracture, tendon, joint, or a combination. Of the total, 570 were hand injuries. An unspecified number were allowed to heal by secondary intention. Infection rates were 4.9%, 6.6%, and 10.2%, respectively, with a significant difference between those receiving either of the antibiotic treatments and those receiving placebo ($P = .046$).

The environment of injury may play a role in antibiotic treatment. Fitzgerald and colleagues[17] reported differences in bacterial isolates from 86 hand injuries, based on environment. Farm-related injuries were colonized by a greater proportion of gram-negative bacteria, most commonly Enterobacter, Clostridium, and Klebsiella species. In contrast, injuries sustained in a home or industry setting showed more gram-positive isolates, most commonly Staphylococcus epidermidis, Staphylococcus aureus, and Streptococcus group D. Although initial cultures do not necessarily predict the infecting organism,[8,12] several reports have identified S aureus as the most common organism isolated in open hand fractures.[8,10,12–15]

Although some think that these compiled reports support foregoing routine antibiotic therapy in the management of all open digital fractures, they are often given in routine treatment of open hand fractures, and many centers continue routine use in open finger wounds as well.

In 2006, Hauser and colleagues[18] published guidelines for antibiotic use in open fractures on behalf of the Surgical Infection Society. These guidelines included administration of a first-generation cephalosporin, or other gram-positive coverage, for 24 to 48 hours to effectively decrease infectious risk in grade I[3,19] open fractures. Forty-eight hours of coverage was supported as efficacious in grade II and III fractures. The guidelines describe insufficient data to support any of the following: routine prolongation of prophylactic antibiotics beyond 24 to 48 hours, the addition of gram-negative coverage in any open fracture, use of culture-specific antibiotics determined either from presentation or operative culture, or addition of penicillin for Clostridium-prone injuries. However, when treating open hand fractures, continued investigation specifically into the nature of hand injuries remains warranted.

In terms of the timing of antimicrobial administration in open hand fractures, it is advocated to initiate treatment as early as possible, preferably within the first 6 hours.[13,16,20] Duration in hand studies ranges from a single intravenous dose on presentation to 5 days of an oral regimen,[12–16] with some including an oral regimen up to 10 days.[20]

TIMING OF RECONSTRUCTION

Segmental bone and soft tissue loss in the hand can be reconstructed either primarily or in a staged fashion. In primary reconstruction, immediate osteosynthesis with corticocancellous bone grafting restores bony length, reestablishes normal muscle tension, and further decreases opportunity for soft tissue contracture. Restored length also decreases infectious risk and edema by eliminating dead space and encouraging resumed venous and lymphatic circulation.[21] The foundation of a stable osseous construct also sets the framework for immediate soft tissue reconstruction. Improved outcomes of primary osseous and soft tissue reconstruction have been described throughout the literature.[21–33]

As an alternative, staged reconstruction is preferred when an extreme degree of contamination makes it difficult to determine tissue viability or when the risk of infection is too high because of injury-related or host-related factors.[23–25,28] The time between stages is variable, depending on the rate of soft tissue healing and the time needed for tissues to be supple and joints mobile. For example, burn, crush, or high-pressure injection injuries usually warrant temporary closure with second look at 48 to 72 hours or more, because tissue viability is difficult to determine during initial debridement. Further excision is often necessary, because questionable tissues commonly declare themselves later.[25,34] In these cases, temporary coverage must still be applied to prevent desiccation, which may be in the form of autografts, allografts, or negative-pressure wound therapy.[25,35–37] While awaiting a clean surgical bed, length may be maintained with use of a mini external fixator or Kirschner wires.[38,39] Results in these cases may be hindered by arthrofibrosis and adhesions, secondary to the prolonged immobilization and multiple procedures inherent to staging of the reconstruction.[23,27,31]

In deciding between primary versus staged reconstruction, perhaps the most important step is the adequacy of the initial surgical debridement.[22,25] This debridement is to be performed by an experienced hand surgeon. Radical and thorough debridement should be performed under tourniquet control. All clearly or marginally devitalized tissues must be excised, intentionally extending beyond the zone of injury, with the goal of converting a contaminated wound to a clean one, suitable for coverage.[24,27,28,30] Temporary tourniquet release following initial debridement should accompany the process, thereby allowing reevaluation of threatened tissue, with further excision as necessary. The debrided wound bed should be free of devitalized tissue and any dead space.[22] If a wound is too heavily contaminated to be prepared for primary closure, any bone grafting or definitive coverage must be delayed until an appropriate wound bed can be achieved.

OPTIONS FOR SOFT TISSUE COVERAGE

Hand trauma often presents with deficits ranging from skin alone to complex defects of the underlying tendons, nerves, vessels, and bone. It is important that the decision of soft tissue reconstruction respects the unique functionality of the hand, and also provides a flexible envelope, durable enough for the intensive therapy that the patient needs.[34]

The options available for soft tissue reconstruction are many, with the number further increasing as microsurgical techniques continue to advance. The concepts of reconstructive ladder and reconstructive triangle[40–43] have now evolved into the reconstructive clockwork, including composite tissue allotransplantation, robotics, and regeneration/tissue engineering.[44] The simplest coverage is not always the most appropriate when a certain degree of form and functionality are goals.

A loss of only superficial skin may be addressed with split-thickness skin grafting (STSG) or full-thickness skin grafting (FTSG), although the risk of contraction and potential for limited flexibility and sensibility must be taken into account, with vascularized flap coverage performed if it is expected to produce a superior outcome, as is the case with exposure of tendon, nerve, bone, ligament, or joint.[41] There is a wide selection of local, regional, and distant flap options. Various reconstructive options for soft tissue coverage are discussed later, excluding fingertip injuries, along with guidelines and a recommendation that the reader refer to our list of references for specific surgical techniques.

Skin Substitutes and Negative-pressure Wound Therapy

Temporary coverage options have been most widely used in burn injuries, although they have been shown to be a useful adjunct for soft tissue deficits of the hand as well. The purposes of temporary coverage are to maintain wound hydration and encourage healing, ideally with the goal of augmenting autologous soft tissue reconstruction. The most commonly used techniques in hand surgery were reviewed by Watt and colleagues[45] and include synthetic bilayer dermal replacements, allogenic acellular skin, and negative-pressure wound therapy.

Integra (Integra LifeSciences, Plainsboro, NJ) is a well-studied example of synthetic bilaminar skin substitutes, which contain various extracellular components to serve as a scaffold for angiogenesis, the formation of granulation tissue, and dermal regeneration, with an overlying removable membrane (typically silicone) to hinder desiccation. This combination is intended to mimic natural skin. These skin substitutes are typically placed for 2 to 4 weeks,[46] after which the outermost layer is discarded, providing a wound bed amenable to STSG or FTSG.[47,48] In addition to ease of use and decreased donor site morbidity, studies (many in burn injuries) have reported benefits of Integra to include a high rate of subsequent STSG take (87%–93%)[49–52]; improved durability, mobility, and cosmesis compared with STSG alone[49]; and tolerance of thinner STSG,[49,53] allowing faster donor site healing.[49] Application of topical negative pressure to Integra has shown decreased time to vascularization and STSG application,[50,51,54] as well as increased take of the Integra graft.[54]

In the hand, Weigert and colleagues[52] reviewed Integra use in 15 traumatic hand wounds with exposed tendon, bone, or joint. Integra application was on day 26 (mean) with STSG after 26 additional days. Mean area covered was 62 cm^2. Thirteen cases showed successful STSG with good mobility and aesthetic scores. Taras and colleagues[48] applied Integra to 21 digits following trauma with exposed bone, tendon, joint, or hardware. After 24 days, FTSG was performed with 4 showing graft loss of 15% to 25%. Improved function and cosmesis, with decreased adhesions, have also been shown following Integra use before STSG for deep hand burns.[55] Successful use has further been reported in deep wound beds following hand tumor resection,[56] in degloving injuries,[47,57] and to enhance free flap donor site coverage.[58]

When using bilaminar skin substitutes, consideration should be given to the risk of altered sensation,[48] increased cost,[46,59] and the additional immobilization time required for dermal regeneration.[45,52]

Temporary application of acellular allogenic dermal matrix has the same goals as synthetic skin substitutes. After various processing and storage techniques, placement of the matrix provides a dermal scaffold, allowing neovascularization and, ultimately, a wound bed suitable for skin grafting. In hand surgery, these have shown successful results mainly in treatment of burn scar contractures.[60,61]

The benefits of negative-pressure wound therapy (wound V.A.C. Therapy, Kinetic Concepts, Inc, San Antonio, TX) include increased perfusion, promotion of angiogenesis, wound area reduction, cellular proliferation, decreased bacterial contamination, and reduction of the inhibitory effects of wound exudate.[62–66] Numerous studies have shown it to be a superior method of skin graft bolstering,[67–75] especially to the various contours of the hand,[68,69,72,74,75] and also to successfully immobilize STSG to microvascular free muscle flaps.[66,76,77] Wound V.A.C. application over pedicled inferior epigastric flap reconstruction of deep dorsal hand and finger burns has shown expedited flap attachment as a result.[63] Improved graft take is secondary to enhanced immobilization of the graft and fluid collection egress, and encouraged contouring to the wound bed.[45,64] As discussed earlier, it has been shown to enhance Integra use for the same reasons.[50,51,54]

Finger Reconstruction (Between the Metacarpophalangeal and Distal Interphalangeal Joints)

The cross-finger and reverse cross-finger flaps are traditional methods of dual-staged coverage for palmar and dorsal defects, respectively.[78] Benefits include ease of dissection, durability, sensibility, and overall patient satisfaction.[78] Disadvantages include flexion contracture of digits at the proximal interphalangeal (PIP) joint, decreased grip strength, cold intolerance, and the 2 surgeries required to achieve the final result.[79] For small palmar-lateral defects, Yam and colleagues[80] described the palmar pivot flap, based on the transverse branches of the digital artery, available for coverage from the PIP joint to the fingertip. Tan[81] described a series of various uses of reverse dorsolateral proximal phalangeal island flaps for defects distal to the PIP joint.

Distally based dorsal metacarpal artery flaps and their subsequent modifications are established options for dorsal digital coverage, including as distal as the fingertip and nail bed if an extended flap is used.[82–86] These flaps are based on native anastomoses between the dorsal and palmar arterial systems (**Figs. 1–3**). Gregory and colleagues[85] described a cutaneous tail modification, whereby the flap is designed with a cutaneous extension that can be closed skin to skin following rotation, completely covering the pedicle and avoiding tunneling. Sebastin and colleagues[87] used 58 metacarpal artery perforator flaps to resurface defects up to the proximal half of the middle phalanx, with flaps based on the second, third, and fourth web space perforators. Ten were performed primarily. Three flaps were completely lost, warranting revision surgery. The first dorsal metacarpal artery (FDMA) flap has been shown to be effective for resurfacing thumb pulp defects.[88–91] Chen and colleagues[92] described their group's results restoring thumb tip sensation after degloving injuries, using a modified FDMA including both dorsal branches of the proper digital nerves.

The adipofascial turnover flap with subsequent skin grafting is another option for defects on the dorsal finger or hand with good cosmesis, single-stage surgery, and minimal donor site morbidity (**Table 1**).[93–95]

Soft Tissue Defects of the Hand

Radial forearm flap

The radial forearm flap has long been a workhorse for hand coverage,[96,97] able to cover most hand wounds, including to the fingertips, with the option

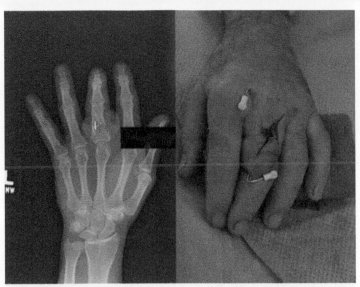

Fig. 1. A 35-year-old patient presented to an outside hospital with a gunshot injury to his left long finger sustaining an open comminuted fracture of the proximal phalanx with bone and soft tissue loss along with laceration of flexor digitorum superficialis and common extensor tendon. He was transferred to our facility following an initial irrigation and temporary K-wire fixation.

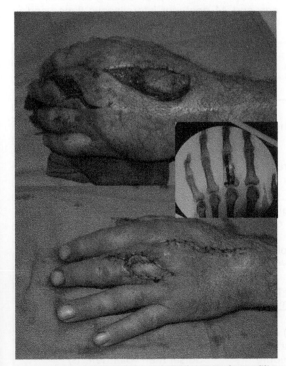

Fig. 2. The patient underwent single-stage bone (iliac crest) and soft tissue reconstruction using second dorsal intermetacarpal artery flap. We routinely use Doppler ultrasound to locate the perforator. This flap can be extended more proximally to the dorsal aspect of the wrist joint based on the same pedicle.

for a variety of composite grafting.[98–100] As originally described, the 2 major disadvantages of the fasciocutaneous flap are donor site healing/cosmetic concerns, and sacrifice of the radial artery. If the Allen test is abnormal, use of the radial forearm flap may not be safe without vein grafting. To improve the donor site appearance and graft acceptance, Chang and colleagues[101] described more than 400 suprafascial flap harvests. In addition to improved cosmesis, sensory dysfunction was also decreased, because the superficial radial nerve and thenar cutaneous branch of the lateral antebrachial cutaneous nerve were preserved. Lutz and colleagues[102] confirmed the superiority of suprafascial dissection after harvesting 95 suprafascial free radial forearm flaps ranging from 24 to 191 cm^2, mean 78.3 cm^2. Other investigators report even better cosmetic results with FTSG[103] and fascia-only harvests.[104]

Chang and colleagues[105] reconstructed 34 hands (19 traumatic) using distally based radial perforator forearm flaps for defects including the volar and dorsal hand, as well as thumb-index space. Nineteen fasciocutaneous flaps and 15 turnover adipofascial flaps were performed with 2 showing less than 10% partial necrosis. Flap length ranged from 9 to 18 cm with length/pedicle ratios of 3:1 to 5:1. Hansen and colleagues[100] reported a small series using a reverse radial forearm fascial flap to cover defects of the dorsal or palmar hand to the proximal phalanges. Ignatiadis and colleagues[106] reported successful use of the radial

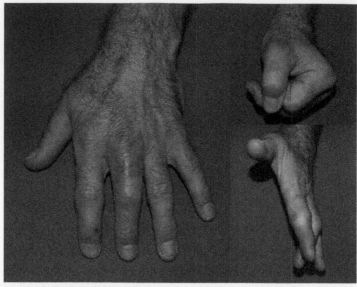

Fig. 3. Nine months after his initial surgery, he underwent hardware removal and a tenolysis procedure. These photographs show his final follow-up at 18 months.

artery perforator flap in 11 severe open hand traumas with 1 requiring revision with a groin flap for 50% necrosis. Limitations of the radial forearm perforator flap include its moderate size and its dependence on an intact volar arch.[107]

Most early perforator flap descriptions were as free flaps.[108,109] Georgescu and colleagues[110] published a large series of local and regional perforator forearm flaps, including 65 radial, 16 ulnar, and 44 posterior interosseous flaps used to

Table 1
Local options for coverage of digital soft tissue loss

	Pros	Cons
Cross-finger/reverse cross-finger flap[70,71,88]	Ease of dissection Ideal donor tissue for finger coverage Functional mobility Ability to cover dorsal (reverse cross-finger) and volar (cross-finger) defects	Two-stage procedure (with interim immobilization) Noticeably reduced motion ($\sim 20°$) Requires grafting to donor site
Dorsal metacarpal artery flaps[74–84,88]	Multiple perforators available for potentially large area of dorsal digital coverage: • Proximal and middle phalanges • Extension to fingertip/nail bed possible • Thumb pulp coverage possible Often can be closed primarily	More unreliable vasculature/possible congenital absence with progression ulnarly (although flap based off perforator still possible) Low-flow system with tenuous venous drainage Careful dissection required
Turnover flaps[85–87]	Single-stage procedure Random (dorsal harvest) and pedicled (volar harvest) options Technically simpler procedure	Requires skin grafting to recipient site Insensate flaps (more suitable for dorsal than volar defects)
Flag flaps[86,89]	Mobility via rotation allows coverage of dorsal or volar proximal phalanges/Metacarpophalangeal joints Good sensibility	Unsuitable for coverage distal to proximal phalanges Typically requires grafting to donor site

cover forearm and hand defects (number of each recipient site not specified). They noted the long pedicles possible with regional flaps, able to achieve a large rotational arc, which is especially useful in coverage of dorsal hand defects. Either local or regional-type perforator flaps may be used as composite flaps. Complete flap survival was reported in 87.8% with only 1 flap completely lost. All 5 osteofasciocutaneous flaps with radial bone segment showed union. Investigators highlight the preservation of major arteries and improved donor site morbidity, and not requiring microvascular anastomosis on transfer.

Ulnar artery perforator flap

Since it was first described,[111] the distal ulnar artery perforator flap has undergone modifications, some including an osseous segment.[112–114] This flap is supplied by the ulnodorsal artery, arising from the ulnar artery, used for the proximal third of the midpalm, hypothenar area, and more than two-thirds of the dorsal hand.[106] Areas up to 180 cm^2 can be covered.[106,114] Unal and colleagues[114] described the use of this transposition flap in 6 patients with hand trauma with no flap complications and good patient satisfaction overall. Ignatiadis and colleagues[106] performed 12 ulnar perforator flaps for hand trauma. Two patients had partial flap loss (25% necrosis). The flap is useful in covering small and medium-sized defects without sacrificing a major artery (**Figs. 4–6**). However, its arc of rotation is limited because of its small pedicle length. The donor site is usually closed primarily leaving a longitudinal scar along the ulnar border of the forearm.[106,114]

Posterior interosseous flap

The posterior interosseous flap arises from the common interosseous artery. Lu and colleagues[115] published a series of 201 patients undergoing posterior interosseous flap coverage of the distal third of the forearm, wrist, and hand, including 27 composite flaps and the remainder fasciocutaneous. Flap areas ranged from 20 cm^2 to 160 cm^2. There was only 1 total flap failure and 16 with partial necrosis. Outcomes were good in general. Function was suboptimal for flexor tendon composite grafts with a recommendation for tenolysis; the extensor tendon composite graft had superior functionality. The investigators described venous congestion in 16 flaps, also noting that donor scars were conspicuous and influenced cosmesis in female patients. In addition to the results of Georgescu and colleagues[110] discussed earlier, other series also support its use for the hand dorsum and palm, able to cover as distal as the proximal phalanges without requiring sacrifice of a major artery (**Figs. 7** and **8**).[116,117]

Distant tissue transfer

If the soft tissue loss is large, free tissue transfer is indicated to replace the deficit. In addition to the surface area requiring coverage, the quality of the transferred skin and donor site morbidity play important roles in selection of the tissue for transfer. Lateral arm flap, anterolateral thigh flap, latissimus dorsi flap, serratus anterior fascial flap,

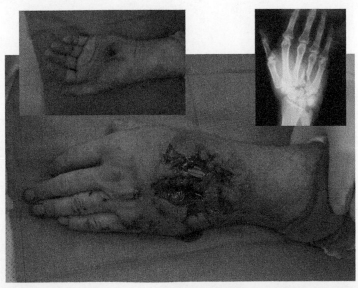

Fig. 4. A 29-year-old patient presented with a gunshot injury sustaining open fracture/dislocations of the third and fourth carpometacarpal (CMC) joints with a dorsal soft tissue defect. Bone loss included the base of the third metacarpal and capitellum.

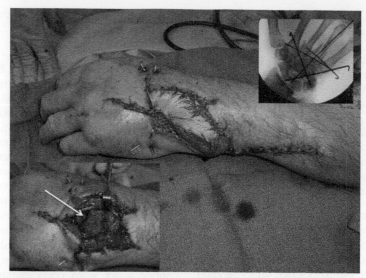

Fig. 5. Following extensive irrigation and debridement, the patient underwent primary bone and soft tissue reconstruction in a single stage. The iliac crest corticocancellous bone graft measuring 1.5 × 3 cm, placed at the CMC joints of the third and fourth digits, can be seen in the left lower corner (*arrow*). Coverage was performed with an ulnar artery perforator flap harvested along the ulnar border of the forearm and rotated 120°. Common extensor tendons of the third and fourth digits were then repaired.

gracilis muscle flap, and temporoparietal fascial flaps are among the commonly used free flaps.[118] Microsurgical combinations thereof have also been described to address more complex injuries, termed chimeric free flaps.[119]

The lateral arm flap, supplied by the posterior radial collateral artery (a branch of the profunda brachii), has the benefit of having predictable vascular anatomy, a more discreet donor site, and no need for major artery sacrifice.[120,121] It may be transferred as a variety of composite grafts, including with vascularized triceps tendon. The flap size may be as large as 8 × 15 cm[98] with primary closure of the donor site possible if

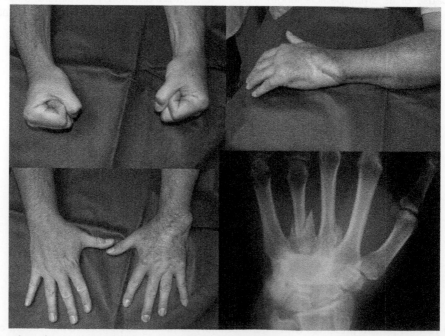

Fig. 6. The patient shows near-complete range of motion and incorporation of the bone graft 6 months after the surgery. Further remodeling and flattening of the flap is expected up to 12 months after the surgery.

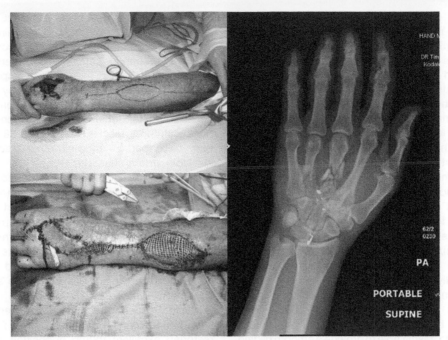

Fig. 7. A 65-year-old gun safety instructor accidentally shot himself, sustaining open fractures of the third and fourth metacarpals with bone and soft tissue loss. Following extensive irrigation and debridement, he underwent iliac crest corticocancellous bone grafting and soft tissue coverage with posterior interosseous flap. Doppler ultrasound is routinely used to locate the perforator, usually at the floor of the fifth dorsal compartment, as marked in the upper left picture.

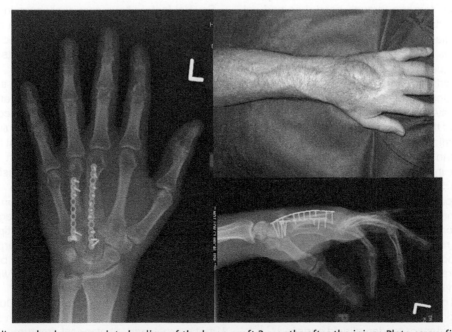

Fig. 8. Radiographs show complete healing of the bone graft 3 months after the injury. Plate-screw fixation was placed across the CMC joints of the third and fourth digits on the hamate and capitate, which did not result in any motion limitation at the wrist.

the width is 5 to 6 cm or less.[122] Lister and Scheker[24] reported on 14 emergency free lateral arm flaps (5 fascia only) with no total failures. Partial failures were limited to the fascia-only flaps. Ulusal and colleagues[123] reported 118 hand defects, including fingers, dorsal hand, and palmar hand wounds, with several variants of the lateral arm flap (mainly fasciocutaneous) with 97.5% survival. The investigators noted poor functional results in the 7 patients with extensor tendon reconstruction via triceps tendon as a composite graft. As the lateral arm flap is more limited than other options in its potential width coverage, Wong and colleagues[122] described a turnaround technique following an extended lateral arm flap, to increase its functional width. In this series of 31 flaps, sizes ranged from 48 to 144 cm^2 (mean 94.6 cm^2) with 100% survival. Twelve patients successfully underwent minor secondary procedures to improve function or for debulking.

Benefits of the anterolateral thigh flap, first described by Song and colleagues,[124] include a long pedicle, fascia able to provide a smooth gliding surface for tendons, versatility of design given perforator anatomy, and minimal donor site morbidity if closed primarily.[118] A width range of 6 to 9 cm is suggested as the limit to primary closure.[43,125] The axial vessel that supplies this flap is the lateral circumflex femoral artery. The available area of this flap is large, with Koshima[126] describing the skin paddle up to dimensions of 35 cm in length and 25 cm in width on a single perforator. In the forearm through hand, Lee and colleagues[127] had partial failure of only 1 of their 7 flaps, with flap areas up to 150 cm^2. In 58 upper extremity flaps (number of hands not specified), Wei and colleagues[125] had 4 partial and no total failures. Other reports support reliable composite use in complex hand and forearm coverage.[128,129] Various methods have been used for addressing the disadvantages of this flap, which include anatomic variation and difficulty with dissection.[125,130]

Ulrich and colleagues[131] presented a series of 9 patients in whom free serratus anterior fascial flaps with STSG were used to cover defects of the hand (palmar and dorsal) and degloved fingers. One flap had less than 10% partial necrosis. The investigators described good functional and cosmetic results with flap areas up to 168 cm^2. Other studies had success with 90 cm^2,[132] although raised flaps of 600 cm^2 (20 × 30 cm) have been reported.[133] Additional articles support Ulrich and colleagues'[131] findings, especially when used for dorsal hand defects with a need for an excellent extensor tendon gliding surface.[132,134]

On analysis of 35 temporoparietal fascial flaps for dorsal or palmar hand tissue loss, Carty and colleagues[135] described excellent long-term mobility, pliability, and contour with minimal bulk, as well as commenting on the inconspicuous donor site scar in patients with overlying hair. The ability of this flap to be applied in a dual-leafed sandwich fashion, thereby providing circumferential gliding surfaces for repaired or reconstructed tendons, is a known benefit.[135–137] Successful free fascial flaps up to 238 cm^2 have been described,[137] although other articles report available area around 120 cm^2.[138]

Given the bulkiness of a myocutaneous gracilis flap, a free muscle transfer with skin grafting is typically used to fill hand defects, particularly for thenar area reconstruction.[139] Engelhardt and colleagues[140] used a free gracilis muscle transfer with skin graft from the foot instep for a central palm defect reconstruction, providing good durability, adherence, and minor deep pressure sensibility. Baker and Watson[141] described free innervated gracilis muscle flap with STSG for thenar reconstruction following traumatic loss in 2 patients, restoring excellent thumb opposition in both. A gracilis perforator flap has also been described, with harvested area up to 270 cm^2.[142] The free muscle gracilis flap has minimal donor site morbidity in an inconspicuous location, excellent vascular supply, and the ability to obliterate dead space and restore function.[138,143]

FACTORS AFFECTING OVERALL OUTCOME

Several factors have commonly been investigated for their influence on outcome in open hand fractures. These factors may be classified as those variables related to the injury itself, its management, and the patient.

The mechanism of injury can have a substantial influence on outcome. Crush injuries can produce large areas of threatened tissue secondary to more proximal vascular injury, requiring wide debridement.[144,145] Likewise, electrical burns can cause adjacent tissue death, which may not initially be demarcated, thereby increasing risk of infection if the degree of injury is underestimated.[146] In addition to threat of compartment syndrome, this warrants careful management of these injuries, which often require multiple procedures, including fasciotomies and carpal tunnel release.[146] Given the stretch of tissue before failure, avulsion injuries are associated with longer segments of neurovascular injury.[147]

With regard to the extent of injury, Duncan and colleagues[9] analyzed 75 patients with 140 open metacarpal and phalangeal fractures and described poorer total active range of motion correlating most highly with increasing grade of injury, as per their modified Gustilo and Anderson classification (**Table 2**). Further, when additional dissection was required for osteosynthesis, patients with grade I, II, or IIIA fractures then had worse motion than their counterparts who did not require further incision. Fractures with associated tendon injury showed more limited mobility than those without, specifically with injuries to extensor zones 3 to 6, flexor zone 2 (which correlates with extensor zones 3–6), or both. Overall, metacarpal fractures recovered best. Finger injuries requiring soft tissue coverage and/or multiple procedures were more likely to have fair or poor outcomes.

Chow and colleagues[11] performed a prospective analysis of 201 patients with 245 open fractures, spanning from the distal quarter of the metacarpals through the middle phalanges, with varying degrees of soft tissue injury. Avulsion fractures, fracture-dislocations, amputations, or injuries requiring revascularization were excluded. Comminuted fractures fared worse, as did proximal phalangeal fractures. Significant soft tissue injuries were defined as injuries to tendons, digital nerves, or skin defects requiring reconstruction. Fifty-one percent of their cohort had significant tissue injury, which fared worse than those without (16.8% good and 52% poor vs 41.7% good and 25.8% poor, respectively). Flexor tendon injuries

were significantly more detrimental then extensor injuries. The investigators concluded that the stiffness following skin grafting was likely secondary to both immobilization and increased susceptibility to adhesions. Following analysis of each of the significant injuries, they proposed a prognostic classification system that allowed incorporation of those components that they had associated with mobility.

Several findings in the two studies discussed earlier have been supported by other reports, specifically including worse outcomes with greater soft tissue injury,[8,148–150] with increased comminution,[8,148–150] and with associated tendon injury.[148,150]

An area of controversy exists as to whether there is a relationship between the degree of soft tissue injury and rate of infection. Although some reports have supported increased risk of infection with increasing degree of soft tissue injury in the hand,[8,9,20] several others have shown a lack of that association.[10,11,21,24,25,151,152] As discussed previously, meticulous surgical debridement is critical in treating open hand injuries, because retained devascularized tissue becomes a nidus for infection. Studies have shown a correlation between initial contamination and subsequent infection.[8,10] However, if appropriate debridement produces a clean wound bed, internal fixation and primary closure in open hand fractures has not been shown to increase infectious risk.[9–11,21,24,25,151]

In terms of the timing of initial treatment, it is important to reestablish the vascular flow if disrupted. Although there are reports of successful digital revascularization at up to 42 hours of warm ischemia[153,154] and 94 hours of cold ischemia,[155] digital replantation is ideally to be performed within 12 hours. If the devascularized portion of the extremity contains muscle, irreversible changes begin to occur beyond 4 hours of ischemia.[156]

Even in the presence of a well-perfused hand, delay in the management of open fractures, particularly when associated with soft tissue loss, may still result in unfavorable outcomes. Swanson and colleagues[10] found an increased risk of infection with delayed treatment of open hand fractures beyond 24 hours from injury. Several reports have shown no significant difference in outcome when treated within 24 hours.[8,9,21,151]

In evaluating host factors, early reports suggested that systemic illness and age older than 50 years portend inferior outcomes for open hand fractures.[10,157] Duncan and colleagues[9] did not find either of these associations in their cohort of 75 patients, although they acknowledged a high

Table 2
Modified Gustilo and Anderson classification system for open hand fractures

Grade	Definition
I	Tidy laceration, <1 cm in length. No contamination. No soft tissue crush, loss, or fracture comminution
II	Tidy laceration, <2 cm in length. No contamination. No soft tissue crush, loss, or fracture comminution
III A	Laceration >2 cm in length. Penetrating or puncturing projectile wound, soft tissue crush, or frankly contaminated
III B	Same as III A, plus any periosteal elevation or stripping
III C	Same as III B, plus neurovascular injury

This system does not take into account injury to flexor or extensor tendons or adjacent musculature, which commonly accompany open hand fractures, given the intimate association of these structures in the low-profile anatomy of the hand.

Modified from Duncan RW, Freeland AE, Jabaley ME, et al. Open hand fractures: an analysis of the recovery of active motion and of complications. J Hand Surg Am 1993;18(3):389; with permission.

proportion of younger, healthier patients in their series. With regard to early reports of stiffness with local flap use in patients older than 50 years, Melone and colleagues,[152] in their series of 150 thenar flaps (31 patients older than 50 years), reported 6 flexion contractures with only 1 older than 50 years. The investigators recommended an evaluation of patients' health and age but did not find support for an age cutoff. Such health evaluations should be encouraged, given the impaired wound healing and compromised infectious resistance that accompany many medical comorbidites (ie, peripheral vascular disease, diabetes, tobacco use), despite the overall lower rate of infectious complications in open hand fractures with proper management. Psychosocial factors such as patient compliance, determination, and outlook also play a role in determining outcome following most hand injuries in general, especially when measures such as return to work are evaluated.

AUTHOR'S PREFERRED METHOD OF MANAGEMENT

In the author's practice, primary reconstruction is the gold standard in the management of open fractures with soft tissue and bone loss, as seen in case examples presented in this article. In small and medium-sized defects of the hand, we prefer to use posterior interosseous or ulnar artery perforator flaps, because these do not sacrifice a major blood supply to the hand. If perforators to these flaps are within the zone of injury, or the flow is not detectable on Doppler examination, a pedicled radial forearm flap or a free flap is considered. If the palmar arch is severed with no back flow through the radial artery, we prefer using a lateral arm free flap, because its positioning and dissection is simple. Skin quality matches well, particularly to the dorsum of the hand. In small and medium-sized defects in which cosmesis is a prime concern, free groin flap is a useful alternative with primary closure of the donor site. In cases of a large soft tissue defect associated with a significant dead space, as seen in thenar or hypothenar muscle loss, free gracilis muscle flap fills the void with minimal donor site morbidity. In addressing the bone loss, we prefer tricortical or cancellous iliac crest bone grafting along with rigid internal fixation and early motion, preferably within 2 days after the surgery.

SUMMARY

Open fractures of the hand require expedited and thorough evaluation. Prospective, randomized controlled trials of prophylactic antibiotic use in this context are less common than in long bone fractures. Reports on the association between antibiotic use and infectious risk are mixed, although many centers continue their routine administration. The initial surgical debridement is important and must be meticulous, because it often guides the decision between primary and staged reconstruction. Given the improved outcomes reported, complete primary reconstruction should be favored when feasible. Reconstructive options for the soft tissue envelope are many, and the decision should be guided by both injury-specific and patient-specific characteristics. Effective augmentation has been shown with the addition of skin substitutes and/or negative-pressure therapy, in the appropriate setting. The literature suggests worse outcomes with greater soft tissue injury, increased comminution, and associated tendon injury. The degree of soft tissue injury and rate of infection have shown a less robust association. In the context of thorough debridement, primary internal fixation with bone grafting as needed and immediate soft tissue reconstruction have been shown to improve patient outcomes without an increased risk of infection.

REFERENCES

1. Burke JF. The effective period of preventive antibiotic action in experimental incisions and dermal lesions. Surgery 1961;50:161–8.
2. Patzakis MJ, Harvey JP Jr, Ivler D. The role of antibiotics in the management of open fractures. J Bone Joint Surg Am 1974;56(3):532–41.
3. Gustilo RB, Anderson JT. Prevention of infection in the treatment of one thousand and twenty-five open fractures of long bones: retrospective and prospective analyses. J Bone Joint Surg Am 1976;58(4):453–8.
4. Patzakis MJ, Wilkins J. Factors influencing infection rate in open fracture wounds. Clin Orthop Relat Res 1989;(243):36–40.
5. Wilkins J, Patzakis M. Choice and duration of antibiotics in open fractures. Orthop Clin North Am 1991;22(3):433–7.
6. Hoffman RD, Adams BD. Antimicrobial management of mutilating hand injuries. Hand Clin 2003; 19(1):33–9.
7. Chappell JE, Mitra A, Weinberger J, et al. Gunshot wounds to the hand: management and economic impact. Ann Plast Surg 1999;42(4): 418–23.
8. McLain RF, Steyers C, Stoddard M. Infections in open fractures of the hand. J Hand Surg Am 1991;16(1):108–12.

9. Duncan RW, Freeland AE, Jabaley ME, et al. Open hand fractures: an analysis of the recovery of active motion and of complications. J Hand Surg Am 1993;18(3):387–94.

10. Swanson TV, Szabo RM, Anderson DD. Open hand fractures: prognosis and classification. J Hand Surg Am 1991;16(1):101–7.

11. Chow SP, Pun WK, So YC, et al. A prospective study of 245 open digital fractures of the hand. J Hand Surg Br 1991;16(2):137–40.

12. Peacock KC, Hanna DP, Kirkpatrick K, et al. Efficacy of perioperative cefamandole with postoperative cephalexin in the primary outpatient treatment of open wounds of the hand. J Hand Surg Am 1988;13(6):960–4.

13. Sloan JP, Dove AF, Maheson M, et al. Antibiotics in open fractures of the distal phalanx? J Hand Surg Br 1987;12(1):123–4.

14. Suprock MD, Hood JM, Lubahn JD. Role of antibiotics in open fractures of the finger. J Hand Surg Am 1990;15(5):761–4.

15. Stevenson J, McNaughton G, Riley J. The use of prophylactic flucloxacillin in treatment of open fractures of the distal phalanx within an accident and emergency department: a double-blind randomized placebo-controlled trial. J Hand Surg Br 2003;28(5):388–94.

16. Madsen MS, Neumann L, Andersen JA. Penicillin prophylaxis in complicated wounds of hands and feet: a randomized, double-blind trial. Injury 1996;27(4):275–8.

17. Fitzgerald RH Jr, Cooney WP 3rd, Washington JA 2nd, et al. Bacterial colonization of mutilating hand injuries and its treatment. J Hand Surg Am 1977;2(2):85–9.

18. Hauser CJ, Adams CA Jr, Eachempati SR, et al. Surgical Infection Society guideline: prophylactic antibiotic use in open fractures: an evidence-based guideline. Surg Infect (Larchmt) 2006;7(4):379–405.

19. Gustilo RB, Mendoza RM, Williams DN. Problems in the management of type III (severe) open fractures: a new classification of type III open fractures. J Trauma 1984;24(8):742–6.

20. Capo JT, Hall M, Nourbakhsh A, et al. Initial management of open hand fractures in an emergency department. Am J Orthop (Belle Mead NJ) 2011;40(12):E243–8.

21. Saint-Cyr M, Miranda D, Gonzalez R, et al. Immediate corticocancellous bone autografting in segmental bone defects of the hand. J Hand Surg Br 2006;31(2):168–77.

22. Godina M. Early microsurgical reconstruction of complex trauma of the extremities. Plast Reconstr Surg 1986;78(3):285–92.

23. Freeland AE, Jabaley ME. Stabilization of fractures in the hand and wrist with traumatic soft tissue and bone loss. Hand Clin 1988;4(3):425–36.

24. Lister G, Scheker L. Emergency free flaps to the upper extremity. J Hand Surg Am 1988;13(1):22–8.

25. Ninkovic M, Deetjen H, Ohler K, et al. Emergency free tissue transfer for severe upper extremity injuries. J Hand Surg Br 1995;20(1):53–8.

26. Rinaldi E. Autografts in the treatment of osseous defects in the forearm and hand. J Hand Surg Am 1987;12(2):282–6.

27. Sundine M, Scheker LR. A comparison of immediate and staged reconstruction of the dorsum of the hand. J Hand Surg Br 1996;21(2):216–21.

28. Scheker LR, Langley SJ, Martin DL, et al. Primary extensor tendon reconstruction in dorsal hand defects requiring free flaps. J Hand Surg Br 1993;18(5):568–75.

29. Stahl S, Lerner A, Kaufman T. Immediate autografting of bone in open fractures with bone loss of the hand: a preliminary report. Case reports. Scand J Plast Reconstr Surg Hand Surg 1999;33(1):117–22.

30. Gupta A, Shatford RA, Wolff TW, et al. Treatment of the severely injured upper extremity. Instr Course Lect 2000;49:377–96.

31. Saint-Cyr M, Gupta A. Primary internal fixation and bone grafting for open fractures of the hand. Hand Clin 2006;22(3):317–27.

32. Kömürcü M, Alemdaroğlu B, Kürklü M, et al. Handgun injuries with metacarpal and proximal phalangeal fractures: early definitive treatment. Int Orthop 2008;32(2):257–62.

33. Stahl S, Lotter O, Stahl AS, et al. Immediate reconstruction of complex hand trauma with iliac crest bone graft and 2 pedicled fasciocutaneous skin flaps: a case report. Eplasty 2010;10:e21.

34. Giessler GA, Erdmann D, Germann G. Soft tissue coverage in devastating hand injuries. Hand Clin 2003;19(1):63–71, vi.

35. Neumeister MW, Brown RE. Mutilating hand injuries: principles and management. Hand Clin 2003;19(1):1–15, v.

36. Tarkin IS. The versatility of negative pressure wound therapy with reticulated open cell foam for soft tissue management after severe musculoskeletal trauma. J Orthop Trauma 2008;22(Suppl 10):S146–51.

37. Lee DL, Ryu AY, Rhee SC. Negative pressure wound therapy: an adjuvant to surgical reconstruction of large or difficult skin and soft tissue defects. Int Wound J 2011;8(4):406–11.

38. Peimer CA, Smith RJ, Leffert RD. Distraction-fixation in the primary treatment of metacarpal bone loss. J Hand Surg Am 1981;6(2):111–24.

39. Haughton D, Jordan D, Malahias M, et al. Principles of hand fracture management. Open Orthop J 2012;6:43–53.

40. Gottlieb LJ, Krieger LM. From the reconstructive ladder to the reconstructive elevator. Plast Reconstr Surg 1994;93(7):1503–4.

41. Vedder NB, Hanel DP. The mangled upper extremity. In: Wolfe SW, Hotchkiss RN, Pederson WC, et al, editors. Green's operative hand surgery. 6th edition. Philadelphia: Churchill Livingstone; 2011. p. 1603–44.

42. Mathes SJ, Nahai F. Reconstructive surgery: principles, anatomy & technique. New York: Churchill Livingstone; 1997. p. 9–36.

43. Spyropoulou A, Jeng SF. Microsurgical coverage reconstruction in upper and lower extremities. Semin Plast Surg 2010;24(1):34–42.

44. Knobloch K, Vogt PM. The reconstructive clockwork of the twenty-first century: an extension of the concept of the reconstructive ladder and reconstructive elevator. Plast Reconstr Surg 2010; 126(4):220e–2e.

45. Watt AJ, Friedrich JB, Huang JI. Advances in treating skin defects of the hand: skin substitutes and negative-pressure wound therapy. Hand Clin 2012;28(4):519–28.

46. Rizzo M. The use of Integra in hand and upper extremity surgery. J Hand Surg Am 2012;37(3):583–6.

47. Azzena B, Amabile A, Tiengo C. Use of acellular dermal regeneration template in a complete finger degloving injury: case report. J Hand Surg Am 2010;35(12):2057–60.

48. Taras JS, Sapienza A, Roach JB, et al. Acellular dermal regeneration template for soft tissue reconstruction of the digits. J Hand Surg Am 2010;35(3): 415–21.

49. Heimbach D, Luterman A, Burke J, et al. Artificial dermis for major burns. A multi-center randomized clinical trial. Ann Surg 1988;208(3):313–20.

50. Molnar JA, DeFranzo AJ, Hadaegh A, et al. Acceleration of Integra incorporation in complex tissue defects with subatmospheric pressure. Plast Reconstr Surg 2004;113(5):1339–46.

51. Park CA, Defranzo AJ, Marks MW, et al. Outpatient reconstruction using integra and subatmospheric pressure. Ann Plast Surg 2009;62(2):164–9.

52. Weigert R, Choughri H, Casoli V. Management of severe hand wounds with Integra dermal regeneration template. J Hand Surg Eur Vol 2011;36(3):185–93.

53. Fang P, Engrav LH, Gibran NS, et al. Dermatome setting for autografts to cover INTEGRA. J Burn Care Rehabil 2002;23(5):327–32.

54. Jeschke MG, Rose C, Angele P, et al. Development of new reconstructive techniques: use of Integra in combination with fibrin glue and negative-pressure therapy for reconstruction of acute and chronic wounds. Plast Reconstr Surg 2004;113(2):525–30.

55. Dantzer E, Queruel P, Salinier L, et al. Dermal regeneration template for deep hand burns: clinical utility for both early grafting and reconstructive surgery. Br J Plast Surg 2003;56(8):764–74.

56. Carothers JT, Brigman BE, Lawson RD, et al. Stacking of a dermal regeneration template for reconstruction of a soft-tissue defect after tumor excision from the palm of the hand: a case report. J Hand Surg Am 2005;30(6):1322–6.

57. Katrana F, Kostopoulos E, Delia G, et al. Reanimation of thumb extension after upper extremity degloving injury treated with Integra. J Hand Surg Eur Vol 2008;33(6):800–2.

58. Murray RC, Gordin EA, Saigal K, et al. Reconstruction of the radial forearm free flap donor site using integra artificial dermis. Microsurgery 2011;31(2): 104–8.

59. Fitton AR, Drew P, Dickson WA. The use of a bilaminate artificial skin substitute (Integra) in acute resurfacing of burns: an early experience. Br J Plast Surg 2001;54(3):208–12.

60. Askari M, Cohen MJ, Grossman PH, et al. The use of acellular dermal matrix in release of burn contracture scars in the hand. Plast Reconstr Surg 2011;127(4):1593–9.

61. Chen SG, Tzeng YS, Wang CH. Treatment of severe burn with DermACELL(®), an acellular dermal matrix. Int J Burns Trauma 2012;2(2):105–9.

62. Mouës CM, Heule F, Hovius SE. A review of topical negative pressure therapy in wound healing: sufficient evidence? Am J Surg 2011;201(4): 544–56.

63. Weinand C. The Vacuum-Assisted Closure (VAC) device for hastened attachment of a superficial inferior-epigastric flap to third-degree burns on hand and fingers. J Burn Care Res 2009;30(2): 362–5.

64. Eisenhardt SU, Schmidt Y, Thiele JR, et al. Negative pressure wound therapy reduces the ischaemia/reperfusion-associated inflammatory response in free muscle flaps. J Plast Reconstr Aesthet Surg 2012;65(5):640–9.

65. Kang GC, Yam A. Vacuum-assisted closure of a large palmar defect after debriding a midpalmar tuberculous abscess. Int Wound J 2008;5(1):45–8.

66. Hanasono MM, Skoracki RJ. Securing skin grafts to microvascular free flaps using the vacuum-assisted closure (VAC) device. Ann Plast Surg 2007;58(5):573–6.

67. Blackburn JH 2nd, Boemi L, Hall WW, et al. Negative-pressure dressings as a bolster for skin grafts. Ann Plast Surg 1998;40(5):453–7.

68. Schneider AM, Morykwas MJ, Argenta LC. A new and reliable method of securing skin grafts to the difficult recipient bed. Plast Reconstr Surg 1998; 102(4):1195–8.

69. Isago T, Nozaki M, Kikuchi Y, et al. Skin graft fixation with negative-pressure dressings. J Dermatol 2003;30(9):673–8.

70. Scherer LA, Shiver S, Chang M, et al. The vacuum assisted closure device: a method of securing skin grafts and improving graft survival. Arch Surg 2002;137(8):930–3 [discussion: 933–4].

71. Moisidis E, Heath T, Boorer C, et al. A prospective, blinded, randomized, controlled clinical trial of topical negative pressure use in skin grafting. Plast Reconstr Surg 2004;114(4):917–22.

72. Llanos S, Danilla S, Barraza C, et al. Effectiveness of negative pressure closure in the integration of split thickness skin grafts: a randomized, double-masked, controlled trial. Ann Surg 2006;244(5): 700–5.

73. Petkar KS, Dhanraj P, Kingsly PM, et al. A prospective randomized controlled trial comparing negative pressure dressing and conventional dressing methods on split-thickness skin grafts in burned patients. Burns 2011;37(6):925–9.

74. Kamolz LP, Lumenta DB. Topical negative pressure therapy for skin graft fixation in hand and feet defects: a method for quick and easy dressing application–The "sterile glove technique". Burns 2013;39(4): 814–5. http://dx.doi.org/10.1016/j.burns.2012.09.019. pii:S0305–4179(12)00308–7.

75. Pyle JW, Holladay J, Molnar JA, et al. Multiple modality treatment regimen in an aggressive resistant fungal hand infection: a case report. Hand (N Y) 2010;5(3):318–21.

76. Eisenhardt SU, Momeni A, Iblher N, et al. The use of the vacuum-assisted closure in microsurgical reconstruction revisited: application in the reconstruction of the posttraumatic lower extremity. J Reconstr Microsurg 2010;26(9):615–22.

77. Bannasch H, Iblher N, Penna V, et al. A critical evaluation of the concomitant use of the implantable Doppler probe and the Vacuum Assisted Closure system in free tissue transfer. Microsurgery 2008; 28(6):412–6.

78. Kappel DA, Burech JG. The cross-finger flap. An established reconstructive procedure. Hand Clin 1985;1(4):677–83.

79. Koch H, Kielnhofer A, Hubmer M, et al. Donor site morbidity in cross-finger flaps. Br J Plast Surg 2005;58(8):1131–5.

80. Yam A, Peng YP, Pho RW. "Palmar pivot flap" for resurfacing palmar lateral defects of the fingers. J Hand Surg Am 2008;33(10):1889–93.

81. Tan O. Reverse dorsolateral proximal phalangeal island flap: a new versatile technique for coverage of finger defects. J Plast Reconstr Aesthet Surg 2010;63(1):146–52.

82. Earley MJ, Milner RH. Dorsal metacarpal flaps. Br J Plast Surg 1987;40(4):333–41.

83. Maruyama Y. The reverse dorsal metacarpal flap. Br J Plast Surg 1990;43(1):24–7.

84. Quaba AA, Davison PM. The distally-based dorsal hand flap. Br J Plast Surg 1990;43(1):28–39.

85. Gregory H, Heitmann C, Germann G. The evolution and refinements of the distally based dorsal metacarpal artery (DMCA) flaps. J Plast Reconstr Aesthet Surg 2007;60(7):731–9.

86. Zhang X, Shao X, Ren C, et al. Coverage of dorsal-ulnar hand wounds with a reverse second dorsal metacarpal artery flap. J Reconstr Microsurg 2012;28(3):167–73.

87. Sebastin SJ, Mendoza RT, Chong AK, et al. Application of the dorsal metacarpal artery perforator flap for resurfacing soft-tissue defects proximal to the fingertip. Plast Reconstr Surg 2011;128(3): 166e–78e.

88. Yang JY. The first dorsal metacarpal flap in first web space and thumb reconstruction. Ann Plast Surg 1991;27(3):258–64.

89. Ege A, Tuncay I, Çetin Ö. Foucher's first dorsal metacarpal artery flap for thumb reconstruction: evaluation of 21 cases. Isr Med Assoc J 2002; 4(6):421–3.

90. Chang SC, Chen SL, Chen TM, et al. Sensate first dorsal metacarpal artery flap for resurfacing extensive pulp defects of the thumb. Ann Plast Surg 2004;53(5):449–54.

91. Tränkle M, Sauerbier M, Heitmann C, et al. Restoration of thumb sensibility with the innervated first dorsal metacarpal artery island flap. J Hand Surg Am 2003;28(5):758–66.

92. Chen C, Zhang X, Shao X, et al. Treatment of thumb tip degloving injury using the modified first dorsal metacarpal artery flap. J Hand Surg Am 2010; 35(10):1663–70.

93. Lai CS, Lin SD, Yang CC, et al. The adipofascial turn-over flap for complicated dorsal skin defects of the hand and finger. Br J Plast Surg 1991; 44(3):165–9.

94. Al-Qattan MM. The adipofascial turnover flap for coverage of the exposed distal interphalangeal joint of the fingers and interphalangeal joint of the thumb. J Hand Surg Am 2001;26(6):1116–9.

95. Deal DN, Barnwell J, Li Z. Soft-tissue coverage of complex dorsal hand and finger defects using the turnover adipofascial flap. J Reconstr Microsurg 2011;27(2):133–8.

96. Chai YM, Lin CZ, Chen HD. The clinical application of distally based neurocutaneous flaps by anastomosis of superficial veins. Zhongguo Xiu Fu Chong Jian Wai Ke Za Zhi 2001;15(4):217–8 [in Chinese].

97. Page R, Chang J. Reconstruction of hand soft-tissue defects: alternatives to the radial forearm fasciocutaneous flap. J Hand Surg Am 2006; 31(5):847–56.

98. Pederson WC. Nonmicrosurgical coverage of the upper extremity. In: Wolfe SW, Hotchkiss RN, Pederson WC, et al, editors. Green's operative hand surgery. 6th edition. Philadelphia: Churchill Livingstone; 2011. p. 1645–720.

99. Vilain R, Dupuis JF. Use of the flag flap for coverage of a small area on a finger or the palm. 20 years experience. Plast Reconstr Surg 1973; 51(4):397–401.

100. Hansen AJ, Duncan SF, Smith AA, et al. Reverse radial forearm fascial flap with radial artery preservation. Hand (N Y) 2007;2(3):159–63.

101. Chang SC, Miller G, Halbert CF, et al. Limiting donor site morbidity by suprafascial dissection of the radial forearm flap. Microsurgery 1996;17(3):136–40.

102. Lutz BS, Wei FC, Chang SC, et al. Donor site morbidity after suprafascial elevation of the radial forearm flap: a prospective study in 95 consecutive cases. Plast Reconstr Surg 1999;103(1):132–7.

103. Davis WJ 3rd, Wu C, Sieber D, et al. A comparison of full and split thickness skin grafts in radial forearm donor sites. J Hand Microsurg 2011;3(1):18–24.

104. Jin YT, Guan WX, Shi TM, et al. Reversed island forearm fascial flap in hand surgery. Ann Plast Surg 1985;15(4):340–7.

105. Chang SM, Hou CL, Zhang F, et al. Distally based radial forearm flap with preservation of the radial artery: anatomic, experimental, and clinical studies. Microsurgery 2003;23(4):328–37.

106. Ignatiadis IA, Mavrogenis AF, Avram AM, et al. Treatment of complex hand trauma using the distal ulnar and radial artery perforator-based flaps. Injury 2008;39(Suppl 3):S116–24.

107. Ho AM, Chang J. Radial artery perforator flap. J Hand Surg Am 2010;35(2):308–11.

108. Gedebou TM, Wei FC, Lin CH. Clinical experience of 1284 free anterolateral thigh flaps. Handchir Mikrochir Plast Chir 2002;34(4):239–44.

109. Allen RJ, Treece P. Deep inferior epigastric perforator flap for breast reconstruction. Ann Plast Surg 1994;32(1):32–8.

110. Georgescu AV, Matei I, Ardelean F, et al. Microsurgical nonmicrovascular flaps in forearm and hand reconstruction. Microsurgery 2007;27(5):384–94.

111. Becker C, Gilbert A. The ulnar flap. Handchir Mikrochir Plast Chir 1988;20(4):180–3.

112. Jihui JU, Liu Y, Hou R. Ulnar artery distal cutaneous descending branch as free flap in hand reconstruction. Injury 2009;40(12):1320–6.

113. Choupina M, Malheiro E, Guimarães I, et al. Osteofasciocutaneous flap based on the dorsal ulnar artery. A new option for reconstruction of composite hand defects. Br J Plast Surg 2004;57(5):465–8.

114. Unal C, Ozdemir J, Hasdemir M. Clinical application of distal ulnar artery perforator flap in hand trauma. J Reconstr Microsurg 2011;27(9):559–65.

115. Lu LJ, Gong X, Lu XM, et al. The reverse posterior interosseous flap and its composite flap: experience with 201 flaps. J Plast Reconstr Aesthet Surg 2007;60(8):876–82.

116. El-Sabbagh AH, Zeina AA, El-Hadidy AM, et al. Reversed posterior interosseous flap: safe and easy method for hand reconstruction. J Hand Microsurg 2011;3(2):66–72.

117. Shahzad MN, Ahmed N, Qureshi KH. Reverse flow posterior interosseous flap: experience with 53 flaps at Nishtar Hospital, Multan. J Pak Med Assoc 2012;62(9):950–4.

118. Yildirim S, Taylan G, Eker G, et al. Free flap choice for soft tissue reconstruction of the severely damaged upper extremity. J Reconstr Microsurg 2006;22(8):599–609.

119. Giessler GA, Schmidt AB, Germann G, et al. The role of fabricated chimeric free flaps in reconstruction of devastating hand and forearm injuries. J Reconstr Microsurg 2011;27(9):567–73.

120. Song R, Song Y, Yu Y, et al. The upper arm free flap. Clin Plast Surg 1982;9(1):27–35.

121. Katsaros J, Tan E, Zoltie N, et al. Further experience with the lateral arm free flap. Plast Reconstr Surg 1991;87(5):902–10.

122. Wong M, Tay SC, Teoh LC. Versatility of the turn-around technique of the lateral arm flap for hand reconstruction. Ann Plast Surg 2012;69(3):265–70.

123. Ulusal BG, Lin YT, Ulusal AE, et al. Free lateral arm flap for 1-stage reconstruction of soft tissue and composite defects of the hand: a retrospective analysis of 118 cases. Ann Plast Surg 2007;58(2):173–8.

124. Song YG, Chen GZ, Song YL. The free thigh flap: a new free flap concept based on the septocutaneous artery. Br J Plast Surg 1984;37(2):149–59.

125. Wei FC, Jain V, Celik N, et al. Have we found an ideal soft-tissue flap? An experience with 672 anterolateral thigh flaps. Plast Reconstr Surg 2002;109(7):2219–26 [discussion: 2227–30].

126. Koshima I. Free anterolateral thigh flap for reconstruction of head and neck defects following cancer ablation. Plast Reconstr Surg 2000;105(7):2358–60.

127. Lee N, Roh S, Yang K, et al. Reconstruction of hand and forearm after sarcoma resection using anterolateral thigh free flap. J Plast Reconstr Aesthet Surg 2009;62(12):e584–6.

128. Meky M, Safoury Y. Composite anterolateral thigh perforator flaps in the management of complex hand injuries. J Hand Surg Eur Vol 2013;38(4):366–70.

129. Yazar S, Gideroglu K, Kilic B, et al. Use of composite anterolateral thigh flap as double-vascularised layers for reconstruction of complex hand dorsum defect. J Plast Reconstr Aesthet Surg 2008;61(12):1549–50.

130. Lee YC, Chiu HY, Shieh SJ. The clinical application of anterolateral thigh flap. Plast Surg Int 2011;2011:127353.

131. Ulrich D, Fuchs P, Bozkurt A, et al. Free serratus anterior fascia flap for reconstruction of hand and finger defects. Arch Orthop Trauma Surg 2010;130(2):217–22.

132. Fassio E, Laulan J, Aboumoussa J, et al. Serratus anterior free fascial flap for dorsal hand coverage. Ann Plast Surg 1999;43(1):77–82.

133. Wintsch K, Helaly P. Free flap of gliding tissue. J Reconstr Microsurg 1986;2(3):143–51.

134. Fotopoulos P, Holmer P, Leicht P, et al. Dorsal hand coverage with free serratus fascia flap. J Reconstr Microsurg 2003;19(8):555–9.

135. Carty MJ, Taghinia A, Upton J. Fascial flap reconstruction of the hand: a single surgeon's 30-year experience. Plast Reconstr Surg 2010;125(3): 953–62.

136. Biswas G, Lohani I, Chari PS. The sandwich temporoparietal free fascial flap for tendon gliding. Plast Reconstr Surg 2001;108(6):1639–45.

137. Brent B, Upton J, Acland RD, et al. Experience with the temporoparietal fascial free flap. Plast Reconstr Surg 1985;76(2):177–88.

138. Neumeister M, Hegge T, Amalfi A, et al. The reconstruction of the mutilated hand. Semin Plast Surg 2010;24(1):77–102.

139. Anastakis DJ. Free functioning muscle transfers. In: Wolfe SW, Hotchkiss RN, Pederson WC, et al, editors. Green's operative hand surgery. 6th edition. Philadelphia: Churchill Livingstone; 2011. p. 1757–74.

140. Engelhardt TO, Rieger UM, Schwabegger AH, et al. Functional resurfacing of the palm: flap selection based on defect analysis. Microsurgery 2012; 32(2):158–66.

141. Baker PA, Watson SB. Functional gracilis flap in thenar reconstruction. J Plast Reconstr Aesthet Surg 2007;60(7):828–34.

142. Peek A, Müller M, Ackermann G. The free gracilis perforator flap: anatomical study and clinical refinements of a new perforator flap. Plast Reconstr Surg 2009;123(2):578–88.

143. Terzis JK, Kostopoulos VK. Free muscle transfer in posttraumatic plexopathies: part III. The hand. Plast Reconstr Surg 2009;124(4):1225–36.

144. Del Piñal F, Pisani D, García-Bernal FJ, et al. Massive hand crush: the role of a free muscle flap to obliterate the dead space and to clear deep infection. J Hand Surg Br 2006;31(6):588–92.

145. Molski M. Replantation of fingers and hands after avulsion and crush injuries. J Plast Reconstr Aesthet Surg 2007;60(7):748–54.

146. Ofer N, Baumeister S, Megerle K, et al. Current concepts of microvascular reconstruction for limb salvage in electrical burn injuries. J Plast Reconstr Aesthet Surg 2007;60(7):724–30.

147. Adani R, Marcoccio I, Castagnetti C, et al. Long-term results of replantation for complete ring avulsion amputations. Ann Plast Surg 2003; 51(6):564–8 [discussion: 569].

148. Pun WK, Chow SP, So YC, et al. A prospective study on 284 digital fractures of the hand. J Hand Surg Am 1989;14(3):474–81.

149. Pun WK, Chow SP, So YC, et al. Unstable phalangeal fractures: treatment by A.O. screw and plate fixation. J Hand Surg Am 1991;16(1):113–7.

150. Shibata T, O'Flanagan SJ, Ip FK, et al. Articular fractures of the digits: a prospective study. J Hand Surg Br 1993;18(2):225–9.

151. Freeland AE, Jabaley ME, Burkhalter WE, et al. Delayed primary bone grafting in the hand and wrist after traumatic bone loss. J Hand Surg Am 1984; 9(1):22–8.

152. Melone CP Jr, Beasley RW, Carstens JH Jr. The thenar flap–An analysis of its use in 150 cases. J Hand Surg Am 1982;7(3):291–7.

153. Inoue G, Nakamura R, Imamura T. Revascularization of digits after prolonged warm ischemia. J Reconstr Microsurg 1988;4(2):131–8.

154. Baek SM, Kim SS. Successful digital replantation after 42 hours of warm ischemia. J Reconstr Microsurg 1992;8(6):455–8 [discussion: 459].

155. Wei FC, Chang YL, Chen HC, et al. Three successful digital replantations in a patient after 84, 86, and 94 hours of cold ischemia time. Plast Reconstr Surg 1988;82(2):346–50.

156. Harris K, Walker PM, Mickle DA, et al. Metabolic response of skeletal muscle to ischemia. Am J Physiol 1986;250(2 Pt 2):H213–20.

157. Strickland JW, Steichen JB, Kleinman WB, et al. Phalangeal fractures–factors influencing performance. Orthop Rev 1982;11:39–50.

Pediatric Hand Fractures

Kate W. Nellans, MD, MPH*, Kevin C. Chung, MD, MS

KEYWORDS

- Pediatric hand fractures • Physeal injuries of the hand • Radiographs • Malunion

KEY POINTS

- Hand fractures in children are common; conservative management is usually sufficient if initiated early.
- Seymour fractures (open physeal fracture of the distal phalanx) should be diagnosed with a good lateral radiograph to ensure timely operative extrication of the nail plate, irrigation and debridement, fracture reduction, and percutaneous pinning.
- Finger malrotation in metacarpal and phalangeal fractures must be assessed clinically, because radiographs may not reveal the deformity.
- Late presentations of displaced distal condylar phalanx fractures may be managed conservatively if well aligned in the coronal radiograph because sagittal malalignment can remodel, even in older children.
- Suspected scaphoid fractures in adolescents may be ruled out using magnetic resonance imaging to decrease the immobilization time. Scaphoid nonunions will require operative fixation and possible bone grafting, but an associated dorsal intercalated segment instability deformity may not improve with restoration of scaphoid anatomy.

EPIDEMIOLOGY

Distinguishing true "pediatric" hand fractures from fractures occurring in skeletally mature adolescents can be difficult if using epidemiologic studies only. Typically, a "pediatric" hand fracture would include children who continue to have open physes and therefore deserve special consideration regarding immobilization, remodeling potential, and surgical indications. Population database studies often use 18 years as a cutoff age for defining these fractures and may overestimate the prevalence of true pediatric hand fractures.

Fifteen percent of all fractures seen in the emergency room setting are hand fractures and nearly half of these fractures are a result either of sports activities or fights.[1,2] In the pediatric population, hand fractures make up 2.3% of all emergency room visits, and the incidence of these fractures varies significantly by age.[3,4] In the United Kingdom, a stratified examination found the number of hand fractures per year within the general pediatric population to be low in toddlers (34/100,000 children) and increased nearly 20-fold after the 10th year to 663 hand fractures each year per 100,000 children ages 11 to 18.[4]

In a comprehensive examination of the 1998 National Hospital Ambulatory Medical Care Survey from US facilities, Chung and Spilson[5] stratified both the injuries and the patients by age and found that in children 5 to 14 the carpal fracture

Supported in part by grants from the National Institute of Arthritis and Musculoskeletal and Skin Diseases and National Institute on Aging (R01 AR062066), the National Institute of Arthritis and Musculoskeletal and Skin Diseases (2R01 AR047328-06), and a Midcareer Investigator Award in Patient-Oriented Research (K24 AR053120) (to Dr Kevin C. Chung).
Section of Plastic Surgery, University of Michigan Health System, University of Michigan, 2130 Taubman Center, SPC 5340, 1500 East Medical Center Drive, Ann Arbor, MI 48109-5340, USA
* Corresponding author.
E-mail address: nellansk@umich.edu

incidence was 131 per 100,000 children, the metacarpal fracture incidence was 250/100,000 children, and the phalangeal fracture incidence was 165.6/100,000 children in this age group. The overall incidence of hand fractures in this high-risk age group was 546/100,000. Cumulatively, these incidence studies suggest emergency room physicians and pediatricians may treat many pediatric hand fractures definitively. In the United Kingdom, the incidence of pediatric hand fractures seen in specialty hand clinics for follow-up was only 264/100,000 children, less than half of the overall incidence found in other studies.[3–5]

Nearly all studies indicate boys suffer hand fractures more frequently than girls, with 65% to 75% of fractures occurring in boys, peaking between the ages of 9 to 14.[1,4,6–8] Phalangeal fractures are more common in the 9- to 12-year age group, whereas metacarpal fractures are most common in older adolescents.[8] The border rays account for most phalangeal and metacarpal fractures, over 75% in one 2006 study.[4]

SPECIAL CONSIDERATIONS IN THE PEDIATRIC POPULATION

Pediatric bone growth occurs through the physeal plate, but because the physis is unmineralized, it is weaker than the surrounding mature bone. Following a fracture, differential growth at the physis and remodeling in the diaphysis can correct for substantial initial fracture displacement. This displacement occurs most reliably in the plane of motion (ie, flexion/extension). In fingers, displacement in the sagittal plane may remodel extensively (**Fig. 1**), but remodeling in the coronal plane occurs less reliably.

The physes are particularly vulnerable in younger children when *shear* forces are applied to the fingers, stressing the attachments of the chondrocytes at the zone of proliferation.[9] In contrast, adolescents tend to place more *compressive* stresses across the metacarpals (in sports or with punching), resulting in metacarpal shaft fractures as the physes remain strong when compressed.[4] Multiple attempts at reduction of physeal fractures can crush and disrupt the layered order of the physis, resulting in an iatrogenic physeal arrest. If a physeal fracture reduction cannot be accomplished in 1 or 2 attempts, it is better to consider open operative reduction to reduce the chance of growth arrest. Physeal arrest can result in difficult-to-treat angular deformities and joint malalignment due to continued growth in adjacent bones. The physis can be a source of confusion if one is accustomed to primarily reading adult imaging. In a large study of pediatric hand fractures, a misdiagnosis rate of 8% was found on the initial radiology interpretation, where 5 of the 11 misdiagnosed fractures were the normal physeal lucency.[8]

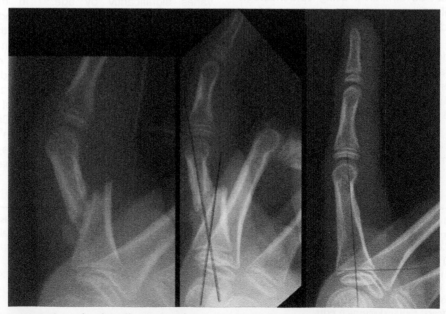

Fig. 1. Late presentation of a dorsally displaced and shortened P1 fracture in an 11-year-old girl demonstrates extensive remodeling in the sagittal plane over 2 years. (*Courtesy of* Dr Jeffrey Lawton.)

SPECIFIC INJURIES
Distal Tuft Fractures from Crush Injuries

The most common injury in toddler and preschool-aged children is a crush injury to the fingertips, resulting in a distal tuft fracture. Tuft fractures account for up to 80% of hand fractures in this age group.[4,10] These injuries can also involve soft tissue lacerations and nail bed injuries in addition to the distal phalangeal fracture, and irrigation and debridement remain the mainstay of initial treatment of these open injuries. Immobilization with a clamshell-type plastic splint for 2 to 3 weeks will help protect the sensitive fingertip.

Although antibiotics are typically included as the standard of care for open injuries, there is evidence in adults that routine antibiotics may not be necessary. In a randomized double-blind study, thorough irrigation and debridement alone had no greater infection rates than those given antibiotics after the irrigation and debridement.[11] It is unclear whether these results may be generalized to the pediatric population. Only rarely do these distal tuft fractures progress to a nonunion, but radiographs may not show signs of union for up to 6 months, so diligence and patience are required when dealing with these injuries (**Fig. 2**).[12,13]

Seymour Fractures (Open Physeal Fracture of the Distal Phalanx)

Originally described in 1966, this open distal phalanx physeal fracture can easily be overlooked as a minor injury to the nail.[14] Even so, Seymour fractures can reliably be identified with a good lateral radiograph and a high degree of suspicion. Although the nail bed laceration itself is usually

not visible, the proximal edge of the nailplate sits on top of the eponychial fold rather than beneath, making the nail appear "too long" in comparison to the other nails (**Fig. 3**).[15]

Occurring often in older children and adolescents, a mallet finger with blood at the nail fold should be considered an open fracture through the distal phalanx physis (Salter Harris I) and/or metaphysis (Salter Harris II) until proven otherwise. A true lateral radiograph of the distal interphalangeal (DIP) joint must be used to confirm the diagnosis (see **Fig. 3**). Seymour fractures may closely mimic true mallet fingers at presentation, but the displacement occurs through the fracture rather than the DIP joint, as the insertion of the extensor tendon on the epiphysis is uninjured. Seymour fractures require operative irrigation and debridement, and a careful exploration to remove the proximal nail plate from the site of incarceration. Once the nail plate is extracted, the fracture can be reduced without difficulty.[12] The nail itself may help to stabilize the reduction and does not need to be routinely removed.[14] In the largest series of these fractures, just more than 20% (5 of 23 acute fractures) remained unstable after operative debridement and reduction.[16] A single k-wire placed from the fingertip through the DIP joint for 4 weeks will allow the fracture to heal in a reduced position.

Late presentations of Seymour fracture often result in infection, growth arrest, and persistent mallet deformity of the distal phalanx.[15] A variant of this injury, reported only in toddlers, is a complete dorsal rotation of the epiphysis in Salter Harris I type fractures.[17–19] At presentation, this is difficult to recognize, as the epiphysis of the distal

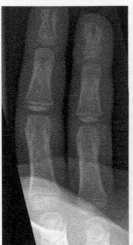
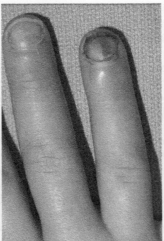
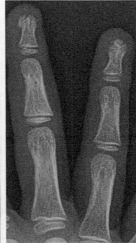

Fig. 2. Six-year-old boy with middle and ring fingertip crush injury and a closed subungal hematoma on the ring finger. The fractures persisted on radiograph 5 months after injury.

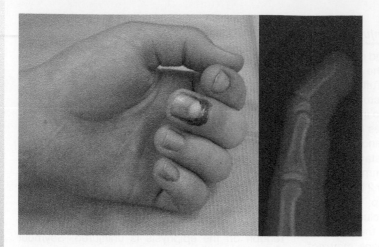

phalanx does not ossify until 18 to 24 months. The completely extruded epiphysis results in extensor mechanism dysfunction and distal phalanx deformity combined with a longitudinal growth arrest. There is no consensus on treatment in these cases and outcomes are generally poor.

Bony Mallet Finger Fractures

A flexion force directed to an actively extended finger will result in a bony mallet injury. The extensor tendon avulses a fragment of the epiphysis, resulting in an intra-articular fracture that may also extend into the metaphysis of the distal phalanx. Bony mallets in adolescents approaching skeletal maturity present similarly to those in adults but should be recognized as a Salter Harris III or IV type fracture. There are no published reports specifically on bony mallets in the pediatric population, but treatment principles are similar to those for adults.[20,21] Fractures involving less than one-third of the joint surface are not usually unstable and can successfully be treated with extension splints, even on late presentation.[22] Fractures with persistent volar subluxation of the distal phalanx, joint incongruity, or fracture fragments larger than 50% of the joint surface should be addressed surgically to restore congruity of the articular surface.[23]

For nonoperative management, adherence to strict splinting is mandatory. Smaller children may have difficulty keeping the extension splint in place because of poor compliance or a poor fit on their plump digit. Some authors suggest that in children who are likely to be noncompliant, it may be more reliable to reduce and pin the fracture operatively.[15] Originally described by Ishiguro and colleagues,[21] extension block pinning is a minimally invasive way to reduce the bony mallet

to the remaining joint surface of the distal phalanx. The bony fragment is prevented from displacing dorsally while the DIP joint is flexed, then the distal phalanx is skewered on a k-wire and reduced up to the fragment by extending the joint and pinning across the DIP joint in extension (**Fig. 4**).

Intra-articular Condylar Split Fractures

The intra-articular condylar split fracture is a problematic fracture, mainly due to its frequent late presentation. A patient's finger may appear normal on an anteroposterior radiograph, but the displaced condyle will create a "double-density" sign on a true lateral radiograph. These fractures result from an avulsion force, a direct axial blow, or a shearing of the subchondral bone from the underlying shaft and perfect reduction is required for the phalangeal condyles to conform to the facets in the middle or distal phalanx. In the pediatric population, these fragments can be tiny, and delays longer than 1 week may result in difficulties achieving an adequate closed reduction. The reduction, if addressed early, can be augmented with a towel clip to close the gap between the condyles and secured with k-wires.[15]

Percutaneous pinning is generally the preferred fixation, rather than other methods of internal fixation, for intracondylar split fractures to prevent tethering of the collateral ligaments. Fortunately, at the distal aspect of phalanx, one does not need to contend with a potential growth disturbance because the physis is located at the proximal aspect of each phalanx. However, if open reduction is required, the soft tissue envelope must be respected to prevent avascular necrosis (AVN).[24] In cases of malunion, attempts to perform an osteotomy to improve alignment should be undertaken with great care to preserve the

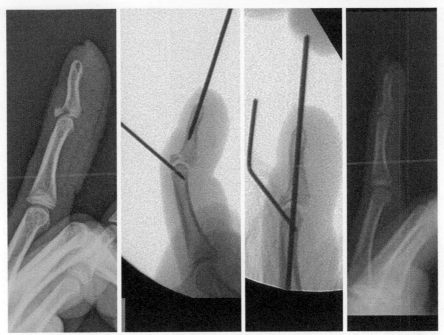

Fig. 4. Fixation of an adolescent bony mallet fracture using Ishiguro extension block technique. (*Courtesy of Dr Steven Haase.*)

surrounding soft tissue attachments to the distal fragment to reduce the risk of AVN.[15] In the setting of a congruous joint with an angular malalignment, an extra-articular osteotomy can be considered (**Fig. 5**).

Phalangeal Neck Fractures

Fractures of the proximal and middle phalanx located distal to the collateral ligament recess are called phalangeal neck fractures, or distal condylar phalangeal (DCP) fracture. These fractures tend to displace into extension with dorsal translation, and if left unreduced, a typical volar spike of bone prevents flexion of the joint. This type of fracture occurs almost exclusively in children and has historically been mistaken for a physeal injury at the distal aspect of the phalanx, despite the proximal location of the physis in the phalanges of the fingers.[25] True lateral radiographs of the affected finger, without overlap of other fingers, must be obtained to determine the most appropriate course of treatment. Many of these fractures can be successfully reduced in a closed manner because they do not involve the articular surface. However, due to the rapid healing in children, if the fracture is more that 1 to 2 weeks old, closed reduction will likely not be possible. For reasons not well understood, conservative treatment carries an additional risk for nonunion in thumb phalangeal neck fractures and avascular necrosis in the small finger.[26]

A classification by Al-Quattan using a case series of 66 of these fractures suggests that non-displaced fractures heal well with splinting alone (type I). The author found that displaced fractures with some remaining bony contact (type II) were most likely to have good outcomes with operative reduction and fixation.[16] Completely displaced DCP fractures with no bony contact (type III) had the worst outcomes ranging from nonunions to digital necrosis and amputation, especially for late presentations (**Fig. 6**). Owing to the poor blood supply and lack of soft tissue attachments to the distal fragment, this fracture usually requires the pins to be left in place for at least 4 weeks.[27]

Controversy remains as to the necessity of an osteotomy for missed, malunited DCP fractures. Recent case series have shown excellent remodeling in the sagittal plane with nonoperative treatment.[15,28,29] It should be noted that little remodeling can be expected in the coronal plane, and coronal deformities need to be addressed surgically. Osteotomy carries the risk of avascular necrosis due to the tenuous collateral blood supply of the distal aspect of the phalanx and must be approached with care.[27]

Proximal Phalanx Fractures

Treatment of fractures along the shaft of the proximal phalanx is dictated by the orientation of the fracture as well as the degree of initial displacement. Management is also guided by clinical

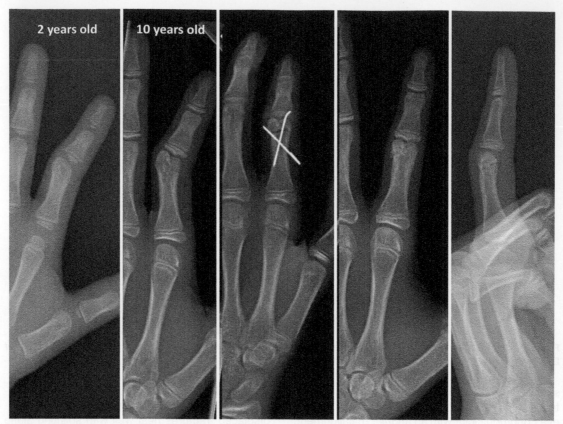

Fig. 5. Two-year-old girl with an unwitnessed injury to her left index finger. She presented 10 months later with an intracondylar proximal phalanx malunion. Due to persistent deformity and inability to form a closed fist, she underwent a corrective osteotomy 8 years later with good final results despite the known risk of AVN. Note lack of remodeling with coronal displacement. (*Courtesy of* Dr Jeffrey Lawton.)

evaluation, as very innocuous-looking fractures can have substantial rotational deformities that can lead to problems forming a tight fist and grip. There are no trials comparing one treatment method to another for phalangeal fractures in children, and the literature is largely limited to retrospective case reports and series. Despite this insufficiency, much can be gleaned from the generations of experience in some of these studies.

For length stable fractures with minimal displacement, buddy taping to an adjacent finger for both support and encouragement of early motion can be an effective treatment until the fracture site is no longer tender, typically from 3 to 4 weeks. Oblique or spiral fractures requiring reduction need more rigid immobilization, such as an ulnar or radial gutter splint or cast. These fractures must be monitored vigilantly for displacement, but this can be difficult to see through casting material. No splint can hold a phalanx fracture "out to length"; it can only control radial and ulnar

deviation, flexion, and extension. Length unstable fractures require operative fixation to maintain the reduction.

Fractures at the base of the proximal phalanx occur when the finger is abducted past the normal range of the metacarpophalangeal joint. These fractures are most common in the small finger where they are known as "extra octave" fractures. These fractures can occur transversely through the physis, or just distal to the physis in the metaphysis.[16,30,31] Owing to their proximity to the physis, significant remodeling can be expected in all but the most displaced fractures.[16] Flexor tendon entrapment, disruption of the collateral ligaments, or fracture comminution can prevent successful closed reduction. As originally described by Beatty and colleagues,[32] using a pencil as a fulcrum in the fourth web space to gain control over the proximal segment of the fifth proximal phalanx fracture can be a useful technique to restore alignment.

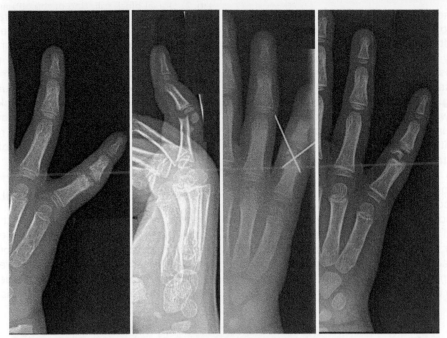

Fig. 6. Three-year-old girl presented 2 weeks after right small finger injury. Radiographs show a small finger DCP fracture, with no bony contact (type III). Despite efforts to reduce and stabilize the fracture, the fracture went on to a nonunion with minimal motion at the proximal interphalangeal joint.

Scaphoid Fractures

Although scaphoid fractures account for only 3% of pediatric fractures of the hand and wrist, they are the most common carpal fracture in this population.[33,34] Diagnosis and treatment in the pediatric population rely heavily on an understanding of the ossification and blood supply of the carpal bones. The scaphoid begins to show an ossific nuclei at 4 to 5 years of age, finishing ossification at 13 to 15 years of age.[35] Fractures are rarely identified before age 6 because they involve cartilage only, but increase in incidence with each subsequent year, peaking at age 15.[36–38]

D'Arienzo[39] proposed a 3-part classification system that considers the age of the child and the presumed degree of ossification. Type 1 lesions are typically seen in children younger than 8 and are purely chondral injuries, occurring just proximal to the ossific nuclei at the waist. These fractures are rare and often require a magnetic resonance imaging (MRI) for diagnosis. In children 8 to 11 years of age, the ossification process has crossed the waist and fractures are osteochondral in nature, and these heal readily if immobilized properly. Type 3 lesions are the most common fractures occurring in adolescents 12 and older. At this age, the scaphoid is nearly completely ossified, and these fractures behave similarly to those in the adult population with a tenuous proximal

blood supply. In a retrospective analysis of 351 pediatric scaphoid fractures, the average patient age was 14.6 years, with 71% of fractures occurring at the waist.[34] Twenty-three percent occurred at the distal pole, whereas only 6% occurred at the proximal pole.

In 13% to 30% of scaphoid fractures, initial radiographs are normal.[33,40] Most authors recommend a thumb spica casting for 2 weeks with repeat imaging to determine the course of treatment.[39–41] There is little consensus on short-arm or long-arm casting; however, if radiographs at 2 weeks are normal and the child has improved symptoms, no further immobilization is recommended.[39–41] MRI may be used to rule out a fracture shortly after the injury. In one study, a negative MRI performed 3 to 10 days after the injury shortened the course of immobilization in 58% of patients.[42]

In the previously described study of 351 scaphoid fractures, the authors reported a 90% union rate for casting acute fractures, whereas only 23% of chronic fractures achieved union with casting alone.[34] With casting only, acute fractures of the distal pole heal most rapidly, taking from 4 to 8 weeks, whereas waist fractures can take 5 to 16 weeks to show radiographic healing.[36,39,43,44] Once a nonunion has been identified, whether due to late presentation, inadequate immobilization, or subsequent fracture displacement, surgical intervention is recommended to improve the union rates. Autologous bone grafting with a volar approach is most commonly used for nonunions and "humpback" deformities, secured with either temporary k-wire fixation or a permanent compression screw (**Fig. 7**). Recently, narrow diameter headless screws have been shown to shorten time to union in older adolescents compared with screws with wider shafts.[34] It is proposed that these narrow screws decrease the amount of disruption to the endogenous blood supply, allowing for faster bony healing.

For reasons not completely understood, dorsal intercalated segment instability (DISI) deformities associated with scaphoid nonunions in children have never been observed to progress to scaphoid nonunion advanced collapse. As opposed to adult scaphoid nonunion surgeries, the DISI deformity in children can persist even after the correction of

the scaphoid anatomy with bone grafting (see **Fig. 7**).[41] One case report discussed the resolution of the DISI deformity over time following surgical fixation, whereas another showed persistent, asymptomatic DISI deformities 4 years after surgery.[45,46] Immediate restoration of the lunate orientation following correction of a humpback deformity may not be possible in adolescents. However, the growing carpus may retain some remodeling capacity, allowing for some correction of the malalignment over time.[47]

CLOSED TREATMENT AND IMMOBILIZATION

The vast majority of phalangeal and metacarpal fractures are minimally displaced, stable fractures. The thick periosteal covering and ability of the bone to plastically deform afford a great deal of stability in incomplete fractures. These fractures require minimal augmentation because of their

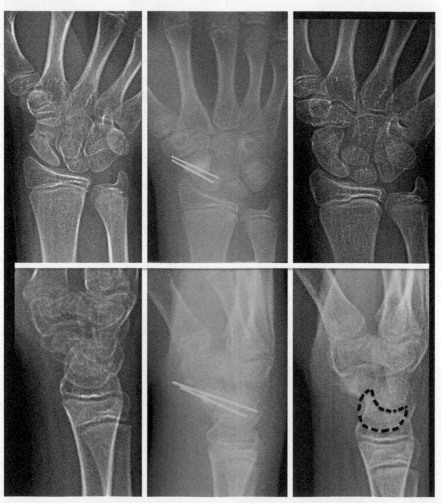

Fig. 7. Scaphoid non-union in 12 year-old female addressed surgically with autologous bone graft and K-wire fixation. Final xrays show a healed scaphoid fracture with a persistent asymptomatic DISI deformity.

inherent stability and rapid fracture healing. The periosteum can be a powerful tool for reduction in children, providing a "hinge" to lever the distal segment on the proximal portion of the bone to attain anatomic alignment.[48]

Nearly all active children will attempt escape from even the best-molded cast, and therefore, compliance should never be assumed. For younger children, long arm casts with just 2 or 3 layers of padding will prevent motion within the cast and stop the cast from slipping distally on the arm. In addition, supracondylar molding of the fiberglass can help to prevent the elbow pulling proximally within the upper portion of the cast. If a fracture must be perfectly immobile to maintain a reduction, augmentation with k-wires is advisable. Most well-aligned fractures do not need to be immobilized for longer than 4 weeks, because most healing at the physis occurs within 3 weeks, with slightly slower healing noted at the diaphysis.[49]

OPERATIVE CONSIDERATIONS

In most pediatric hand fractures, closed reduction and percutaneous pinning remain the mainstay of operative treatment for acute displaced fractures that cannot be closed reduced and held in position with splinting alone. A limited open approach may be used to extract interposed tissue, usually either a tendon or the volar plate in phalangeal fractures. A k-wire may be gently inserted into the fracture site and be used to create leverage for reduction once any interposed tissue is removed.[26,29] A fracture may be secured with multiple wires, but care must be taken not to create a pivot point at the fracture site by crossing the pins. Ideally, the pins should diverge at the fracture site to optimize stability, but can be difficult to achieve in very small children. Fortunately, most fractures have a robust soft tissue envelope to aid stability.

Once k-wires are in place, they must be protected at all times with a cast or brace if left outside the skin for later removal, and rarely do these wires need to stay in place longer than 3 to 4 weeks. The length of percutaneous k-wire fixation does not appear to correlate to rates of infection; therefore, routine antibiotics are not necessary.[50] If the wire ends are capped and out of the skin, even toddlers usually tolerate removal of the pins in the office. If a longer period of immobilization is desired, as in a scaphoid nonunion, pins may be cut below the skin for convenience, but then require a return to the operating room for removal. If a skin incision closure is required, absorbable sutures (such as 4-0 chromic) must be used to prevent tedious suture removal on a screaming child.

REFERENCES

1. Landin LA. Epidemiology of children's fractures. J Pediatr Orthop 1997;6(2):79–83.
2. Worlock P, Stower M. Fracture patterns in Nottingham children. J Pediatr Orthop 1986;6(6):656–60.
3. Worlock P, Stower M. The incidence and pattern of hand fractures in children. J Hand Surg Br 1986;11(2):198–200.
4. Vadivelu R, Dias JJ, Burke FD, et al. Hand injuries in children: a prospective study. J Pediatr Orthop 2006;26(1):29–35.
5. Chung KC, Spilson SV. The frequency and epidemiology of hand and forearm fractures in the United States. J Hand Surg Am 2001;26(5):908–15.
6. Mahabir RC, Kazemi AR, Cannon WG, et al. Pediatric hand fractures: a review. Pediatr Emerg Care 2001;17(3):153–6.
7. Bhende MS, Dandrea LA, Davis HW. Hand injuries in children presenting to a pediatric emergency department. Ann Emerg Med 1993;22(10):1519–23.
8. Chew EM, Chong AK. Hand fractures in children: epidemiology and misdiagnosis in a tertiary referral hospital. J Hand Surg Am 2012;37(8):1684–8.
9. Salter RB, Harris WR. Injuries involving the epiphyseal plate. J Bone Joint Surg 1963;45(3):587–622.
10. Rajesh A, Basu AK, Vaidhyanath R, et al. Hand fractures: a study of their site and type in childhood. Clin Radiol 2001;56(8):667–9.
11. Stevenson J, McNaughton G, Riley J. The use of prophylactic flucloxacillin in treatment of open fractures of the distal phalanx within an accident and emergency department: a double-blind randomized placebo-controlled trial. J Hand Surg Br 2003;28(5):388–94.
12. Al Qattan M, Hashem F, Helmi A. Irreducible tuft fractures of the distal phalanx. J Hand Surg Br 2003;28(1):18–20.
13. DaCruz D, Slade R, Malone W. Fractures of the distal phalanges. J Hand Surg Br 1988;13(3):350–2.
14. Seymour N. Juxta-epiphysial fracture of the terminal phalanx of the finger. J Bone Joint Surg Br 1966;48(2):347–9.
15. Cornwall R, Waters PM. Remodeling of phalangeal neck fracture malunions in children: case report. J Hand Surg Am 2004;29(3):458–61.
16. Al-Qattan M. Extra-articular transverse fractures of the base of the distal phalanx in children and adults. J Hand Surg Br 2001;26(3):201–6.
17. Waters PM, Benson LS. Dislocation of the distal phalanx epiphysis in toddlers. J Hand Surg Am 1993;18(4):581–5.
18. Keene JS, Engber WD, Stromberg W. An irreducible phalangeal epiphyseal fracture-dislocation. A case report. Clin Orthop Relat Res 1984;186:212–5.

19. de Jong A, Haddad B, Wood M. Irreducible dorsal epiphyseal fracture dislocation of the distal phalanx: a case report. Hand 2013;8(2):235–8.

20. Wehbe M, Schneider L. Mallet fractures. J Bone Joint Surg Am 1984;66(5):658–69.

21. Ishiguro T, Itoh Y, Yabe Y, et al. Extension block with Kirschner wire for fracture dislocation of the distal interphalangeal joint. Tech Hand Up Extrem Surg 1997;1(2):95–102.

22. Kalainov DM, Hoepfner PE, Hartigan BJ, et al. Nonsurgical treatment of closed mallet finger fractures. J Hand Surg Am 2005;30(3):580–6.

23. Pegoli L, Toh S, Arai K, et al. The Ishiguro extension block technique for the treatment of mallet finger fracture: indications and clinical results. J Hand Surg Br 2003;28(1):15–7.

24. Topouchian V, Fitoussi F, Jehanno P, et al. Treatment of phalangeal neck fractures in children: technical suggestion. Chir Main 2003;22(6): 299–304.

25. Puckett BN, Gaston RG, Peljovich AE, et al. Remodeling potential of phalangeal distal condylar malunions in children. J Hand Surg Am 2012; 37(1):34–41.

26. Al-Qattan M. Nonunion and avascular necrosis following phalangeal neck fractures in children. J Hand Surg Am 2010;35(8):1269–74.

27. Yousif N, Cunningham M, Sanger J, et al. The vascular supply to the proximal interphalangeal joint. J Hand Surg Am 1985;10(6 Pt 1):852–61.

28. Hennrikus W, Cohen M. Complete remodelling of displaced fractures of the neck of the phalanx. J Bone Joint Surg Br 2003;85(2):273–4.

29. Mintzer C, Waters P, Brown D. Remodelling of a displaced phalangeal neck fracture. J Hand Surg Br 1994;19(5):594–6.

30. Fischer MD, McElfresh EC. Physeal and periphyseal injuries of the hand. Patterns of injury and results of treatment. Hand Clin 1994;10(2):287–301.

31. Leclercq C, Korn W. Articular fractures of the fingers in children. Hand Clin 2000;16(4):523–34.

32. Beatty E, Light T, Belsole R, et al. Wrist and hand skeletal injuries in children. Hand Clin 1990;6(4): 723–38.

33. Christodoulou A, Colton C. Scaphoid fractures in children. J Pediatr Orthop 1986;6(1):37–9.

34. Gholson JJ, Bae DS, Zurakowski D, et al. Scaphoid fractures in children and adolescents: contemporary injury patterns and factors influencing time to union. J Bone Joint Surg Am 2011;93(13):1210–9.

35. Stuart HC, Pyle SI, Cornoni J, et al. Onsets, completions and spans of ossification in the 29 bone-growth centers of the hand and wrist. Pediatrics 1962;29(2):237–49.

36. Mussbichler H. Injuries of the carpal scaphoid in children. Acta Radiol 1961;56:361–8.

37. Toh S, Miura H, Arai K, et al. Scaphoid fractures in children: problems and treatment. J Pediatr Orthop 2003;23(2):216–21.

38. Bloem J. Fracture of the carpal scaphoid in a child aged 4. Arch Chir Neerl 1971;23(1):91–4.

39. D'Arienzo M. Scaphoid fractures in children. J Hand Surg Br 2002;27(5):424–6.

40. Evenski AJ, Adamczyk MJ, Steiner RP, et al. Clinically suspected scaphoid fractures in children. J Pediatr Orthop 2009;29(4):352–5.

41. Anz AW, Bushnell BD, Bynum DK, et al. Pediatric scaphoid fractures. J Am Acad Orthop Surg 2009;17(2):77–87.

42. Johnson KJ, Haigh SF, Symonds KE. MRI in the management of scaphoid fractures in skeletally immature patients. Pediatr Radiol 2000;30(10): 685–8.

43. Gamble JG, Simmons SC III. Bilateral scaphoid fractures in a child. Clin Orthop Relat Res 1982; 162:125–8.

44. Vahvenen V, Westerlund M. Fracture of the carpal scaphoid in children: a clinical and roentgenological study of 108 cases. Acta Orthop Scand 1980;51(6):909–13.

45. Suzuki K, Herbert TJ. Spontaneous correction of dorsal intercalated segment instability deformity with scaphoid malunion in the skeletally immature. J Hand Surg Am 1993;18(6):1012–5.

46. Mintzer C, Waters P, Simmons B. Nonunion of the scaphoid in children treated by Herbert screw fixation and bone grafting. A report of five cases. J Bone Joint Surg Br 1995;77(1):98–100.

47. Hamdi MF, Khelifi A. Operative management of nonunion scaphoid fracture in children: a case report and literature review. Musculoskelet Surg 2011;95(1):49–52.

48. Charnley J. The closed treatment of common fractures. New York: Cambridge University Press; 2003.

49. Rang M. Injuries of the epiphysis, growth plaste and perichondrial ring. Children's fractures. Philadelphia: JB Lippincott; 1983. p. 10–25.

50. Battle J, Carmichael KD. Incidence of pin track infections in children's fractures treated with Kirschner wire fixation. J Pediatr Orthop 2007;27(2):154–7.

Treatment of Pathologic Fractures

Steven C. Haase, MD

KEYWORDS

- Hand fractures • Pathologic fractures • Enchondroma

KEY POINTS

- Fractures due to minor trauma may be pathologic in nature, so a high degree of suspicion is warranted.
- Pathologic fractures are usually due to benign bone tumors, but other metabolic causes and malignancy need to be ruled out.
- The underlying pathologic diagnosis should guide treatment.
- In cases involving benign lesions, treatment can be conducted after the fracture has healed.
- In cases involving malignant lesions, more urgent treatment may be required.

INTRODUCTION

Pathologic fractures occur because the bone in question has been weakened by a disease process. Often, these injuries result from minor trauma, which might not otherwise cause a fracture in healthy bone. Fractures that result from a fall from standing height or less, or in the absence of any notable trauma, are often referred to as fragility fractures.[1] These fractures typically occur at the neck of the femur, the vertebral bodies, and the distal radius; they are uncommon in the hand. In the absence of another pathologic diagnosis, fragility fractures are thought essentially diagnostic of osteoporosis.

In the hand, pathologic fractures are most commonly associated with benign bone tumors, but a wide range of other possibilities exist. Some of these pathologic diagnoses have subtle x-ray findings, so a high degree of suspicion is warranted for any fracture that occurs unexpectedly from minor trauma. Because these fractures can be attributed to a wide range of processes, it is important to make the correct diagnosis, so that the correct treatment can be selected.

ETIOLOGY AND EPIDEMIOLOGY

A review of a Scottish bone tumor registry found that 23% of bone tumors in the hand presented with pathologic fracture.[2] The average age of the patients was 37 years old. The most common bone affected was the proximal phalanx (51% of cases); the fifth ray was involved in 44%. Of the 53 cases identified, 43 (81%) of pathologic fractures were due to enchondromas.

Solitary enchondroma is the most common bone tumor of the hand, typically afflicting the small tubular bones and more commonly involving the ulnar digits.[3] More than half of these benign tumors present with pathologic fractures.[4] Because of this strong association, much of the scientific literature on pathologic hand fractures focuses on the management of fractures associated with enchondromas. A careful search of the literature, however, reveals many more causes of pathologic fractures, although many are rare.

Aneurysmal bone cysts have been well described in the hand. Metacarpal lesions are more common than phalangeal or carpal lesions. Due to the eccentric nature of most of these cysts,

Section of Plastic Surgery, Department of Surgery, University of Michigan Health System, 2130 Taubman Center, SPC 5340, 1500 East Medical Center Drive, Ann Arbor, MI 48109, USA
E-mail address: shaase@umich.edu

Hand Clin 29 (2013) 579–584
http://dx.doi.org/10.1016/j.hcl.2013.08.010
0749-0712/13/$ – see front matter © 2013 Elsevier Inc. All rights reserved.

hand.theclinics.com

pathologic fracture is uncommon.[5] Most studies suggest that aneurysmal bone cysts present with pathologic fracture in only 10% of cases.[6–8]

Giant cell tumor of bone is an uncommon hand lesion but can rarely present as a pathologic fracture.[6] At the Mayo Clinic, a 50-year review of patient records revealed only 14 cases of this tumor in the bones of the hand, and only one of these cases presented with pathologic fracture.[9]

Epidermal inclusion cysts of bone are also uncommon and are usually associated with previous trauma.[10,11] In Beasley's textbook, he reports on an unusual case of pathologic fracture due to an epithelial inclusion cyst, which occurred in an old pin tract.[12] It is thought that epidermal elements driven into the bone during percutaneous pin fixation can lead to the development of these cysts. As minimally invasive procedures become more widespread, there is some concern these lesions may become more common.[13]

Fibrous dysplasia of bone is rare in the hand, with fewer than 10 cases reported.[14,15] Apparently, only one case of fracture associated with this lesion has been described.[2] Similarly, Paget disease is also rare in the hand, with few reports of pathologic fracture.[16]

Pathologic fractures due to malignancy accounted for only 15% of the total in the bone tumor registry study (discussed previously).[2] This subset of patients had a 5-year mortality rate of 25%, however, reflecting the aggressiveness of these lesions. The most common malignancy leading to pathologic fracture in this study was chondrosarcoma, with one case of Ewing sarcoma also reported. Pathologic fracture due to subungual melanoma has also been described and had a similarly poor prognosis.[17] Metastatic tumors to the hand are uncommon[18,19] but may rarely present with pathologic fracture.

Inflammation and infection have also been implicated, as fractures have been noted in advanced cases of gout[20] and microparticulate synovitis.[21] Osteomyelitis can be a cause of pathologic fractures in weight-bearing long bones[22] but seems rare as a cause of pathologic hand fractures.

Ironically, some of the treatments directed at eradicating bone lesions can lead to increased incidence of pathologic fracture after treatment. Cryosurgery, when used as an adjunct in the treatment of aneurysmal bone cysts and giant cell tumors, has been shown to increase the rate of fractures after treatment.[6,23] There is some evidence that the risk of postcryosurgery fracture can be decreased by the use of bone grafting or cement to fill the tumor defect.[24] It seems this risk is mainly for weight-bearing bones, however, and cryosurgery-related fractures in the hand are uncommon.[25,26]

Radiation therapy has also been implicated in pathologic fractures after treatment of non-Hodgkin lymphoma of bone,[27] Ewing sarcoma, aneurysmal bone cysts,[7] and soft tissue sarcoma. It is rare for this problem to occur in the hand, however. In a series of 26 patients who received surgery plus radiation for sarcoma of the hand, only a single pathologic fracture occurred 7 years after treatment.[28] Although this is a rare problem, it is worth noting that experimental evidence suggests healing of postradiation pathologic fractures can be augmented with deferoxamine.[29]

DIAGNOSTIC TESTS

Arriving at the correct diagnosis is of critical importance to selecting the correct treatment option for these fractures. Many common lesions, such as enchondromas and Paget disease, have characteristics that make them easily identifiable on plain radiographs (**Fig. 1**). If all evidence points to a benign lesion, surgical extirpation can often be delayed or deferred. If the presentation, patient history, or radiologic studies suggest anything other than a benign bone lesion, open biopsy to determine the exact diagnosis is warranted.

Imaging may be able to differentiate primary from metastatic bone tumors in cases of pathologic fracture. Specifically, plain radiographs and CT scans were found most helpful, demonstrating a higher incidence of lytic bone cortex, mineralization, and a soft tissue mass in fractures associated with primary bone tumors compared with those found with metastatic bone tumors.[30] MRI was not as helpful in characterizing these lesions.

TREATMENT
Fractures due to Enchondromata

In clinical practice, the most common pathologic hand fracture encountered is one associated with a solitary enchondroma.[31] Despite the frequent occurrence of this fracture, there is still some debate regarding optimum treatment. Specifically, opinions differ regarding the need for, the timing of, and the type of surgical intervention.

Regardless of the treatment selected for the enchondroma, the fracture should be managed with the intent to obtain the best possible outcome. Any significant malalignment should be corrected, and fixation used as necessary to maintain an adequate reduction. If the treatment of the fracture requires an open approach, immediate treatment of the enchondroma should be entertained. If the fracture can be treated nonoperatively, or with percutaneous fixation, clinicians may choose to allow the fracture to heal prior to enchondroma

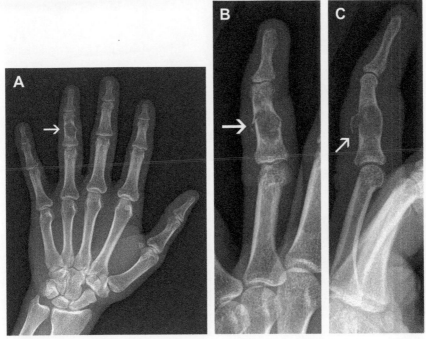

Fig. 1. (*A*) Posteroanterior, (*B*) oblique, and (*C*) lateral radiographs of pathologic fracture of the left ring finger middle phalanx (*white arrows*).

treatment. Once the fracture is healed, and rehabilitation is completed, the enchondroma is typically removed using curettage. The bony defect can be left alone or filled with bone graft or bone graft substitute. Most clinicians feel this treatment is indicated to prevent refracture at the enchondroma site.

Natural history and long-term follow-up studies do not exist, however, for this clinical scenario, so the real risk of a second fracture after treatment is unknown. An early review of 40 enchondroma cases, in which 63% presented with pathologic fractures, concluded, "the group with the most satisfactory outcome is that where surgery was avoided."[32] Granted, the nonoperative group only contained 5 patients with fractures, but all 5 were graded as "good" or "excellent" results at short-term follow-up. The lack of robust evidence to support treatment, as well as the potential morbidity of surgery, has motivated some hand surgeons to simply observe these lesions after fracture healing is complete.

Regarding the timing of surgery, there is reasonable evidence to suggest that delayed treatment is better. Ablove and colleagues[33] reviewed 16 pathologic fractures associated with enchondromata and found a higher complication rate with immediate curettage and bone grafting (67%) compared with delayed treatment after fracture healing (10%). Complications consisted mainly of issues

related to loss of motion and fracture displacement. In their opinion, the only disadvantage to delayed treatment was an extended period of disability. Other studies suggest this added disability is not significant. Sassoon and colleagues[4] evaluated immediate versus delayed treatment of these fractures and found that despite additional immobilization time in the delayed group, the two groups had similar range-of-motion results, and the time to full motion was identical between groups. Finally, Whiteman and colleagues[34] reported a prospective study using curettage plus demineralized bone powder for enchondroma and cyst defects in the hand. In the one pathologic fracture treated acutely, tenolysis was required later. Those fixed in a delayed fashion had quick return to normal motion.

With regard to the type of surgery performed, there is general agreement that curettage should be the minimum intervention (**Fig. 2**). After waiting for fractures to heal, Tordai and colleagues[35] proposed curettage alone should be considered, because the risk of recurrence leading to reoperation was low (2%). The review by Sassoon and colleagues[4] reported no difference in healing time or final range of motion between curettage alone, use of allograft, or use of autograft. Given these findings, it seems prudent to avoid autograft in most cases, both to minimize morbidity and to avoid inadvertent tumor seeding at the bone graft donor site.

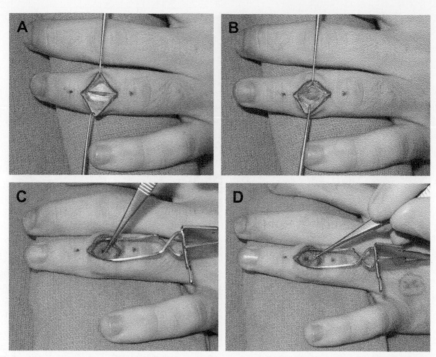

Fig. 2. (*A*) A dorsal, tendon-splitting approach is used to expose the tumor shown in **Fig. 1**. (*B*) The tumor is exposed at the point where it had ruptured through the dorsal cortex. (*C*) Curettage is performed to remove the tumor. (*D*) This shows the typical appearance of tumor substance removed from an enchondroma.

Various formulations of bone cement have been used by some investigators, with the apparent goal of minimizing disability or immobilization. Yasuda and colleagues[36] reported that calcium phosphate bone cement worked well but was harder to handle in acute fracture treatment cases; delayed treatment after fracture healing was recommended. Bickels and colleagues[37] described use of curettage plus fixation with a custom bent wire form and cement for fractures treated early (within 10 days). They reported significant stiffness in most patients, possibly due to the extensive dissection performed or postoperative adhesions. Based on the studies available, the use of cement does not seem to add any additional benefit, and delayed treatment seems preferred to immediate intervention when possible. Furthermore, chemical cauterization, which is discussed in some early reports, is not indicated.

Fractures due to Other Causes

Pathologic fractures associated with other disease states are far less common than those associated with enchondromata and may be treated with a wide range of surgical and nonsurgical options, underscoring the importance of establishing the correct diagnosis before proceeding with treatment (**Box 1**).

Fractures associated with aneurysmal bone cysts, which typically expand the margins of the bone, may be allowed to heal before proceeding with surgical treatment of the cyst. Occasionally, spontaneous healing of these cysts has been reported,[38] and it has been suggested that fractures involving the lesion or surgical biopsy of the lesion may actually stimulate this healing to occur.[39]

Fractures associated with giant cell tumors of bone may be an indication for more aggressive

---

Box 1
Pathology tip

Some investigators recommend first obtaining a small specimen of tumor and awaiting frozen section diagnosis prior to completing excision.[41] In my practice, I am hesitant to make important decisions based on frozen section pathology, and most patients are not consented for possible amputation before this type of surgery. Therefore, it is more cost effective to simply send the specimen for permanent sectioning rather than waste valuable operating room time on frozen sections. In a rare case of a malignancy discovered on the final pathology analysis, I prefer to discuss options with both the institutional tumor board and the patient before additional definitive treatment.

treatment. Athanasian[6] advises en bloc resection, rather than intralesional therapy for tumors with pathologic fractures, to reduce the risk of recurrence. In a study of giant cell tumors treated with cryosurgery, Marcove and colleagues[26] reported a post-treatment fracture in the hand that "spontaneously healed"; no other details were given.

Epidermal inclusion cysts and fibrous dysplasia of bone rarely lead to pathologic fractures, and little can be derived from the literature about how best to treat these entities. Given that they are benign, managing associated fractures should probably follow guidelines similar to those for enchondromata.

Paget disease of bone may rarely result in pathologic hand fractures, but this lesion does not require excision. These fractures should be treated as indicated with appropriate reduction and immobilization until healed, but no surgical resection of the disease is indicated.[16] Similarly, gout may respond to medical treatment without the need for surgery, and associated fractures should heal with proper care.[20]

Malignancy-related fractures carry a poor prognosis, even with aggressive surgery (eg, amputation) and appropriate adjuvant therapy.[2] For chondrosarcoma associated with fracture, it is likely the entire field is contaminated with tumor, and amputation is advisable, unless a thorough wide resection can be carried out.[40] Ewing sarcoma should ideally be treated with preoperative chemotherapy plus surgery and/or radiation for local control. In one reported case of a pathologic hand fracture associated with Ewing sarcoma, postoperative chemotherapy was performed, but metastatic disease eventually led to the patient's demise.[2]

Metastatic disease is unusual in the hand; the most common primary tumors implicated are lung, breast, and kidney. For extensive or distal lesions, amputation can be considered, but intralesional surgery with curettage, internal fixation, and/or cementation is often adequate treatment of palliation of symptoms.[40]

SUMMARY

Although enchondromas are the most common cause of pathologic fracture, many other causes have been reported. In general, fractures associated with benign lesions may be allowed to heal before definitive treatment of the tumor. After curettage, there is no convincing evidence that adding autograft or cement improves the final result. Fractures associated with aggressive or malignant tumors may require more urgent management of the underlying disease, and these patients have increased risks for both morbidity and mortality.

REFERENCES

1. Recommendations for enhancing the care of patients with fragility fractures. [AAOS Position Statement]. 2009. Available at: http://www.aaos.org/about/papers/position/1159.asp. Accessed February 19, 2013.
2. Shenoy R, Pillai A, Reid R. Tumours of the hand presenting as pathological fractures. Acta Orthop Belg 2007;73(2):192–5.
3. Gaulke R. The distribution of solitary enchondromata at the hand. J Hand Surg Br 2002;27(5):444–5.
4. Sassoon AA, Fitz-Gibbon PD, Harmsen WS, et al. Enchondromas of the hand: factors affecting recurrence, healing, motion, and malignant transformation. J Hand Surg Am 2012;37(6):1229–34.
5. Capanna R, Campanacci DA, Manfrini M. Unicameral and aneurysmal bone cysts. Orthop Clin North Am 1996;27(3):605–14.
6. Athanasian EA. Aneurysmal bone cyst and giant cell tumor of bone of the hand and distal radius. Hand Clin 2004;20(3):269–81, vi.
7. Campanacci M, Capanna R, Picci P. Unicameral and aneurysmal bone cysts. Clin Orthop Relat Res 1986;(204):25–36.
8. Ramirez AR, Stanton RP. Aneurysmal bone cyst in 29 children. J Pediatr Orthop 2002;22(4):533–9.
9. Athanasian EA, Wold LE, Amadio PC. Giant cell tumors of the bones of the hand. J Hand Surg Am 1997;22(1):91–8.
10. Ruchelsman DE, Laino DK, Chhor KS, et al. Digital intraosseous epidermoid inclusion cyst of the distal phalanx. J Hand Microsurg 2010;2(1):24–7.
11. Kurosawa K, Kobayashi R, Takagishi K. Distal phalangeal reconstruction for recurrent intraosseous epidermoid cyst of the finger-a case report. Hand Surg 2011;16(3):375–7.
12. Beasley R. Beasley's surgery of the hand. New York: Thieme Medical Publishers, Inc; 2003. p. 152–3.
13. Farrer AK, Forman WM, Boike AM. Epidermal inclusion cysts following minimal incision surgery. J Am Podiatr Med Assoc 1992;82(10):537–41.
14. Borys D, Canter R, James MA. Monostotic fibrous dysplasia of the distal phalanx: case report. J Hand Surg Am 2010;35(8):1294–6.
15. Amillo S, Schweitzer D, San Julian M. Monostotic fibrous dysplasia in the hand: a case report. J Hand Surg Am 1996;21(2):290–2.
16. Ogilvie-Harris DJ, Fornasier VL. Pathologic fractures of the hand in Paget's disease. Clin Orthop Relat Res 1979;(143):168–70.
17. Gregorcyk S, Shelton RM, Ladaga LE, et al. Pathologic fracture secondary to subungual melanoma. J Surg Oncol 1996;61(3):230–3.

18. Amadio PC, Lombardi RM. Metastatic tumors of the hand. J Hand Surg Am 1987;12(2):311–6.

19. Kerin R. Metastatic tumors of the hand. A review of the literature. J Bone Joint Surg Am 1983;65(9):1331–5.

20. Yaegashi Y, Nishida J, Oyama K. Gouty tophus of the second metacarpal simulating a malignancy with pathologic fracture. J Hand Surg Am 2013;38(1):208–9.

21. Peimer CA, Taleisnik J, Sherwin FS. Pathologic fractures: a complication of microparticulate synovitis. J Hand Surg Am 1991;16(5):835–43.

22. Belthur MV, Birchansky SB, Verdugo AA, et al. Pathologic fractures in children with acute Staphylococcus aureus osteomyelitis. J Bone Joint Surg Am 2012;94(1):34–42.

23. Marcove RC, Weis LD, Vaghaiwalla MR, et al. Cryosurgery in the treatment of giant cell tumors of bone. A report of 52 consecutive cases. Cancer 1978;41(3):957–69.

24. Marcove RC, Sheth DS, Takemoto S, et al. The treatment of aneurysmal bone cyst. Clin Orthop Relat Res 1995;(311):157–63.

25. Meals RA, Mirra JM, Bernstein AJ. Giant cell tumor of metacarpal treated by cryosurgery. J Hand Surg Am 1989;14(1):130–4.

26. Marcove RC, Lyden JP, Huvos AG, et al. Giant-cell tumors treated by cryosurgery. A report of twenty-five cases. J Bone Joint Surg Am 1973;55(8):1633–44.

27. Stokes SH, Walz BJ. Pathologic fracture after radiation therapy for primary non-Hodgkin's malignant lymphoma of bone. Int J Radiat Oncol Biol Phys 1983;9(8):1153–9.

28. Rohde RS, Puhaindran ME, Morris CD, et al. Complications of radiation therapy to the hand after soft tissue sarcoma surgery. J Hand Surg Am 2010;35(11):1858–63.

29. Donneys A, Weiss DM, Deshpande SS, et al. Localized deferoxamine injection augments vascularity and improves bony union in pathologic fracture healing after radiotherapy. Bone 2013;52(1):318–25.

30. Soldatos T, Chalian M, Attar S, et al. Imaging differentiation of pathologic fractures caused by primary and secondary bone tumors. Eur J Radiol 2013;82(1):e36–42.

31. Jacobson ME, Ruff ME. Solitary enchondroma of the phalanx. J Hand Surg Am 2011;36(11):1845–7.

32. Noble J, Lamb DW. Enchondromata of bones of the hand. A review of 40 cases. Hand 1974;6(3):275–84.

33. Ablove RH, Moy OJ, Peimer CA, et al. Early versus delayed treatment of enchondroma. Am J Orthop (Belle Mead NJ) 2000;29(10):771–2.

34. Whiteman D, Gropper PT, Wirtz P, et al. Demineralized bone powder. Clinical applications for bone defects of the hand. J Hand Surg Br 1993;18(4):487–90.

35. Tordai P, Hoglund M, Lugnegard H. Is the treatment of enchondroma in the hand by simple curettage a rewarding method? J Hand Surg Br 1990;15(3):331–4.

36. Yasuda M, Masada K, Takeuchi E. Treatment of enchondroma of the hand with injectable calcium phosphate bone cement. J Hand Surg Am 2006;31(1):98–102.

37. Bickels J, Wittig JC, Kollender Y, et al. Enchondromas of the hand: treatment with curettage and cemented internal fixation. J Hand Surg Am 2002;27(5):870–5.

38. Malghem J, Maldague B, Esselinckx W, et al. Spontaneous healing of aneurysmal bone cysts. A report of three cases. J Bone Joint Surg Br 1989;71(4):645–50.

39. Cottalorda J, Bourelle S. Current treatments of primary aneurysmal bone cysts. J Pediatr Orthop B 2006;15(3):155–67.

40. Weber K. Pathologic Fractures. In: Bucholz R, Heckman J, Court-Brown C, et al, editors. Rockwood & Green's fractures in Adults. 6th edition. Philadelphia: Lippincott Williams & Wilkins; 2006. p. 652.

41. O'Connor MI, Bancroft LW. Benign and malignant cartilage tumors of the hand. Hand Clin 2004;20(3):317–23, vi.

Rehabilitative Strategies Following Hand Fractures

Peyton L. Hays, MD, Tamara D. Rozental, MD*

KEYWORDS

- Rehabilitative strategies • Hand fractures • Hand therapy • Management

KEY POINTS

- Collaboration between surgeon, therapist and patient is critical in the management of hand fractures.
- Efforts to minimize edema improve patient comfort and early range of motion.
- Range of motion modalities may be active, active-assisted, passive and resisted. These may be combined with tendon gliding exercises to maximize recovery.
- Multiple splinting modalities exist to overcome joint stiffness following fracture.
- Potential treatment algorithms are provided to guide post-injury care and rehabilitation.

INTRODUCTION

The importance of rehabilitation in the management of hand fractures cannot be overstated. The breadth of rehabilitative strategies ranges from heat and range-of-motion exercises to more complex splinting and tendon gliding modalities. The goals, however, are clear: control pain; limit soft tissue swelling; provide support for fracture healing; restore motion, strength, and function; and enable return to work and daily activities.[1,2]

One of the keys to successful rehabilitation is communication. Effective management of hand fractures depends on collaboration among the surgeon, therapist, and patients. A period of immobilization is commonly required during the acute healing phase. Once fracture stability permits motion, the small joints of the hand are frequently stiff. The surgeon must communicate with the therapist both the radiologic and clinical evaluations, fracture management decisions, assessment of fracture stability, and need for further protection or immobilization. In turn, therapy progress and the individual concerns identified by the hand therapist should be discussed with the treating physician. Complicated injuries and contractures typically require a combination of rehabilitative strategies skillfully selected by the therapist.

The patients' goals and expectations should remain at the center of these discussions. Patients should be encouraged to engage with the surgeon and therapist in directing care. With a better understanding of the injury, patients should be informed of the risks and benefits of management options and their implications for the duration of care. Realistic expectations and outcomes must be clearly addressed, and individual patient circumstances or limitations must be considered. On initiation of hand therapy, the short- and long-term goals of the therapeutic plan should be outlined. As therapy progresses, all 3 parties should remain in close communication to ensure appropriate adjustments are made as needed from the patients', therapist's and surgeon's perspectives.

Funding Sources: Dr Rozental: Orthopaedic Research and Education Foundation, American Society for Surgery of the Hand; Dr Hays: Nil.
Conflict of Interest: Dr Rozental: Guest Faculty for Arthrex; Dr Hays: Nil.
Harvard Medical School - Beth Israel Deaconess Medical Center, Department of Orthopaedic Surgery, 330 Brookline Avenue, Stoneman 10, Boston, MA 02215, USA
* Corresponding author.
E-mail address: trozenta@bidmc.harvard.edu

Hand Clin 29 (2013) 585–600
http://dx.doi.org/10.1016/j.hcl.2013.08.011
0749-0712/13/$ – see front matter © 2013 Elsevier Inc. All rights reserved.

Collaboration and clearly defined goals lay the cornerstone for maximized rehabilitative benefit, return of function, prevention of long-term disability and secondary surgical procedures, an efficient rehabilitative course, reduced health care costs, and meaningful return to work and recreation.[1,2] The purpose of this discussion is to familiarize the hand practitioner with the vast therapeutic strategies available for the treatment of hand fractures. The most common of these include thermal agents, electrotherapeutic devices, differential motion exercises, and splint applications.[1,3-5]

THERAPEUTIC MODALITIES

Following hand fractures, 4 phases of therapy have been described: protective, restorative, strengthening, and functional.[2] During the initial protective phase, motion is limited and aggravating activities, such as dynamic joint loading, grip, and pinch, are avoided in an effort to minimize pain and control swelling and inflammation. As the fracture demonstrates radiographic signs of healing, or following early operative fixation, the restoration of active and passive range of motion may begin. With greater fracture stability and soft tissue healing, patients are advanced to the strengthening and endurance phase. Finally, the functional phase of therapy prepares patients for return to work and hobby with exercises aimed at integrating work- or life-specific skills into the rehabilitative program.[2]

Heat

Heat and ice have been used to treat early injury, pain, and stiffness for centuries. The application of heat, also known as *thermotherapy*, is directed at multiple aspects of the rehabilitative process beginning with early edema control and extending to restoration of motion.[2,5-9] Heat may be delivered via multiple routes, including heating pads, moist heat, water or paraffin baths, heating lamps, and ultrasound. The optimal range for thermotherapy is 41°C to 45°C. Heating modalities are also characterized by the depth of the heat delivered. Traditionally, superficial heat (pads, moist towels, baths) is considered at a depth of less than 3 cm, whereas deep heating (ultrasound, microwave therapy) reaches tissues beyond this level. Because the anatomic tissue layers and capsuloligamentous structures of the hand are more superficial than those of other parts of the body, simple topical heat options are quite effective and most commonly used.[8]

The physiologic effects of heat therapy have been broadly studied. During the early inflammatory phase of fracture healing, heat application increases local circulatory volume with a vasodilatory effect on small capillary beds. Increased blood flow assists in reducing local edema and the presence of soft tissue pain mediators. Furthermore, the effect of thermotherapy on the viscoelastic properties of collagen and tissue extensibility aid in the recovery of joint range of motion.[8] At temperatures of more than 40°C, collagen extensibility is increased by as much as 25%.[3] Heat, when combined with stretching, generates a greater effect on collagen fibril reorganization in a shorter period of time than either modality on its own.[5,9] The extent of improved joint range of motion following heat and preconditioning may also indicate the need for more aggressive splinting interventions.[7]

Ice

Similar to heat, ice (cryotherapy) may be used to address pain and soft tissue swelling. Examples include ice packs, cold-water baths, cooling units, and gel wraps. The desired therapeutic range is 10°C to 25°C. Physiologically, short exposure to cryotherapy (less than 15 minutes) alters vascular permeability. This modality is especially effective during the acute inflammatory phase when cold application induces vasoconstriction and decreases local tissue blood flow. These changes in turn lead to decreased histamine and prostaglandin synthesis, reduced swelling, and transiently elevated pain thresholds. Cryotherapy may also reduce muscle spasticity. Additionally, the alternation of cold and hot contrast baths promotes local blood flow and control of tissue edema.[2,6,8] In general, though, the selection of heat or cold therapy by the hand therapist is often based on patient-specific responses.

Ultrasound

Ultrasound delivers therapeutic heat to deeper tissue layers by altering cell membrane permeability. The ultrasound waves are administered in either a continuous (thermal)[6,10,11] or low-intensity, pulsed (nonthermal) manner.[12,13] Enhanced tissue penetration of continuous ultrasound effectively targets the capsuloligamentous tissues of the hand and digit addressing pain and mobility.[10,11] Tissue extensibility increases with temperature elevation to 40°C to 45°C. Tissue heating depths range from 0.8 to 1.6 cm using 3-MHz ultrasound to 2.5 to 5.0 cm at 1 MHz.[11] When combined with topically applied agents, such as triamcinolone or dexamethasone, ultrasound phonophoresis may be used to address hypertrophic scar formation.[6,14-16] Although thermal ultrasound is a frequently used modality before the initiation of therapeutic exercise, its application parameters and clinical effectiveness in the rehabilitation of patients with hand fractures requires further study.

Electrical Stimulation

Just as ultrasound has assumed a role in hand fracture rehabilitation, electrical stimulation has also become a frequently used therapeutic modality. Electrical stimulation targets not only pain but also neuromuscular response.[2,6,8,10,17,18] Therapeutic pain modulation is termed *transcutaneous electrical nerve stimulation* (TENS). Well-controlled studies are lacking, and there are mixed results present in the literature. However, there is evidence to support the use of TENS to treat acute and chronic pain.[17,18] When applied at a frequency that is just tolerable to patients, the electrical stimulus produces a local tingling sensation and elevates the pain threshold. Neuromuscular electrical stimulation (NMES), on the other hand, directly generates contraction of specific motor units and may be used to preserve motor recruitment and functional capacity of innervated muscles following injury as well as to strengthen muscles after prolonged disuse.[6,10] The application of NMES in the rehabilitation of patients with hand injuries is largely derived from mixed results observed in animal and human studies for other conditions. Additional well-powered clinical studies would enhance our understanding of the full therapeutic benefit of electrical stimulation in the treatment of patients with hand fractures.

Edema Control

Edema control following injury and surgical intervention is critical to patient comfort, restoration of early joint motion, and overall functional outcome.[2,3,5,6,19,20] Swelling is considered an indirect measure of inflammation and may be objectively quantified using a water volumeter or with wrist and digit circumference measurements. The simplest intervention to reduce edema is extremity elevation. With the hand positioned above the level of the heart, local tissue swelling is reduced by way of increased central venous return.

Wrapping and compressive techniques are also commonly used and easily performed by patients in between therapy visits. In the authors' hand therapy clinic, 1-in Coban (3M, St Paul, MN) is frequently used, starting distally and wrapping proximally (**Fig. 1**). String wrapping may also be used. Patients should be instructed to avoid over-wrapping multiple layers at the base of the digit to avoid creating a tourniquet effect. Range-of-motion exercises may then proceed, further enhancing edema control.[5,6] Compression gloves

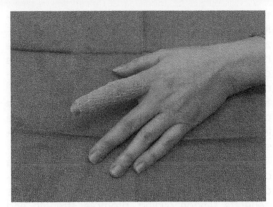

Fig. 1. Digital wrapping with Coban from distal to proximal is an inexpensive and easily applied technique to control postinjury edema.

or sleeves may also be provided for edema control and may be more easily manipulated by patients. Pneumatic compression sleeves are adjuncts to control edema, which work via controlled inflation and deflation of the garment.[21,22] Many certified hand therapists are also trained in therapeutic massage and lymphatic drainage techniques, which have been demonstrated to optimize the effect when combined with other edema control measures.[20,22] The combination of wrapping and massage has also been demonstrated to reduce edema more significantly than either modality on its own.[23]

Scar massage applies direct compression to edematous tissues during the postoperative period. Once the surgical incision is adequately healed (usually around 10 days), sutures may be removed and massage initiated. The primary benefit of scar massage, however, is its ability to disrupt fibrous tissue adhesions, which naturally occur as tissues heal. The therapist and surgeon should instruct patients on daily scar massage therapy in an attempt to enhance tissue compliance and minimize the formation of tendon adhesions. Mild lotion may also be incorporated for patient comfort and to address dry skin. Scar massage also contributes to desensitization of the incision.[3,5] The literature supports the use of desensitization exercises implementing textured dowels and hand immersion to alter the central nervous system's interpretation of nonpainful stimuli.[6] Contrast baths alternating warm and cold water also serve a similar purpose. In general, the effects of scar massage and desensitization therapy may be seen as late as 6 months following surgery.[3]

Motion

In addition to elevation and direct compression, early range of motion is one of the most effective therapeutic modalities aimed at reducing extremity edema.[24] Although a period of initial immobilization may be necessary to protect fracture healing, multiple studies demonstrate the benefits of early rehabilitation and range of motion, especially for high-energy and open fractures.[3,25] Several types of joint motion are described as part of the rehabilitative process. These types include active, active-assisted, passive, and resisted motions.[2,24]

Active motion is under direct patient control via cortical processing and activation of musculotendinous units.[19] Active range-of-motion exercises generate tendon gliding, promote strength and endurance, and enhance lymphatic drainage. In the digit, active range of motion generates a local compressive effect to the surrounding skin, subcutaneous tissues, and lymphatic system.[5,19,24]

Active-assisted motion combines active muscle recruitment with patient- or therapist-assisted motion. This type of exercise is especially useful in hesitant or guarding patients. A low-load, passively applied force is used to enhance the patients' own active contribution.[19,24]

Passive motion consists of a short, externally applied, high load across a joint. The therapist or patient applies a steady load to the point of maximum tissue resistance. Flexion bands may be used to place and hold flexion across the affected joint (**Fig. 2**). With tissue relaxation, the force is continued in the same manner as long as gentle gains continue. However, excessive force to the point of increased patient discomfort or pain should be avoided because this may generate tissue injury. Tissue response typically depends on the amount of time since the injury occurred as well as the period of immobilization. Generally, as fracture healing allows, resisted motion is incorporated into the therapy regimen as a means of further enhancing motion while restoring strength and endurance to the injured hand.[19,24]

Several important physiologic distinctions exist between active and passive range-of-motion exercises. Regarding tendon adherence, active motion promotes tendon excursion proximal to the site of scar tissue formation. Passive motion, on the other hand, targets motion distal to the site of adhesions. Specifically, active motion promotes tendon gliding through muscle contraction, whereas passive motion does not. Furthermore, gains via active range-of-motion exercises are more likely to contribute to improvement of the passive motion arc.[19]

Tendon Gliding

Tendon gliding promotes the motion of tendons through their sheaths and prevents soft tissue adherence. Blocking techniques are performed with the interphalangeal (IP) and metacarpophalangeal (MCP) joints differentially blocked (**Fig. 3**). Isolated gliding of the flexor digitorum superficialis (FDS) tendon occurs with flexion of the proximal IP (PIP) joint while holding the MCP joint extended. Alternatively, the flexor digitorum profundus (FDP) tendon is isolated by flexing the distal IP (DIP) joint while maintaining MCP and PIP joint extension. Blocking and tendon glide exercises may be performed with the aid of the uninjured hand or with a blocking splint fabricated by the hand therapist.[1–3,6,19,24]

The utility of blocking exercises is based on the fact that the digital flexor tendons, as they cross the MCP and IP joints, preferentially flex the digit in a proximal-to-distal manner along the path of least resistance. For example, if the IP joint is stiff following injury and the MCP joint is supple, the flexion force is primarily transmitted across the MCP joint at the expense of the stiff IP joint. In this case, the therapist may selectively block the MCP joint in extension while encouraging active motion across the IP joint. With the MCP joint blocked, the excursion force generated along the flexor tendons is directed across the stiff IP joint.[1–3,19,24] Digit extension requires 20 mm of extensor mechanism glide: 14 mm across the MCP joint and 6 mm across the PIP joint.[26]

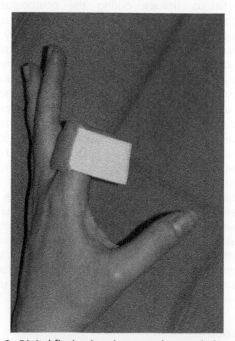

Fig. 2. Digital flexion bands are used to maximize passive range-of-motion gains via constant load application across the affected joint.

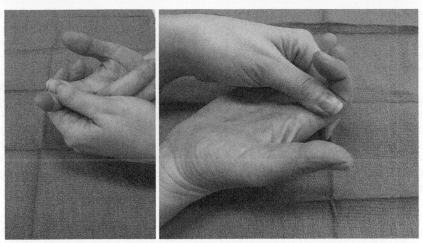

Fig. 3. Digital blocking exercises enhance tendon glide and prevent tissue adherence. Isolated motion across the distal IP joint with the proximal IP (PIP) joint extended promotes flexor digitorum profundus motion (*left image*). In contrast, motion across the PIP joint with the metacarpophalangeal joint extended isolates flexor digitorum superficialis gliding (*right image*).

Adhesions and scar formation may occur along either joint. However, the effect of adherence at the PIP joint is proportionately greater than that at the MCP joint. The PIP joint is, therefore, more susceptible to stiffness resulting from impaired tendon excursion.[26] As extension becomes limited across the PIP joint, the digit seeks to compensate for this loss via hyperextension at the MCP joint. The combination of a PIP joint extensor lag with MCP joint hyperextension is known as a *pseudo-claw deformity*.[27]

Differential gliding between the long flexor tendons, FDS and FDP, is necessary during the rehabilitation period to prevent adhesions between soft tissues and underlying bone. Only 1 to 2 mm of tendon motion is necessary to prevent adhesion.[28] Flexor tendon gliding exercises are performed in 3 distinct hand positions: the hook fist, the full fist, and the straight fist (**Fig. 4**). The hook fist is formed with the MCP joints held extended and the IP joints flexed. This position maximizes gliding between the two long flexor tendons. The full fist involves flexion of all 3 joints and promotes maximal FDP excursion relative to the surrounding tissues. Lastly, with the MCP and PIP joints maintained in flexion and the DIP joint

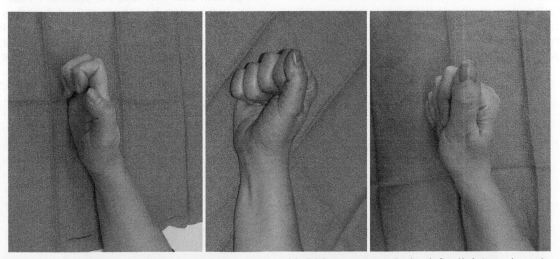

Fig. 4. Tendon gliding is further enhanced with place and hold fist exercises. The hook fist (*left image*) emphasizes motion between the superficial and deep flexor tendons. The full fist (*middle image*) maximizes deep flexor excursion. In contrast, the straight fist (*right image*) maximizes superficial flexor motion.

extended, the straight fist maximizes excursion between the FDS and local tissues.[19]

Targeted gliding of the extrinsic extensor tendons and intrinsic extensor mechanism may also be performed. For the extensor digitorum communis tendons, patients flex and extend the MCP joints while maintaining the IP joints in a flexed position. Alternatively, intrinsic muscles are activated by holding the MCP joints in flexion while flexing and extending the IP joints. Another intrinsic exercise consists of placing the palm flat on a table and then elevating the digit off of the table (the contralateral hand should stabilize the MCP joint on the table, thereby avoiding hyperextension). In general, blocking and tendon gliding exercises should lead to improved motion within several weeks of initiation. Therapy putty may also be incorporated to promote hand strength and endurance. If insufficient motion is gained despite adequate therapy, surgical tenolysis may be considered.[1–3,6,19]

Strengthening

Once fracture healing has occurred and range of motion has been restored, progressive strengthening exercises may be incorporated into the therapy regimen. Muscle strengthening further enhances soft tissue glide and range of motion, thereby preventing late adhesion formation. In the authors' clinic, strengthening exercises using putty is an effective and inexpensive modality (**Fig. 5**). NMES may also be used to supplement motor strengthening exercises, especially when disuse atrophy has developed following prolonged immobilization.[1,2,5,6]

Splinting

Splinting and cast immobilization during the acute phase of injury may limit the local inflammatory response and protect injured tissues and bones. As swelling resolves, splints or casts should be monitored for appropriate fit and changed as necessary to maintain adequate immobilization. As rehabilitation progresses, different types of splints may be fabricated to address hand stiffness that persists despite other conservative rehabilitation modalities and range-of-motion exercises.[2,4–6,19,24,29,30] The following 4 types of splints are commonly described: static, serial static, dynamic, and static progressive. A thorough understanding of these splints and their therapeutic applications is critical to the rehabilitative strategies of hand therapists and surgeons.

Static

Static splints maintain the hand or digit in a single fixed position. These splints are easily fabricated and commonly applied during the early inflammatory phase following acute injury or surgery. Static splints protect injured tissues, maintain fracture reduction and alignment, and assist in the resolution of local inflammation and swelling. They may be constructed with removable platforms designed to allow early joint blocking and tendon gliding exercises under the direction of the hand therapist. Static splints should not immobilize joints for periods longer than 3 to 4 weeks.[2–5,24]

The practitioner should be mindful of the position of the small joints of the hand when applying static splints. A position of safe immobilization has been described based on anatomic joint considerations. This classic position maintains the MCP joint in approximately 70° to 90° of flexion with the IP joints fully extended (**Fig. 6**). MCP joint flexion effectively maintains ligament length and prevents extension contracture by splinting the joint with the capsuloligamentous structures taut. This position also minimizes the potential intrasynovial space where hematoma or joint fluid may promote joint swelling and compensatory extension.[4] In contrast to the MCP joints, extension across the IP joints maintains the collateral

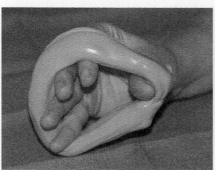
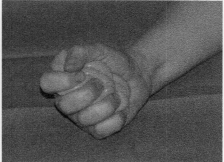

Fig. 5. Putty exercises (*left and right images*) promote not only strengthening but also tendon glide and range of motion. This simple and effective modality is easily incorporated into the home exercise regimen.

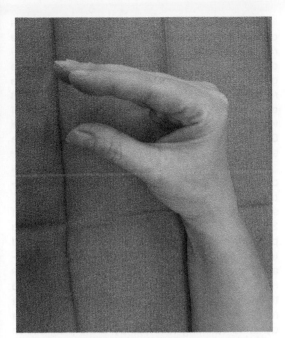

Fig. 6. Splinting of the IP joints in extension and the MCP joints in approximately 70° flexion maintains tension across the small joint collateral ligaments. This position of safe immobilization should be considered when immobilization of the hand and digits is necessary.

ligaments, volar plate, and associated soft tissue structures in a stretched position, which helps prevent contracture.

The range-of-motion demands of the MCP joint are less than that of the IP joints because of the compensatory small joint motion. As a result, contractures of the MCP joint, when present, are typically better tolerated than contractures of the IP joints. The IP joints are unforgiving of injury and prolonged periods of immobilization. The associated capsuloligamentous structures are highly sensitive to trauma and prone to forming thick collagenous bands of scar tissue along the volar aspect of the joints. Simple rehabilitative strategies, such as splinting, edema control, and early motion, are typically sufficient in managing MCP joint contractures. On the other hand, IP joint stiffness often demands more technical splinting modalities over a longer treatment period to restore IP joint motion.[4,31]

Serial static
Serial static splints or casts are useful in the management of digit contractures and early stiffness, especially of joints with hard end points of motion.[5] A stiff joint is splinted at the end range of its motion near its soft tissue elastic deformation limit.[4] Low-load force across the joint promotes

tissue relaxation and lengthening.[7] Although serial casting may also address noncompliant splint wear, casts require regular removal and reapplication because tissues relax under prolonged stretch.[4] A longer duration of cast or splint wear theoretically leads to greater difficulty regaining joint motion after removal. However, in a prospective study comparing serial casting methods for PIP joint contractures, Flowers and LaStayo[7] found that a longer duration of cast wear (6 days vs 3 days before cast change) resulted in greater motion gains. The recommended duration of wear generally varies throughout the literature.

Dynamic
In contrast to static splinting modalities, dynamic splints are fabricated to deliver controlled, continuous force across a mobile joint.[4,5,19,29] Load application is typically via elastic traction bands or springs. Dynamic splints, such as the 3-point LMB finger extension splint (DeRoyal, Powell, TN), are especially useful in treating stiff joints that are responsive to passive stretch or joints with soft motion end points (**Fig. 7**).[5] Dynamic splints may also be intermittently removed to focus on range-of-motion and gliding activities. This therapeutic modality demands greater patient understanding and commitment.

The effectiveness of dynamic splinting in the treatment of stiff joints has been reported. In a prospective case series of PIP joint flexion contractures, the dynamic splint wear of 8 to 12 hours per day over an average of 4 months led to an average gain of 18° extension.[31] Several factors are associated with improved outcomes following dynamic splinting, including shorter time between injury and initiation of therapy, flexion deficits, and the presence of greater pretreatment motion.[29,30]

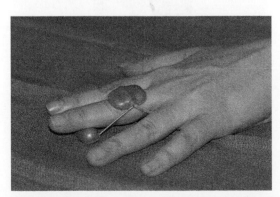

Fig. 7. Dynamic splints, such as the 3-point LMB finger extension splint, deliver controlled, constant load across the joint. Dynamic splints may be removed for further range-of-motion exercises.

There is some evidence to suggest that longer duration of wear on a daily basis leads to greater motion gains; however, this is not completely resolved in the literature.[7,30,31]

Static progressive
Static-progressive splints address joint stiffness by the application of 3 points of force across the joint. Similar to serial static splints, the force is applied at the soft tissue limit of joint motion. The force generated by static-progressive splints may be incrementally adjusted by patients or the therapist (**Fig. 8**).[19] Several types of static-progressive splints are available commercially.[5] This splinting strategy is best suited for joints that are minimally responsive to passive range of motion and is a preferred modality in the authors' clinic. Such devices are commonly used to regain full joint extension following PIP and DIP joint injuries or contractures. The duration of static-progressive splint wear necessary to achieve therapeutic goals is directly related to the time between injury and the initiation of splinting.[19] In general, serial, dynamic, and static-progressive splinting modalities should be continued so long as patients demonstrate improvement. The duration of treatment may range from several weeks to several months. Once motion gains plateau, splinting should be discontinued.[4,5]

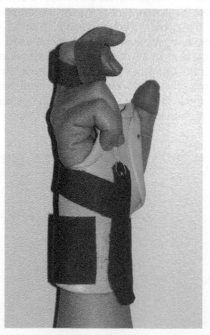

Fig. 8. Static-progressive splinting is a commonly used modality in the authors' clinic. In this example, a stiff PIP joint is effectively mobilized with progressive, incremental adjustments to joint force and position.

The work of Flowers[32] suggests a splinting modality algorithm based on the improvement of the range of motion before and following heat and pre-conditioning. If the range of motion improves greater than 20°, the authors recommend active range-of-motion exercises without splinting. Gains of 15° to 20° are treated with static splints. Lastly, when range of motion improves by only 5° to 10° or 0° to 5°, dynamic splinting and static-progressive splinting, respectively, is recommended.[32]

The effectiveness of splinting modalities in overcoming digit stiffness is well reviewed in the literature. Weeks and colleagues[33] reported an 87% success rate following nonoperative treatment of 212 patients (789 stiff MCP and PIP joints). Among patients with MCP joint stiffness, 82% responded to nonoperative modalities within 2 weeks of initiating therapy. Active range-of-motion improvement ranged from 21° to 40° for the second through fifth digits. For patients requiring splint management, the authors recommend daytime dynamic splinting followed by static-progressive splinting at night. In the same series, patients treated for PIP joint stiffness demonstrated an 87% improvement with nonoperative modalities. The range-of-motion gains ranged from 32° to 42° for the second through fifth digits.[33]

FRACTURE MANAGEMENT
The rehabilitation of hand fractures relies greatly on communication between the treating surgeon and hand therapist. This phase of the patients' treatment is characterized as a fine balance between fracture stability and healing, on the one hand, and early motion and avoidance of stiffness on the other. Depending on the fracture location and stability, the surgeon may choose to recommend nonoperative or operative intervention for the injury. Nondisplaced fractures and fractures that are stable following closed reduction may be amenable to nonoperative management with a period of cast or splint immobilization to provide stability as the fracture heals. Displaced, comminuted, or unstable fractures are more likely treated by operative means, including percutaneous pin, lag screw, tension band, and plate constructs. Although nonoperative management avoids potential complications associated with surgery (ie, superficial or deep infection, wound healing, hardware failure, and local soft tissue injury), a more prolonged period of immobilization is necessary as bridging callus forms and the fracture heals. The consequences of extended immobilization are tissue adherence and joint stiffness. Operative management with internal fixation theoretically provides early stability to the healing bone and

allows early or immediate range-of-motion exercises.[26,34,35] Therefore, the goal of operative intervention, when pursued, is to provide adequate fracture stability to allow early hand motion.

Conservative Fracture Management

Whether treated by closed or open means, the general progression of hand fracture rehabilitation follows a similar pattern. Variability exists within the literature and among practitioners regarding splint selection, the period of immobilization, initiation of range of motion, and progression of activity.[1,3,25,26,34–38] **Tables 1–5** provide treatment algorithms based on the authors' clinical approach to common fractures. Initial immobilization promotes a stable healing environment during the early inflammatory stage of injury. With conservative management, this period of casting or splinting is continued until signs of callus formation suggest a healing fracture. At this point, patients may be transitioned to a splint removable for therapy and hygiene. Active range-of-motion exercises may begin under the supervision of the hand therapist and usually continues for a period of 1 to 2 weeks as motion improves. Patients are also instructed on tendon gliding and joint blocking exercises during this time. Patients continue to wear the protective splint at night and when not performing exercises. With further radiographic evidence of fracture healing, the therapist may introduce passive range-of motion exercises, usually around 4 to 6 weeks following injury or surgery. Strengthening activities may begin with restoration of motion and continued fracture healing. Adjunct modalities are also incorporated into the regimen as the hand therapist sees fit. The progression of therapeutic exercise depends in large part on evidence of bony healing. Throughout this process, the surgeon and hand therapist should communicate not only clinic and therapy progress notes but also impressions of radiographic fracture consolidation and concerns regarding an individual's therapeutic progress.

Operative Fracture Management

The goal of operative management of hand fractures is the establishment of stability allowing early range of motion. Patients typically leave the operating theater in a bulky splint for protection and immobilization as initial inflammation subsides. When patients return for the first postoperative clinic visit, the splint is removed, the wound is evaluated, and a protective splint is fashioned for wear when not performing therapeutic exercises. Scar massage and desensitization modalities should begin following suture removal. In the authors'

practice, when plate or lag screw constructs are used for fracture fixation, they allow immediate range of motion under the supervision of the hand therapist. Fixation using Kirschner wires typically provides only limited stability and should be approached in a manner more similar to conservative treatment measures.[3,36] Critical to early motion is the surgeon's intraoperative evaluation of fracture construct stability. At the authors' institution, once fracture reduction and fixation has been achieved, they prefer to perform an examination under fluoroscopic imaging to determine the safe motion arc parameters for therapy. As active range of motion is restored and with continued evidence of fracture healing, progression to passive motion exercises is allowed. Additional modalities are implemented to enhance motion gains, and strengthening exercises are introduced with improved motion around 6 weeks following surgery.

MEASURES OF REHABILITATION PROGRESS

Thorough documentation of the rehabilitation process is instrumental to the treating therapist and surgeon. A variety of measures, both clinical and patient reported, may be recorded and followed throughout the recovery period. In the rehabilitation of hand fractures, the most commonly followed parameters are range of motion and strength. Patient-based outcome measures are also important indicators of return to function and daily activities, satisfaction, and coping.

Accurate and reproducible measurement of joint motion enables meaningful interval comparison throughout a patient's rehabilitation. Range of motion is best measured with a metal digital goniometer placed along the dorsum of the digit. Measurements are taken at each joint with the hand in full composite flexion and likewise in full extension. Total active motion is recorded as the sum of total flexion across the MCP, PIP, and DIP joints in composite flexion *minus* the sum of any extension deficits present across these joints. Total passive motion is similarly measured with the small joints placed in maximum passive flexion and extension. If full composite flexion of the hand is lacking, the distance of the fingertip from the distal palmar crease should also be measured and recorded.[39]

Motor strength testing is a useful measure of hand functional recovery, especially as patients prepare to return to work and recreational activities. In the authors' clinic, grip and pinch strength is measured using specific dynamometers. Reproducible grip-strength measurements are taken with the shoulder in $0°$ adduction, elbow at $90°$ flexion, and the forearm in neutral. The right and

Table 1
Management of metacarpal shaft fractures

Metacarpal Shaft	Immobilization	AROM	PROM	Strengthening	Considerations
Nondisplaced, stable	Forearm-based radial/ulnar gutter splint in safe position IP joints free Removable for therapy	Immediate as tolerated Buddy tape to neighboring digit	~4 wk with radiographic evidence of healing	~6–8 wk with evidence of healing	—
Closed reduced, stable	Forearm-based radial/ulnar gutter cast in safe position ~3–4 wk IP joints free	~3–4 wk Transition to removable radial/ulnar gutter splint	~5–6 wk with radiographic evidence of healing	~6–8 wk with evidence of healing	—
CRPP	Initially, bulky volar resting splint Then, forearm-based radial/ulnar gutter cast in safe position IP joints free	~3–4 wk Transition to removable radial/ulnar gutter splint	~5–6 wk with radiographic evidence of healing	~6–8 wk with evidence of healing	Removal of hardware ~4–6 wk with evidence of healing
ORIF	Initially, bulky volar resting splint Then, forearm-based radial/ulnar gutter splint in safe position IP joints free	Begin at first follow-up visit Radial/ulnar gutter splint for protective and nighttime wear	~3–4 wk as tolerated	~6–8 wk with evidence of healing	Scar massage Tissue gliding

Abbreviations: AROM, active range of motion; CRPP, closed reduction percutaneous pinning; ORIF, open reduction internal fixation; PROM, passive range of motion.

Table 2
Management of proximal phalanx shaft fractures

Proximal Phalanx Shaft	Immobilization	AROM	PROM	Strengthening	Considerations
Nondisplaced, stable Closed reduced, stable	Hand-based radial/ulnar gutter splint in safe position ~3–4 wk Removable for therapy	Immediate as tolerated Buddy tape to neighboring digit Composite ROM and blocking ~3–4 wk	~4–6 wk with radiographic evidence of healing	~6–8 wk with evidence of healing	Edema control Tissue gliding Joint blocking NMES for tendon excursion Dynamic splint for stiffness
CRPP	Initially, bulky volar resting splint Then, hand-based radial/ulnar gutter splint in safe position ~3–4 wk	~3–4 wk Transition to removable radial/ulnar gutter splint Progress to composite ROM and blocking	~5–6 wk with radiographic evidence of healing	~6–8 wk with evidence of healing	Removal of hardware ~4–6 wk with evidence of healing Modalities as previously discussed
ORIF	Initially, bulky volar resting splint Then, hand-based radial/ulnar gutter splint in safe position	Begin at first follow-up visit Radial/ulnar gutter splint for protective and nighttime wear	Early vs delayed, depends on intraoperative stability	~6–8 wk with evidence of healing	Scar massage Modalities as previously discussed

Abbreviations: AROM, active range of motion; CRPP, closed reduction percutaneous pinning; ORIF, open reduction internal fixation; PROM, passive range of motion.

Table 3
Management of middle phalanx shaft fractures

Middle Phalanx Shaft	Immobilization	AROM	PROM	Strengthening	Considerations
Nondisplaced, stable	Hand-based radial/ulnar gutter splint in safe position vs buddy taping to neighboring digit	Immediate as tolerated Buddy tape to neighboring digit Composite ROM and blocking ~3–4 wk	~4–6 wk with radiographic evidence of healing	~6–8 wk with evidence of healing	Edema control Tissue gliding Joint blocking NMES for tendon excursion Dynamic splint for stiffness
Closed reduced, stable	Hand-based radial/ulnar gutter splint in safe position ~3–4 wk Removable for therapy	~3–4 wk Buddy tape to neighboring digit Composite ROM and blocking ~3–4 wk	~4–6 wk with radiographic evidence of healing	~6–8 wk with evidence of healing	Modalities as previously discussed
CRPP	Initially, bulky volar resting splint Then, hand-based radial/ulnar gutter splint in safe position ~3–4 wk	~3–4 wk Transition to removable radial/ulnar gutter splint Progress to composite ROM and blocking	~5–6 wk with radiographic evidence of healing	~6–8 wk with evidence of healing	Removal of hardware ~4–6 wk with evidence of healing Modalities as previously discussed
ORIF	Initially, bulky volar resting splint Then, hand-based radial/ulnar gutter splint in safe position	Begin at first follow-up visit Radial/ulnar gutter splint for protective and nighttime wear	Early vs delayed, depends on intraoperative stability	~6–8 wk with evidence of healing	Scar massage Modalities as previously discussed

Abbreviations: AROM, active range of motion; CRPP, closed reduction percutaneous pinning; ORIF, open reduction internal fixation; PROM, passive range of motion.

Table 4
Management of distal phalanx tuft fractures

Distal Phalanx Tuft	Immobilization	AROM	PROM	Strengthening	Considerations
Nondisplaced, stable Closed reduced, stable	Digital splint (AlumaFoam) ~3–4 wk	Immediate as tolerated	~4 wk with radiographic evidence of healing	~4–6 wk with evidence of healing	Desensitization exercises Edema control Joint blocking
CRPP	Digital splint (AlumaFoam) ~3–4 wk	Following removal of hardware	Following removal of hardware with improving AROM	Following removal of hardware and restoration of AROM/PROM	Removal of hardware ~4–6 wk with evidence of healing Modalities as previously discussed

Abbreviations: AROM, active range of motion; CRPP, closed reduction percutaneous pinning; PROM, passive range of motion.

left sides are sequentially tested a total of 3 times, and the average for each side is recorded. The literature suggests a difference in strength of 5% to 10% between the dominant and nondominant hands[40]; however, many patients have nondominant hand strength equal to or greater than that of their dominant side.[41] Similarly, pinch strength is measured for the injured and uninjured hands. Three types of pinch strength are typically tested. These types include lateral key pinch (thumb pulp to index finger middle phalanx), 3-point or chuck pinch (thumb pulp to index and middle finger pulps), and fingertip pinch (thumb tip to index finger tip), listed in order of decreasing strength.[42]

Table 5
Management of common injuries of the PIP joint

Avulsion Fracture	Immobilization	AROM	PROM	Strengthening	Considerations
Volar plate avulsion Nondisplaced, stable	Buddy tape to neighboring digit	Immediate	Advance as tolerated	~4 wk with improved motion	—
Middle phalanx dorsal avulsion Nondisplaced, stable	Hand-based volar splint with PIP joint in extension and DIP joint free ~4 wk	~4 wk with radiographic evidence of healing	~5–6 wk with return of AROM	Initiate once fracture is healed and motion returned	Anatomic reduction and healing are necessary to prevent late boutonniere deformity
Middle phalanx dorsal avulsion Displaced, unstable CRPP/ORIF	Hand-based volar splint with PIP joint in extension ~3–4 wk	~2–3 wk (ORIF) ~4 wk (CRPP, after pin removal) Slowly advance flexion with guided therapy	~4–6 wk with radiographic evidence of healing	Initiate once fracture is healed and motion returned	—

Abbreviations: AROM, active range of motion; CRPP, closed reduction percutaneous pinning; ORIF, open reduction internal fixation; PROM, passive range of motion.

As work and hobby functional activities are integrated into the therapy regimen, the Baltimore Therapeutic Equipment Work Stimulator (Baltimore Therapeutic Equipment, Hanover, MD, USA) may be used to mimic the varying resistance encountered among different tools and instruments.[6,42] The addition of work hardening exercises to the rehabilitative process is critical in maximizing functional outcome while promoting safe and effective return to work.

Numerous patient-reported outcome measures are available to the surgeon and therapist and serve as useful, standardized instruments in the assessment of patient recovery following hand injury. The most widely used and well-validated measures include the general Medical Outcomes Study 36-Item Health Survey; the extremity-specific Disabilities of the Arm, Shoulder, and Hand (DASH) and Quick DASH; and the hand-specific Michigan Hand Outcomes Questionnaire.[42]

SUMMARY

Patient satisfaction following hand therapy depends on several outcomes. Patients who report improvement in pain and other symptoms also note greater satisfaction with the general rehabilitation process. Similarly, improved strength, range of motion, and restoration of function all enhance patient satisfaction.[43] Total active range of motion correlates with functional recovery.[3] Meeting preoperative expectations is also important, further emphasizing the utility of evaluating and addressing patients' expectations of their care. The aesthetics and overall alignment of the injured hand may also influence patient satisfaction. Psychosocial factors, such as depression or poor coping skills, on the other hand, have been demonstrated to negatively affect patients' perception of rehabilitation outcomes.[43]

Adherence to the hand-therapy regimen is critically important to the successful recovery of function following hand fractures. Multiple factors influence patients' ability or willingness to engage in therapy, including convenience of access to the therapist's office, social support, visit costs and copays, and travel limitations. Both the surgeon and therapist must understand an individual patient's needs or limitations when initiating therapy. The practitioner must also address patients' expectations of therapy. If patients' expectations are unrealistically high, they may become discouraged early, limiting the full therapeutic potential. Conversely, patients entering with low expectations may plateau early and fail to progress to the maximum benefit. Social issues, such as depression and anxiety, are also common following hand injuries.[44,45] Patients suffering from depression may lack the motivation necessary to meaningfully participate in an intensive hand-therapy regimen, especially one continued at home. Similarly, anxious patients may guard during range-of-motion or stretching exercises or withhold effort at home for fear of causing further damage to the hand or digit.[46] Positive feedback provides encouragement to patients, especially over a prolonged and difficult recovery.

Studies suggest that patients who trust their providers and understand the goals of therapy and the aspects of their home exercise program are more likely to complete the regimen.[24,46] A home program complete with explicit instructions and easily understood illustrations enhances patient compliance.[5] A home exercise program should be customized to the individual patient. Wakefield and McQueen[47] found that adequate instruction from the therapist enhances the

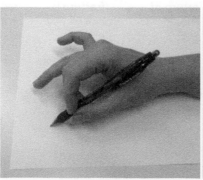 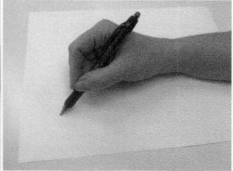

Fig. 9. As therapy progresses, specific exercises are introduced to address common work and recreational activities. Therapist feedback may be used to correct improper hand position and technique (*left image*) as demonstrated during this handwriting exercise in which the patient is reminded to maintain ring and small finger flexion (*right image*).

effectiveness of the home regimen. Comparing conventional physical therapy combined with a home exercise program to a home regimen alone, the investigators observed no significant difference in outcomes between patient groups.[47] The therapeutic regimen should also incorporate exercises with direct relevance to patients' everyday activities. Therapist feedback regarding hand position during seemingly mundane tasks, such as handwriting (**Fig. 9**), opening bottles and jars, typing, and gripping objects, encourages safe and effective hand position during use. In addition to the basic activities of daily living, it is highly important to incorporate activities applicable to patients' work and recreational demands.[6,46]

The joints of the hand are prone to stiffness and disability following injury. Optimal rehabilitation of hand fractures depends on numerous factors directed by the surgeon, therapist, and patients alike. The importance of adopting a team approach when managing the rehabilitation of hand fractures is critical. Many therapeutic strategies are available to the practitioner. A working understanding of these modalities and their clinical applications enhances the successful management of hand fractures.

REFERENCES

1. Gallagher KG, Blackmore SM. Intra-articular hand fractures and joint injuries: part II – therapist's management. In: Skirven TM, Osterman AL, Fedorczyk J, et al, editors. Rehabilitation of the hand and upper extremity. 6th edition. Philadelphia: Elsevier Mosby; 2011. p. 417–38.

2. Michlovitz SL. Principles of hand therapy. In: Berger RA, Weiss AC, editors. Hand surgery. 1st edition. Philadelphia: Lippincott Williams and Wilkins; 2003. p. 105–22.

3. Hardy MA, Freeland AE. Hand fracture fixation and healing: skeletal stability and digital mobility. In: Skirven TM, Osterman AL, Fedorczyk J, et al, editors. Rehabilitation of the hand and upper extremity. 6th edition. Philadelphia: Elsevier Mosby; 2011. p. 361–76.

4. Shin AY, Amadio PC. The stiff finger. In: Wolfe SW, Hotchkiss RN, Pederson WC, et al, editors. Green's operative hand surgery. 6th edition. Philadelphia: Elsevier Churchill Livingstone; 2011. p. 355–88.

5. Trumble TE. Hand therapy. In: Trumble TE, editor. Principles of hand surgery and therapy. 1st edition. Philadelphia: WB Saunders; 2000. p. 603–20.

6. Dorf E, Blue C, Smith BP, et al. Therapy after injury to the hand. J Am Acad Orthop Surg 2010;18:464–73.

7. Flowers K, LaStayo P. Effect of total end range time on improving passive range of motion. J Hand Ther 1994;7:150–5.

8. Hartzell TL, Rubinstein R, Herman M. Therapeutic modalities – an updated review for the hand surgeon. J Hand Surg 2012;37A:597–621.

9. Lentell G, Hetherington R, Eagan J, et al. The use of thermal agents to influence the effectiveness of a low-load prolonged stretch. J Orthop Sports Phys Ther 1992;16:200–7.

10. Michlovitz SL. Is there a role for ultrasound and electrical stimulation following injury to tendon and nerve? J Hand Ther 2005;18:292–6.

11. Nussbaum E. The influence of ultrasound on healing tissues. J Hand Ther 1998;11:140–7.

12. Bashardoust TS, Houghton P, MacDermid JC, et al. Effects of low-intensity pulsed ultrasound therapy on fracture healing: a systematic review and meta-analysis. Am J Phys Med Rehabil 2012;91:349–67.

13. Watanabe Y, Matsushita T, Bhandari M, et al. Ultrasound for fracture healing: current evidence. J Orthop Trauma 2010;24:S56–61.

14. Byl N, McKenzie A, Halliday B, et al. The effect of phonophoresis with corticosteroids: a controlled pilot study. J Orthop Sports Phys Ther 1993;18:590–8.

15. Huys S, Gan BS, Sherebrin M, et al. Comparison of effects of early and late ultrasound treatment on tendon healing in the chicken limb. J Hand Ther 1993;6:58–9.

16. Lampe KE. Electrotherapy in tissue repair. J Hand Ther 1998;11:131–9.

17. Cheing GL, Luk ML. Transcutaneous electrical nerve stimulation for neuropathic pain. J Hand Surg 2005;30B:50–5.

18. Johnson M, Martinson M. Efficacy of electrical nerve stimulation for chronic musculoskeletal pain: a meta-analysis of randomized controlled trials. Pain 2007;130:157–65.

19. Colditz JC. Therapist's management of the stiff hand. In: Skirven TM, Osterman AL, Fedorczyk J, et al, editors. Rehabilitation of the hand and upper extremity. 6th edition. Philadelphia: Elsevier Mosby; 2011. p. 894–921.

20. Howard SB, Krishnagiri S. The use of manual edema mobilization for the reduction of persistent edema in the upper limb. J Hand Ther 2001;14:291–301.

21. Griffin JW, Newsome LS, Stralka SW, et al. Reduction of chronic posttraumatic hand edema: a comparison of high voltage pulsed current, intermittent pneumatic compression, and placebo treatments. Phys Ther 1990;70:279–86.

22. Villeco JP. Edema: a silent but important factor. J Hand Ther 2012;25:153–62.

23. Flowers KR. String wrapping versus massage for reducing digital volume. Phys Ther 1988;68:57–9.

24. Michlovitz SL, Harris BA, Watkins MP. Therapy interventions for improving joint range of motion: a systematic review. J Hand Ther 2004;17:118–31.

25. Feehan LM, Bassett K. Is there evidence for early mobilization following an extraarticular hand fracture? J Hand Ther 2004;17:300–8.

26. Freeland AE, Hardy MA, Singletary S. Rehabilitation for proximal phalangeal fractures. J Hand Ther 2003;16:129–42.

27. Evans R, Thompson D. An analysis of factors that support early active short arc motion of the repaired central slip. J Hand Ther 1992;5:187–201.

28. Zhao C, Amadio PC, Momose T, et al. Effect of synergistic wrist motion on adhesion formation after repair of partial flexor digitorum profundus tendon lacerations in a canine model in vivo. J Bone Joint Surg Am 2002;84A:78–84.

29. Glasgow C, Tooth LR, Fleming J, et al. Dynamic splinting for the stiff hand after trauma: predictors of contracture resolution. J Hand Ther 2011;24:195–206.

30. Glasgow C, Fleming J, Tooth LR, et al. The long-term relationship between duration of treatment and contracture resolution using dynamic orthotic devices for the stiff proximal interphalangeal joint: a prospective cohort study. J Hand Ther 2012;25:38–47.

31. Prosser R. Splinting in the management of proximal interphalangeal joint flexion contracture. J Hand Ther 1996;9:378–86.

32. Flowers KF. A proposed decision hierarchy for splinting the stiff joint, with an emphasis on force application parameters. J Hand Ther 2002;15:158–62.

33. Weeks P, Wray R, Kuxhaus M. The result of nonoperative management of stiff joints in the hand. Plast Reconstr Surg 1978;61:58–63.

34. Cannon NM. Rehabilitation approaches for distal and middle phalanx fractures of the hand. J Hand Ther 2003;16:105–16.

35. McNemar TB, Howell JW, Chang E. Management of metacarpal fractures. J Hand Ther 2003;16:143–51.

36. Feehan LM. Extra-articular hand fractures, part II: therapist's management. In: Skirven TM, Osterman AL, Fedorczyk J, et al, editors. Rehabilitation of the hand and upper extremity. 6th edition. Philadelphia: Elsevier Mosby; 2011. p. 386–401.

37. Day CS, Stern PJ. Fractures of the metacarpals and phalanges. In: Wolfe SW, Hotchkiss RN, Pederson WC, et al, editors. Green's operative hand surgery. 6th edition. Philadelphia: Elsevier Churchill Livingstone; 2011. p. 239–90.

38. Merrell G, Slade JF. Dislocations and ligament injuries in the digits. In: Wolfe SW, Hotchkiss RN, Pederson WC, et al, editors. Green's operative hand surgery. 6th edition. Philadelphia: Elsevier Churchill Livingstone; 2011. p. 291–332.

39. Seftchick JL, Detullio LM, Fedorczyk JM, et al. Clinical examination of the hand. In: Skirven TM, Osterman AL, Fedorczyk J, et al, editors. Rehabilitation of the hand and upper extremity. 6th edition. Philadelphia: Elsevier Mosby; 2011. p. 55–71.

40. O'Driscoll SW, Horii E, Ness R. The relationship between wrist position, grasp size, and grip strength. J Hand Surg 1992;17A:169–77.

41. Petersen P, Petrick M, Connor H, et al. Grip strength and hand dominance: challenging the 10% rule. Am J Occup Ther 1989;43:444–7.

42. Fess EE. Functional tests. In: Skirven TM, Osterman AL, Fedorczyk J, et al, editors. Rehabilitation of the hand and upper extremity. 6th edition. Philadelphia: Elsevier Mosby; 2011. p. 152–62.

43. Marks M, Herren DB, Vlieland TP, et al. Determinants of patient satisfaction after orthopedic interventions to the hand: a review of the literature. J Hand Ther 2011;24:303–12.

44. Niekel MC, Lindenhovius AL, Watson JB, et al. Correlation of DASH and QuickDASH with measures of psychological distress. J Hand Surg 2009;34A:1499–505.

45. Vranceanu AM, Jupiter JB, Mudgal CS, et al. Predictors of pain intensity and disability after minor hand surgery. J Hand Surg 2010;35A:956–60.

46. O'Brien L. The evidence on ways to improve patient's adherence in hand therapy. J Hand Ther 2012;25:247–50.

47. Wakefield A, McQueen M. The role of physiotherapy and clinical predictors of outcome after fracture of the distal radius. J Bone Joint Surg Br 2000;82B:972–6.

Complications of Hand Fractures and Their Prevention

Andrew D. Markiewitz, MD[a,b,*]

KEYWORDS

• Complications • Osteotomy • Malunions • Osteomyelitis • Stiffness

KEY POINTS

- Match patient needs with the intervention.
- Match patient expectations with the surgeon's ability to deliver care.
- Mobilize as soon as possible based on fracture stability.
- Nonoperative treatment can be a satisfactory intervention.
- Identify complications early and intervene promptly.

INTRODUCTION: NATURE OF THE PROBLEM

Regardless of the clinician's technical skill, the results of the treatment of hand fractures are not always optimal. Potentially compromised by open injuries, surgical approaches violate tissue planes with scarring producing adhesions and motion deficits. However, surgery may be necessary to improve the results. Nonsurgical treatment may allow angulation or displacement if motion precedes healing. Close communication with therapists may help reduce complications. One way to consider outcome failures or complications is to determine the following: failure of technique, failure of rehabilitation, and failure caused by patient disease. Despite optimal care after presentation, the outcome depends on the initial injury.[1]

Multiple techniques and implants have been described. Matching the patient's problem with an intervention represents the major task confronting a surgeon. Operating when observing would be better suited for the patient and the comorbidities can lead to a good radiograph and a less satisfying functional outcome. Common in hand trauma, open injuries require irrigation, stabilization, and coverage, although complications still persist.[1–4] Even in the presence of a complication, clinicians should assess the patient's function, commitment, and participation. If they are not committed to steps to improve the results, heroic measures to improve the position and function may be unsatisfying.

Injuries to the hand can affect its function. However, treatment can increase this impact. A stable fracture pattern is essential; how it is achieved seems to matter less.[1] However, the care does not stop at that step. The steps to regaining motion and strength may be equally important. As shown in **Table 1**, complications typically span the spectrum of care and the tissue type. Every complication can impair the final result. Thus providers should be aware of their impact from diagnosis to release from care.

The key decision for treating any fracture is whether to operate or not operate. A closed reduction may obtain a stable pattern. If the fracture has a tendency to angulate or shorten, close observation with clinical/radiographic evaluation on

Disclosures: None.
[a] Department of Orthopaedic Surgery, University of Cincinnati, 231 Albert Sabin Way, P.O. Box 670558, Cincinnati, OH 45267-0558, USA; [b] Department of Surgery, Uniformed Services University of the Health Services, 4301 Jones Bridge Road, Bethesda, MD 20814, USA
* 10700 Montgomery Road, Suite 150, Cincinnati, OH 45242.
E-mail address: amarkiewitz@handsurg.com

Hand Clin 29 (2013) 601–620
http://dx.doi.org/10.1016/j.hcl.2013.08.012
0749-0712/13/$ – see front matter © 2013 Elsevier Inc. All rights reserved.

Table 1
Complications by site

Bone	Nonunion, malunions, delayed union, avascular necrosis, osteomyelitis, amputation
Soft tissue	Stiffness/motion loss, instability, laxity, poor durability, lack of coverage, contracture, flexion/extension loss
Tendon	Adhesions, lag, tightness
Nerve	Numbness, hypersensitivity, complex regional pain (reflex sympathetic dystrophy)
Vascular	Ischemia, congestion
Other	Vibration and temperature sensitivity, chondrolysis, acute pain, joint laxity

Data from Refs.[5–11]

a weekly basis should be done. Casting or splinting may be used after evaluating the patient. Splinting may help the therapist preempt stiffness with a concomitant crush injury. If the site is hard to evaluate or rotation is a concern, the clinician should remove the cast and reexamine. The patient should be aware that surgery may stabilize the fracture but has intrinsic risks. Depending on patient factors, a fracture may be healed enough to tolerate gentle rehabilitation within 3 to 4 weeks, which requires clinical experience.

Fractures may have problems with union, stiffness, avascular necrosis, instability, pain, swelling, posttraumatic arthritis, chondrolysis, dystrophy, and infection. Surgery for fracture treatment or the complications of fracture care have all the same risks plus iatrogenic injury and implant

failure. All surgeons hope for success with surgical management but, despite optimal techniques, poor outcomes occur. Clinicians need to use the optimal fixation to allow healing in a stable fashion. Despite the allure of modern plating techniques, not all fracture patterns need expensive implants for the optimal result. Sirota and colleagues[12] found equal biomechanical stability in a unicondylar phalanx fracture regardless of screw or K-wire fixation.

COMPLICATIONS OF TREATMENT

Regardless of treatment, complications occur, as detailed in **Table 2**. Specific complications are more common depending on the initial injury and, to a lesser amount, to the treatment used. The incidence of complications is hard to define because many surgeons are reluctant to disclose their poor outcomes. Those who document their failures should be commended because they help educate others on what to avoid.[1,3,10,13,14]

Use of Kirschner wire fixation can be demanding. Because they are limited in their fixation, patient compliance can produce complications. Fixing a fracture requires clinicians to think in 3 dimensions, which is a learned skill. Stahl and Schwartz[10] noted that residents need supervision to avoid technical failure. Their study replicated Botte and colleagues[13] study from 1992, which encouraged meticulous pin placement, discerning evaluation of operative placement, and compliance. Although documenting an 18% complication rate, they did not find permanent effects in most cases.[13] It is typically recommended that pins be buried if expected to be left exposed for more than 6 weeks. Phalangeal fractures should heal within 4 weeks; thus, Botte and colleagues[13] found aseptic loosening and infection

Table 2
Recent articles documenting complications relating to fixation methods

K-wire fixation	Stahl & Schwartz,[10] 2001	Osteomyelitis, loosening, migration, tendon rupture, nerve injury
	Botte et al,[13] 1992	Infections (7%), loosening (4%), loss of reduction, pin migration, nonunion, tendon/nerve/artery injury
Screw and miniplate treatment	Page & Stern,[3] 1998	Stiffness, nonunion, plate prominence, infection, tendon rupture
	Duncan et al,[1] 1993	Stiffness, contracture, adhesions, nonunions, infection (deep and superficial), delayed union, reflex sympathetic dystrophy, osteomyelitis, late amputations
	Kurzen et al,[14] 2006	Stiffness, plate loosening, infection, chronic pain syndromes

to be more common if pins had to be maintained for as long as 8 weeks.

Page and Stern[3] noted that complications were more frequent with phalangeal fractures and open fractures. Metacarpal fractures and closed fractures regained more than 220° of total active range of motion (76% vs 67%).[3] Only 11% of phalangeal and only 24% of open fractures regained that degree of motion.[3] These investigators suggested that surrounding damage may bias the results with plate fixation being used in complex injuries. These results parallel those of Duncan and colleagues,[1] who cautioned that infection and amputation were related to wound severity. Kurzen and colleagues[14] did not find increased complications with open fractures, soft tissue injuries, occupation, or phalanx level despite using miniplate fixation.

TIMING OF INTERVENTION

Selecting the time to intervene remains controversial. Malalignment, whether rotational or angular, should be addressed in a timely fashion. However, there may not a large amount of bone stock with which to work. Thus, clinicians may want to wait for union before intervention. Prolonged immobilization may lead to stiff joints above and below the injury site. Clinicians may find it better to allow therapy to obtain some function at these joints before addressing alignment. Some patients find that therapy minimizes their perceived disability and choose against surgery.

Each bone and each deformity produce different functional impairments. If the bone has united, a round of therapy may uncover a deficit, if one is present. If little impairment exists, surgery to correct a radiographic appearance may be counterproductive. Phalangeal malalignment can be addressed at the phalanx level or at the metacarpal level. Correction at the metacarpal level is limited to improvement in finger rotation or metacarpal angulation. Freeland and Lindley[8] noted that 1 mm of metacarpal derotation corrects 1 cm of fingertip overlap.

If the malalignment is appreciated early, clinicians can recreate the fracture line. Also known as a nascent malunion, clinicians can use fluoroscopy, a periosteal freer, and judicious use of an osteotome to track the line. However, redevelopment of the fracture should be avoided if the fragments are too small to fix.

DETERMINING THE TREATMENT OF COMPLICATIONS

When considering surgical management, the surgeon should match implants with mobilization needs. Patient comorbidities and compliance also affect success. K-wire stabilization as a construct may not be stable enough to allow early uncontrolled mobilization, but it does have its place with small fractures, especially condylar fragments.[15] A skilled therapist may be able to allow therapy while maintaining stability for healing. In addition, Kirschner wire fixation has known complications up to 18%.[13] Surgeon skill and patient compliance were of concern.[10,13] Osteomyelitis may lead to failures and require repeat surgeries or prolonged intravenous antibiotic treatment.[2,3,13]

If loss of fixation is identified, clinicians should consider whether the fracture is compromised. If not, remove the loose wire and splint if needed. Therapy may only need to be limited for a short period. If compromised, revision surgery is necessary.

The development of smaller implants including miniplates has allowed more flexibility in malunion and nonunion treatment.[8,9,16–18] Although radiographs may look more anatomic, surgical manipulation can induce scarring and stiffness. Surgeon need to use implants with which they are comfortable and that match the characteristics of the fracture. Working within the soft tissue sleeve limits further scarring.[17]

Key to the management of complications is communication with patients and their families or caregivers. Informed consent starts at the initial evaluation. Complications of any care plan are expected and do not represent malpractice.

MALUNIONS

Defined as an abnormal alignment of a healed bone, malunions do not necessitate treatment. Before considering operative intervention, the clinician should work to mobilize the hand. As tendon balance and joint motion return, seemingly significant issues may become unnoticeable. Puckett and colleagues[15] noted significant remodeling in children (aged 2–14 years) with distal condylar malunions of the phalanges. They found complete correction in the sagittal plane and near-complete coronal plane correction.[15] With none of their malunions producing functional issues, they recommended nonsurgical management.[15] Management of parental expectations may be time consuming.

In adults, if a problem is suspected early in treatment, operative intervention on a nascent malunion may allow the clinician to follow the fracture line and recreate the injury. However, if the fragments are too small to fix, patience is warranted. Likewise, manipulating a small fragment or one with a tenuous blood supply may lead to avascular necrosis and potentially a suboptimal outcome. Ring[9] recommended early treatment of articular malunions before bony remodeling occurs.

METACARPAL MALUNION TREATMENT

Freeland and Lindley[8] presented options for malunion management of the phalanges and metacarpals based on degree (**Table 3**). They found that surgery was frequently necessary in the following cases: middle and proximal phalanx sagittal malunions exceeding 15°, articular incongruity, metacarpal sagittal angulation exceeding 30°, and metacarpal rotation exceeding 10°.[8] As Freeland and Lindley[8] noted, additional issues arise with malunions: muscle fatigue, cramping, pseudoclaw deformity, deformity, and prominent metacarpal heads in the palm. Because the index and middle fingers are more fixed than other fingers, they tolerate shortening or angulation worse than the ring and little metacarpals.[8] However, if the angulation is significant, any metacarpal malunion may need treatment (**Fig. 1**).

To address the controversy of accepting 70° of angulation, Ali and colleagues[25] studied the biomechanical effect of angulation on boxer's fractures and found that 30° of angulation resulted in 92% of normal strength and 78% of normal motion. Although they noted that adaptation may alter functional results, they recommended reduction if angulation exceeded 30°.[25]

Meunier and colleagues[26] found that metacarpal shortening affected strength, with 2 mm of shortening producing a minimal 8% loss of power and 10 mm of shortening producing a 45% loss of power from the dorsal interossei. Low and colleagues[27] found that flexion and extension forces were diminished with shortening of more than 3 mm or dorsal angulation greater than 30° in cadaver hands without the ability to adapt. As reviewed in a single cadaver metacarpal, the power of adaptation and sarcomere absorption could not be determined and may not play as dramatic a role.[26,27] Strauch and colleagues[28] found 7° of extensor lag with every 2 mm of metacarpal shortening, possibly affecting flexor power.[19]

Seitz and Fromison[18] noted that rotational deformities produce significant overlap, with 10° of metacarpal rotation producing 2 cm of overlap at the fingertips. Thus, on presentation, alignment should be checked with the fingers extended as well as flexed. As with any fracture management, they recommended that the soft tissues be respected to minimize scarring, adhesions, and contractures.[18] Pichora and colleagues[23] noted that transverse metacarpal osteotomy does not fully correct scissoring from phalangeal malunions. They recommended using a step-cut osteotomy at the site of malunion. Jawa and colleagues[21] thought that a modified step-cut osteotomy at the metacarpal level healed and was successful at derotating both metacarpal and phalangeal malunions. Stable fixation at this level allows early therapy, minimizing stiffness. Metaphyseal-level osteotomies seem to heal better than diaphyseal osteotomies.[8,16] Gross and Gelberman[20] found that metacarpal base osteotomies can correct deformities in the index, middle, and ring fingers of up to 20° and the small finger up to 30°. Because of a lax connection between phalanx and metacarpal,

Table 3		
Potential osteotomies to correct angulation and rotational deformities		
Proximal Phalangeal Fractures		
Rotational malunion	Transverse extra-articular osteotomy at the base	20° index, middle, ring 30° small
Angular malunion	Step cut, opening or closing wedge osteotomies	Dorsal tendon splitting or lateral approach
Metacarpal Fractures		
Angular malunion	Transverse osteotomy at base	—
Angular ± rotational	Closing or opening wedge osteotomy, step cut osteotomy	Wedge design based on length Adjust if rotational deformity present
Articular malunion	Transverse extra-articular osteotomy at the base, osteotomy at the site with sliding osteotomy, or extra-articular osteotomy	—

Data from Refs.[8,13,15,19–24]

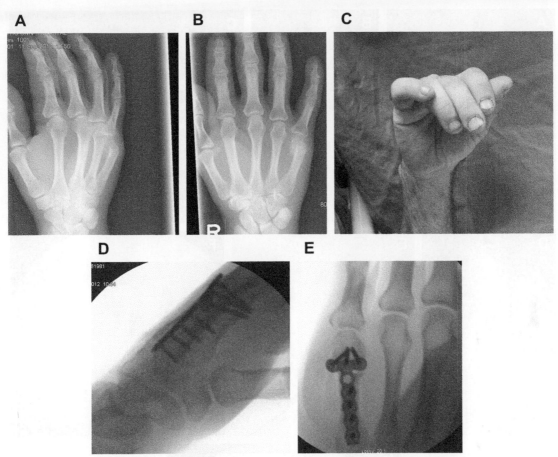

Fig. 1. Individuals can adapt to minor metacarpal deformities because of carpometacarpal motion. However, significant flexion deformities or rotation may need a corrective osteotomy. (*A*) Fifth metacarpal deformity. (*B*) Clinical tenodesis showing scissoring; (*C*, *D*) osteotomy and fixation; (*E*) scissoring corrected. (*Courtesy of* P.J. Stern, MD, Cincinnati, OH.)

they made a key note that metacarpal rotation does not produce the same rotation in the proximal phalanx.[20]

Intra-articular injuries may be hard to define. If one is suspected, a Brewerton view (ball catcher view) may be useful. However, a computed tomography (CT) scan may be of use (**Fig. 2**). Exposure is preformed dorsally, which may require an arthrotomy through the ulnar sagittal band. The joint can be opened, allowing good visualization of the head to place screws outside the articular surface. The band should be repaired on closure and protected for 4 weeks using a P1 blocking splint.

Not every fracture or every digit responds similarly to malunions. A recent European review by Westbrook and colleagues[29] found no difference between surgical and nonsurgical results for neck and shaft fractures of the fifth metacarpal. The Disabilities of the Arm, Shoulder, and Hand (DASH) scores were better for nonsurgical management.

However, neck fractures function differently from shaft fractures.[16,26,27]

PHALANGEAL MALUNION TREATMENT

Proximal phalangeal fractures typically produce a volar apex angulation because of tension on the central slip distally and the lumbrical proximally.[30] With angulation comes shortening, which affects position and function and is significant when more than 15°.[30–33] Coonrad and Pohlman[31] noted that phalanx angulation of more than 25° in older children and adults produced losses in both flexion and extension. Vahey and colleagues[33] noted that shortening by 1 mm produced a resulting extensor lag at the proximal interphalangeal (PIP) joint of 12°. As angulation increased from 16° to 46°, the PIP lags in a cadaver model increased from 10° to 66°.[33] Adhesions may amplify these results. Buchler and colleagues[34] found that 50% of corrective phalangeal osteotomies required

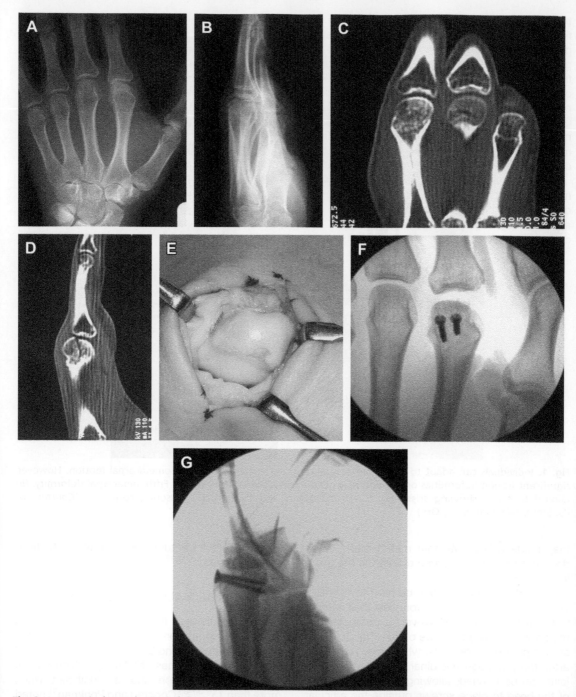

Fig. 2. Intra-articular malunion of the metacarpal head suspected on plain radiographs and caused by failure of therapy. (*A, B*) Plain radiographs. (*C, D*) CT evaluation showing the step-off on the lateral view. (*E*) Intraoperative view showing step-off. (*F, G*) Reduction and fixation with 2 screws that avoid impingement. (*Courtesy of* T.R. Kiefhaber, MD, Cincinnati, OH.)

concurrent tenolysis. Patients with only bony involvement had a 96% rate of good to excellent results. If other structures were involved, the success rate decreased to 64%.[13] Although the osteotomy options are shown in **Table 3**, they

recommended that phalangeal malalignment be treated at the phalanx rather than metacarpal level.[13]

Changes in force at the PIP are also transmitted to the distal interphalangeal (DIP) joint. Based on the pull of the central slip versus the pull of the flexor digitorum superficialis (FDS), middle phalangeal fractures angulate dorsally with fractures proximal to the (FDS) insertion and volarly with fractures distal to the FDS insertion.[8,30] By taking down adhesions at the site rather than working proximally at the metacarpal, Trumble and Gilbert[24] had success with in situ phalanx osteotomies, gaining 10° of motion at the PIP and 10° of motion at the DIP joint. Early motion of the stable construct minimized extensor tendon adhesions.

If a bone spike limits motion, a simple ostectomy may be sufficient. Articular malunions may produce early arthritic damage. Thus, joint replacement or fusion needs to be considered if correction is unfeasible.[8]

When discussing malunion surgery with patients, clinicians must be clear that surgery may be done in stages: malunion correction followed by motion correction. Any surgical approach should protect the soft tissue envelope to avoid compounding the problem. Clinical tenodesis should be done during initial fixation to avoid basing reduction/rotation confirmation on radiographs (**Fig. 3**). Rigid fixation may allow early motion through therapy to minimize scarring and reduce the potential for tenolysis or capsulotomy. Miniplates have allowed rigid fixation using low-profile devices (**Fig. 4**).[8,16] Lag screws can also be used if the spiral fracture line is long enough to accommodate screws (**Fig. 5**). A closing wedge osteotomy can only be used if length has been

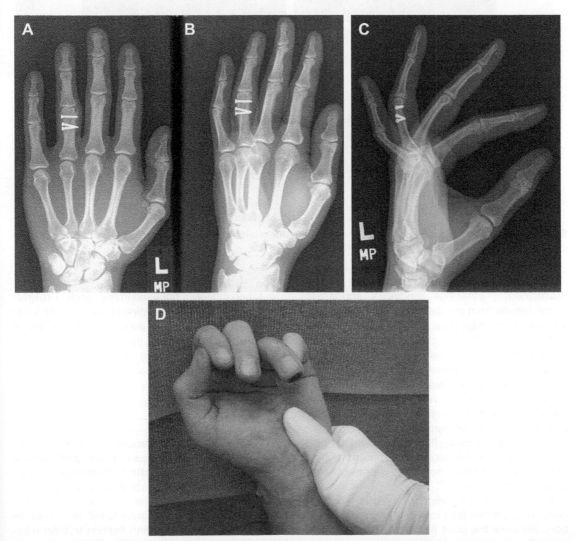

Fig. 3. Rotation; the width of the proximal and distal fragments do not match. (*A*) Posteroanterior view. (*B*) Oblique view with evidence of rotation despite fixation. (*C*) Lateral view with good articular profile. (*D*) Clinical view with obvious rotation. (*Courtesy of* P.J. Stern, MD, Cincinnati, OH.)

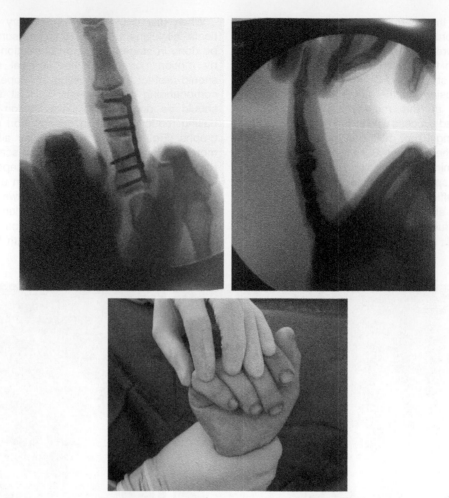

Fig. 4. Surgery to correct rotation done at the site of malunion with takedown of prior hardware and application of new fixation allowing early rehabilitation.

maintained,[18] otherwise tendinous shortening, which results from an opening wedge osteotomy, will create an imbalance of forces (**Fig. 6**). Thus with a shortened bone, clinicians should perform an opening wedge osteotomy.[18] Regardless, once the bone is broken again, healing must be solid enough to allow motion or a nonunion or pseudoarthrosis will result. Potenza and colleagues[35] reported on their outcomes with osteotomy for proximal phalanx malunions. Operating within 6 weeks of injury, they rigidly fixed the fractures at the site. Although posttraumatic arthritis may not be avoided, motion, grip strength, and appearance improved.[35]

The pull of the flexor digitorum profundus at the distal phalanx can lead to shortening and angulation. Because the bone fragments may be small, reduction may require K wires and immobilization until healed (see **Fig. 6**; **Figs. 7** and **8**). Condylar fractures are notoriously unstable and should be watched closely if not fixed immediately. Proximal migration can lead to joint instability, an intra-articular step-off, and angulation (see **Fig. 8**; **Fig. 9**). To avoid arthritis, the joint needs to be leveled. If the fragment is too small, the articular fragment should be elevated and supported by a plate and bone graft.[8]

NONUNIONS

A nonunion can be atrophic or hypertrophic. Atrophic nonunions require bone graft and a healthy bed. A hypertrophic nonunion needs stability to heal. Although controversial, the use of an ultrasound-based bone stimulator has shown bony union after bone graft failed in a phalanx treated with osteotomy and fixation to treat a hyperextension malunion (see **Fig. 6**).

Ring[9] noted that amputation or arthrodesis were useful treatment options, especially if the

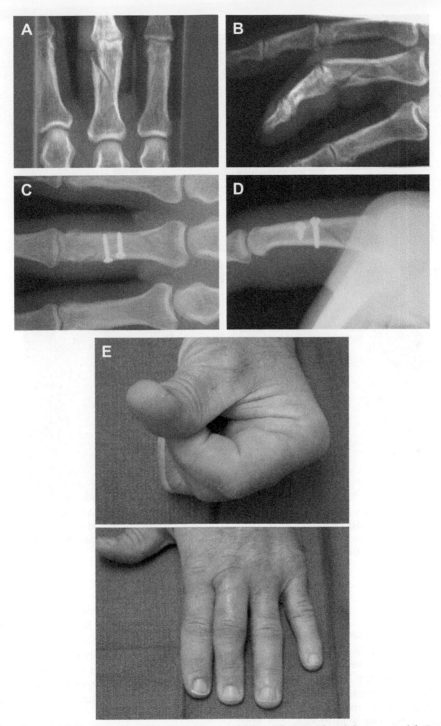

Fig. 5. (*A*) Proximal phalanx fracture with malalignment (*B*) lateral view of malalignment. (*C*) Osteotomy and fixation with screws. (*D*) Lateral view of reduced fracture. (*E*) Clinical views of osteotomy.

associated soft tissue components were compromised. Surgery for nonunions or malunions improved alignment and stability but resulted in modest motion improvement.[9]

Soft tissue trauma, smoking, and infection can also lead to nonunion. The nonunion may need to be debrided and grafted. Secure fixation allows early mobilization in a protected splint (**Fig. 10**).

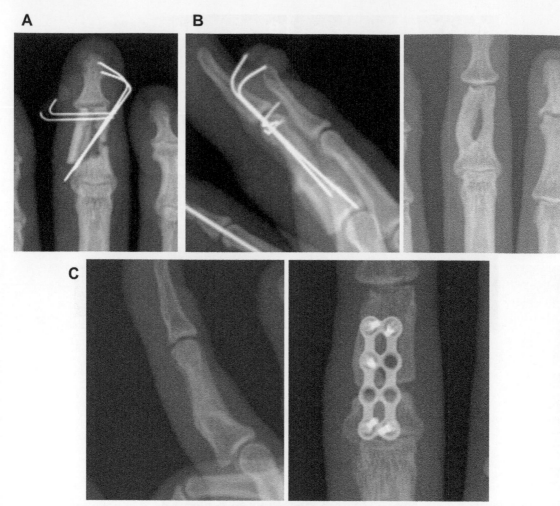

Fig. 6. Near amputation with significant open injuries leading to K-wire fixation. Although healed, a malunion resulted. Surgery to correct the malunion led to a nonunion. Plate fixation required a second surgery with bone grafting and a bone stimulator to get union. (*A*) Initial reduction. (*B*) Healed malunion in extension. (*C*) After osteotomy. (*D*) Nonunion with bone graft. (*E*) Union after bone stimulation.

STIFFNESS

A common misstep is prolonged immobilization while waiting to see bony remodeling. Phalanx fractures heal within 4 weeks, although radiographic incorporation may be delayed. Therapy can be advanced when tenderness starts to disappear. By encouraging motion, the patient's swelling, which interferes with motion, can start to decrease. Judicious use of a splint allows the patient to be active in controlled environments.

Adjusting therapy to fit fixation and injury optimizes the patient's outcome. However, it is not guaranteed. Crush injuries damage every structure from skin to bone. Early motion is better than immobilization in minimizing adhesions. However, fracture fixation or healing must withstand these

efforts. Ring[9] recommended large implants to allow early motion to limit the potential for stiffness. Limiting immobilization to the affected digit may help. Staging intervention is important. Clinicians should aim for a stable fracture fixation or healing before attempting a tenolysis or capsulotomy. The soft tissue should be pliable as swelling results from releases.

Despite literature by Young and colleagues[11] predicting improvement by up to 70°, restoration of normal motion is incomplete. A major point they mention in passing was that 608 patients out of 749 had satisfactory results with therapy and only 61 of the 141 unsatisfied patients had surgery.[11] The PIP joints were more involved. Their technique is described in **Table 4**. A K wire was

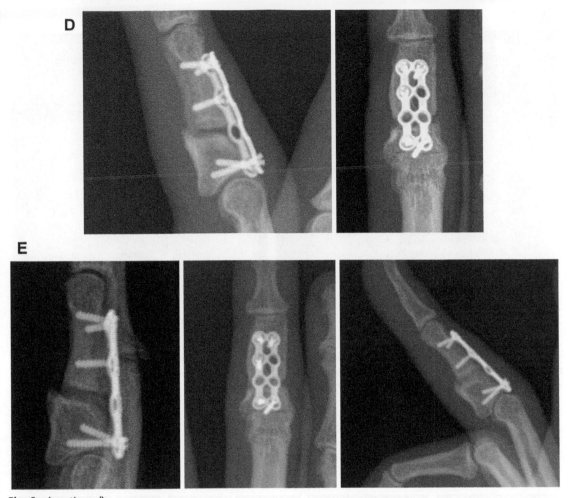

Fig. 6. (*continued*)

used for 2 weeks to immobilize the joint in extension if a flexion deformity was present in Young and colleagues'[11] study. Regardless of the stiffness, therapy was started intensively within days of surgery.

Gould and Nicholson[36] found that functional improvement exceeded motion gains of less than 20°. Patient expectations should match probabilities to avoid disappointment. Using stringent exclusion criteria, Creighton and Steichen[6] reviewed the result of extensor tenolysis. Their indication for tenolysis was an active extensor lag in a supple digit after appropriate therapy (**Fig. 11**).[6] Dorsal capsulotomy was added if passive flexion was limited despite extensor tenolysis.[6] Those digits with an extensor tenolysis alone improved in total active motion (TAM) by 54° and in active extensor lag by 8°.[6] When an additional dorsal capsulotomy was needed, TAM improved by 34° and active extensor lag worsened by 4°.[6]

Faruqui and colleagues[7] noted that extra-articular cross pinning or transarticular pinning of proximal third phalangeal fractures had equal results but nearly 30% of patients had a fixed flexion contracture (at least 15°) at the PIP joint. Although pinning limited soft tissue injury with an open technique, the complication rate remained high, with 8 patients requiring secondary procedures.[7]

Freeland and Orbay[16] noted that results of open reduction and internal fixation with miniplates and small screws provided satisfactory stability and similar results to K-wire fixation. To avoid tendon adhesions over the lateral plate or screws, they recommended excising the lateral band and oblique fibers of the extensor mechanism on the same side.[16] Even small amounts of flexor glides limited postoperative adhesions.[16,37,38]

Requiring a delicate balance between ligaments, bone, and tendon functions, joint dynamics

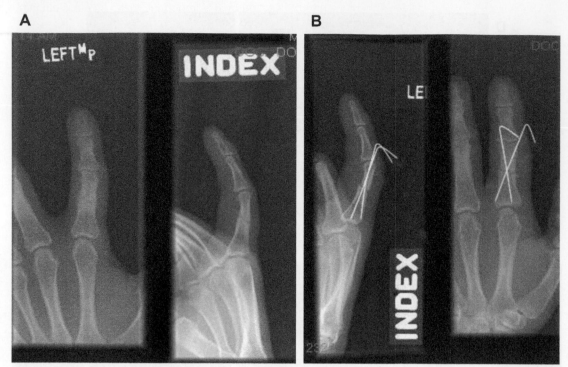

Fig. 7. (*A*) Preoperative films of a proximal phalanx malunion. (*B*) Postoperative films after reduction and fixation with crossed K wires. (*Courtesy of* P.J. Stern, MD, Cincinnati, OH.)

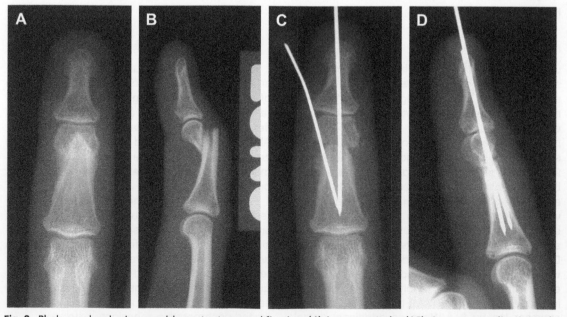

Fig. 8. Phalangeal malunion requiring osteotomy and fixation. (*A*) Anteroposterior (AP) view not revealing joint abnormality. (*B*) Lateral view showing deformity. (*C*) AP view showing osteotomy and correction with divergent K wires to prevent rotation. (*D*) Lateral view showing restoration of alignment. (*Courtesy of* P.J. Stern, MD, Cincinnati, OH.)

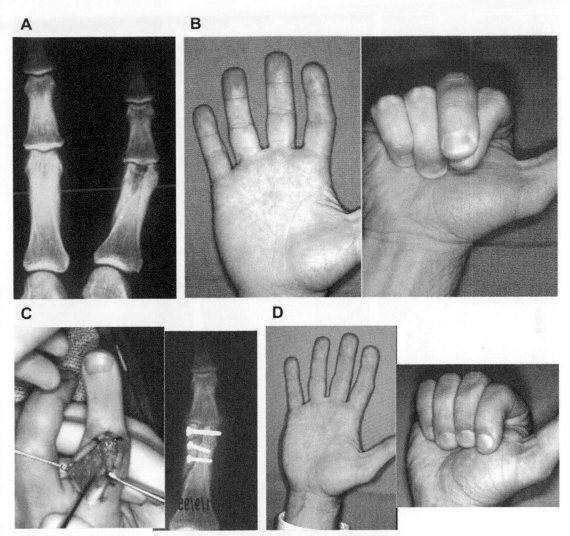

Fig. 9. (*A*) An intra-articular phalanx fracture with malunion and angulation. (*B*) Scissoring. (*C*) Intraoperative view as the fracture line is identified and recreated while being fixed with screws. (*D*) Motion improvement. (*Courtesy of* P.J. Stern, MD, Cincinnati, OH.)

are easily disrupted by a variety of injuries. Even without injury, these structures become less pliable with immobilization and thus produce a stiff finger (**Fig. 12**). This tendency highlights why unaffected joints need to be kept mobile, immobilization time limited, and the joints placed in a safe position.[37,38] Although all digits matter, stiffness in a central digit affects the hand's function to a larger degree. Some distal gliding must be allowed in the extensor system, if possible with DIP blocking exercises.[38] Proximal adhesions in the extensor mechanism can produce a PIP extensor lag.[33,37] A flexion contracture at the PIP joint can produce a compensatory hyperextension metacarpophalangeal (MCP) deformity that may respond to dorsal blocking splinting with stretching and strengthening.[38]

LAXITY

Although similar to stiffness, lag produces limits in motion secondary to disruption of the delicate balance of extensor and flexor forces across the hand.[30,38] Tendon balance remains essential to move 3 joints at the finger level while maintaining stability. Proximal phalanx fractures can disrupt this balance by shortening or angulation.[38] Using a cadaveric study for extensor lag at the PIP joint, Beekman and colleagues[32] recommended release of the extensor digitorum communis (EDC) from the MCP capsule, release of juncturae tendinae, and transfer of the sagittal bands to the EDC.

Bony injuries to the base of the proximal phalanx can disrupt the balance of the collateral ligaments because the joint balance between these

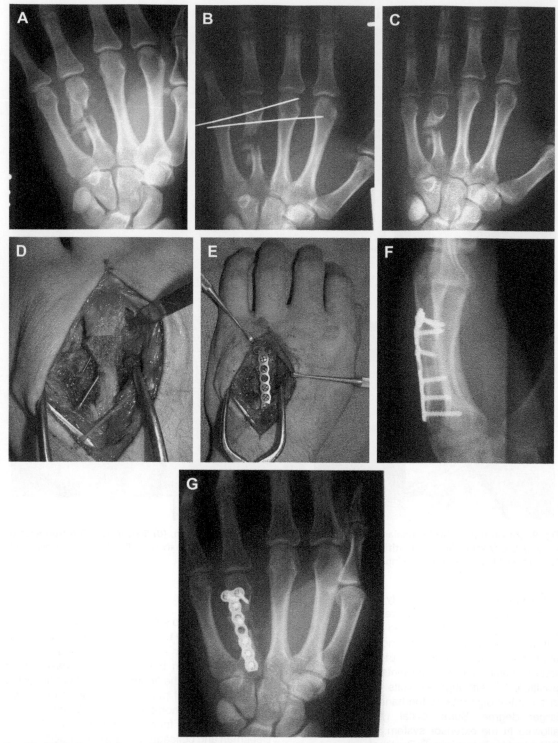

Fig. 10. (*A*) Rollover injury with open metacarpal fracture in a smoker. (*B*) After irrigation and debridement of devitalized tissue. (*C*) After antibiotic treatment of osteomyelitis, showing nonunion. (*D*) Bone graft and provisional fixation after infection has been cleared. (*E*) Fixation. (*F, G*) Healed construct. (*Courtesy of* P.J. Stern.)

Table 4
Recommended approaches to releasing stiff joints

Stiff Joint	Sequence of Release
MP stiff in extension	Release (1) skin and extensor from capsule, (2) dorsal capsule, (3) articular surface and volar pouch, (4) dorsal half of collateral ligaments
MP stiff in flexion	Release (1) skin, (2) adhesions of long flexors, (3) volar plate, (4) volar half of the collateral ligaments
PIP stiff in extension	Release (1) skin, (2) extensor from capsule (preserve central slip), (3) dorsal capsule, (4) dorsal third to half of collateral ligaments
PIP stiff in flexion	Release (1) skin, (2) retinacular ligaments, (3) adhesions of long flexors, (4) volar half of the collateral ligaments, (5) volar plate

Abbreviation: MP, metatarsophalangeal joint.
Data from Refs.[6,11,34]

structures, the capsule, and tendons is precarious.[38] Although a bony injury may heal, a residual laxity or a joint step-off may persist. Because the PIP joint is essential to hand function,[38] disrupting a central digit interferes with hand use. An intraarticular osteotomy may need to be considered. Early treatment of a nascent malunion makes the osteotomy easier than allowing it to remodel before osteotomy. Adhesions around the PIP joint and hyperextension deformities may affect the DIP as well.[38] Hyperextension at the PIP or metatarsophalangeal (MP) joint may be rebalanced with a splint at times.[38]

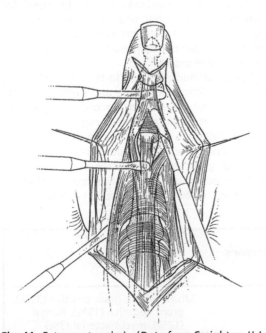

Fig. 11. Extensor tenolysis. (*Data from* Creighton JJ Jr, Steichen JB. Complications in phalangeal and metacarpal fracture management: results of extensor tenolysis. Hand Clin 1994; 10(1):112.)

INFECTION

Infections can be superficial or deep. A superficial infection may result from K-wire loosening. Removal of the causative agent and a short course of oral antibiotics may be sufficient. A deep infection resulting in osteomyelitis or an abscess requires prompt surgical management. If the fixation is stable, debridement and intravenous antibiotic up to 6 weeks in duration may be needed. Pan culture is important to define the causative organism and tailor the treatment (**Table 5**). If the fixation is unstable, it should be removed, external fixation should be considered, and it should be treated as discussed earlier. Once the site is clean, fixation may be done or salvage procedures may be necessary (see **Figs. 10** and **11**). Because open fracture has a higher rate of infections and poor outcomes,[1,3,39–41] patients and families should be aware that an infection is not a complication as much as an expected result. McClain and colleagues[39] found an infection rate of 0% for type 1 fractures, 9% for type 2 fractures, and 14% for type 3 fractures. Duncan and colleagues[1] postulated that surgery converted lower grade types to higher grade injuries with dissection. Reviewing the literature, Gonzalez and colleagues[40] noted that prompt and thorough irrigation and debridement of an open fracture might allow a more judicious use of antibiotics. Debridement is important with osteomyelitis. Packing or the use of antibiotic beads minimizes dead space. The alignment and space can be maintained with K wires and/or external fixation devices[40] until the soft tissues tolerate reconstruction, fixation, or flap coverage.

Aggressive surgical care and appropriate antibiotic use may not result in a functional finger (see **Fig. 10**; **Fig. 13**). Although dated, Reilly and colleagues[4] found the amputation rate to be 39%, especially if multiple procedures were

A   **B**

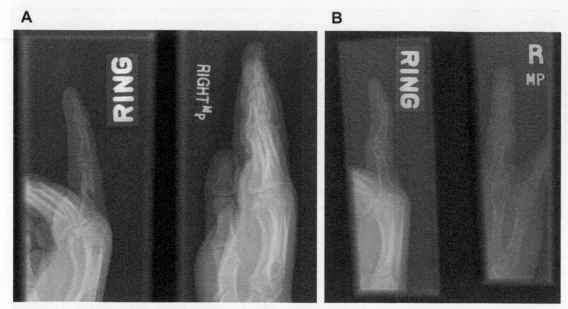

Fig. 12. The balance between bone length and position affects tendon function. Thus allowing a phalanx to heal in distraction leads to stiffness. (*A*) Position of initial immobilization after K wires were removed at another facility. (*B*) Phalanx has healed but the patient is stiff on presentation 1 year later, requiring a tenolysis that allowed full motion.

necessary or care was delayed. Regardless of negative studies, one should follow their clinical judgement in providing care as indicated. Cultures were positive 74% of the time.[4] Comorbidities included vascular insufficiency or immunocompromise. Gonzalez and colleagues[40] and Honda and McDonald[2] presented an approach to management based on the source, noting a difference in organism type depending on bites, source of contamination, postprocedure, or hematogenous spread. They recommended a combined approach of surgical debridement and culture and a medical approach of tailored antibiotic delivery for 4 to 6 weeks.

PAIN

Acute pain represents the normal response of the body to injury. When it persists, causative issues need to be considered from nerve injury, instability, or stiffness. Injury alters the perception of self and may be a major factor in the patient's ability to recover. Narcotics should not be used casually or for extended periods of time. Nonsteroidal antiinflammatory medications can be used for pain relief and to decrease swelling. However, long-term use may interfere with healing because the initial stages of bone healing depend on an inflammatory response.[41,42]

Despite administrative efforts to quantify pain, it remains difficult to define and treat. Clinicians must be careful to discern a slightly exaggerated pain response from a complex regional pain syndrome. Although their existence and diagnosis remain controversial, it is desirable to avoid the cycle of pain, swelling, disuse, and stiffness that can occur with even minor injuries. Therapy becomes a key step once healing allows

Table 5		
Studies reviewing causes and causative agents for infections		
Study	**Causation**	**Organism**
Reilly et al,[4] 1997	Posttraumatic (57%), postoperative (15%), hematogenous (13%), contiguous spread (9%)	Mixed (35%), gram positive (35%), gram negative (15%), fungal (12%), mycobacterial (3%)
Honda & McDonald,[2] 2009	Penetrating trauma, soil or water contamination	Depends on source

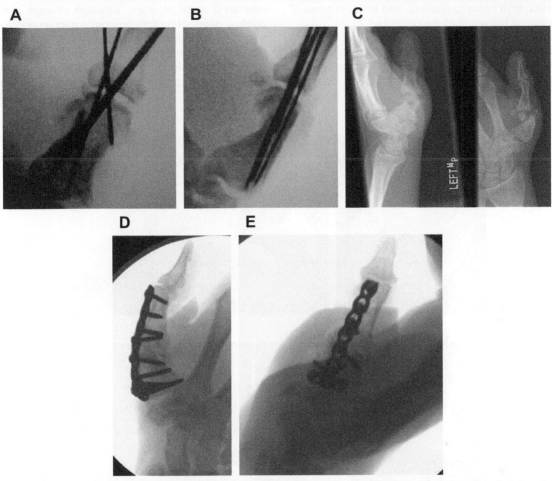

Fig. 13. (*A, B*) Fixed head of a proximal phalanx. (*C*) Collapse secondary to infection. (*D, E*) An arthrodesis for stable thumb. (*Courtesy of* P.J. Stern, MD, Cincinnati, OH.)

intervention.[8,16,18,37] If a patient provides a history of risk, the clinician might consider limiting immobilization. Surgery with early motion is an option if the fracture is displaced. If nondisplaced, the clinician may try to mobilize adjacent joints and digits to minimize swelling and stiffness. Once healed, the use of stress loading and contrast baths has a place in the therapist's tools. Some physicians have found the use of a transcutaneous electrical nerve stimulation unit to be helpful in short-circuiting the patient's perception of pain. With less pain, patients can participate with therapy and break the cycle of pain and stiffness.

If nerve injury/compression is suspected as the source, the cause should be addressed if possible. Gabapentin or pregabapentin medications may help patients with their pain perception and function but should be provided as part of multimodality care monitored by a pain management specialist. Vascular spasticity may benefit from

low-dose calcium channel blockers, such as norvasc 2.5 or 5 mg nightly, especially with cold weather or cold temperature exposure. Joint injury can produce an ache that worsens with heavy use[38]; expected to decrease over the first year, persistence of pain may indicate degeneration and arthritis.[38]

ROLE OF THERAPY

Although discounted by many outside of medicine (possibly by the patient as well), appropriate therapy can make a significant difference in a patient's outcome. Surgeons understand the key role that therapists play in optimizing a patient's results. The motivated individual may succeed without a therapist's guidance. However, a therapist can guide most patients and advance them safely to coordinate fracture stability with intervention. Seitz and Fromison[18] noted that appropriate therapy is mandatory. However, insurers limit or prohibit visits, shift costs to patients, and limit the types of covered therapy that are permitted.

Hardy[37] promoted a 3-step process: maintain fracture stability for healing, mobilize soft tissue while maintaining integrity, and remodel any restrictive scar. He detailed therapy for fractures over an 8-week program, although strength and passive range of motion programs may extend to a year. In addition, he recommended different exercises and splints to avoid common problems of stiffness, lag, and deformities. It is paramount to restrict immobilization and to position the hand in

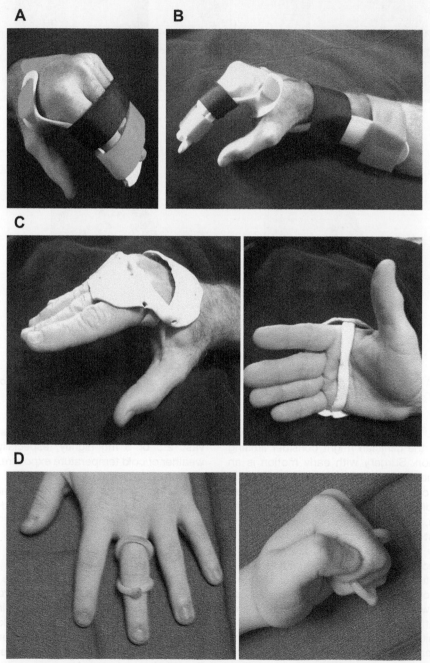

Fig. 14. Therapy and splinting allow patients to focus their efforts on rebalancing joint forces as well as avoiding being placed in an unacceptable position. (*A, B*) Resting hand splint to keep balance while doing therapy out of splint. (*C*) MP flexion splint blocking the MCP joint but allowing full PIP and DIP motion. (*D*) Figure-of-eight or dorsal blocking splints at the PIP help restore MP and DIP balance. (*Courtesy of* O.T. Robert Schneider, CHT, Cincinnati, OH.)

a safe position. As Agee[30] noted, appropriate splinting limits joint stiffness, which allows focused therapy (**Fig. 14**). Therapy also works to control edema. Swelling prevents motion and engenders stiffness: a vicious cycle. Edema management can include reversed isotoner gloves, a warm-up to start therapy, and a cool-down to prevent rebound swelling. Although theoretically interfering with bone growth, nonsteroidal antiinflammatory medications can help limit scarring and its resultant stiffness[37,43] and may be used after healing begins. Duncan and colleagues[1] defined their program as elevation to reduce edema, active range of motion until healed, and strengthening once healed.

SUMMARY

Complications occur when hand fractures are treated, whether surgically or nonsurgically. Open fractures, a common occurrence, have more complications than closed injuries. A surgeon should not assume that a complication equals a failure of skill. However, ignoring the problem does not help the patient. Matching the treatment with the problem and to the patient helps to improve an outcome. A perfect radiograph does not correlate with a perfect result. Therapy helps to minimize issues like swelling and adhesions, which impair function and satisfaction.

REFERENCES

1. Duncan RW, Freeland AE, Jabaley ME, et al. Open hand fractures: an analysis of the recovery of active motion and of complications. J Hand Surg 1993;18: 387–94.
2. Honda H, McDonald JR. Current recommendations in the management of osteomyelitis of the hand and wrist. J Hand Surg 2009;34(6):1135–6.
3. Page SM, Stern PJ. Complications and range of motion following plate fixation of metacarpal and phalangeal fractures. J Hand Surg 1998;23:827–32.
4. Reilly KE, Linz JC, Stern PJ, et al. Osteomyelitis of the tubular bones of the hand. J Hand Surg Am 1997;22(4):644–9.
5. Balaram AK, Bednar MS. Complications after the fractures of metacarpal and phalanges. Hand Clin 2010;26(2):169–77.
6. Creighton JJ Jr, Steichen JB. Complications in phalangeal and metacarpal fracture management: results of extensor tenolysis. Hand Clin 1994;10(1): 111–6.
7. Faruqui S, Stern PJ, Kiefhaber TR. Percutaneous pinning of fractures in the proximal third of the proximal phalanx: complications and outcomes. J Hand Surg 2012;37(7):1342–8.
8. Freeland A, Lindley SG. Malunions of the finger metacarpals and phalanges. Hand Clin 2006;22(3): 341–55.
9. Ring D. Malunion and nonunion of the metacarpals and phalanges. Instr Course Lect 2006;55: 121–8.
10. Stahl S, Schwartz O. Complications of K-wire fixation of fractures and dislocations in the hand and wrist. Arch Orthop Trauma Surg 2001;121(9):527–30.
11. Young VL, Wray RC Jr, Weeks PM. The surgical management of stiff joints in the hand. Plast Reconstr Surg 1978;62(6):835–41.
12. Sirota MA, Parks BG, Higgins JP, et al. Stability of fixation of proximal phalanx unicondylar fractures of the hand: a biomechanical study. J Hand Surg 2013;38(1):77–81.
13. Botte MJ, Davis JL, Rose BA, et al. Complications of smooth pin fixation of fractures and dislocations in the hand and wrist. Clin Orthop Relat Res 1992;(276):194–201.
14. Kurzen P, Fusetti C, Bonaccio M, et al. Complications after plate fixation of phalangeal fractures. J Trauma 2006;60(4):841–3.
15. Puckett BN, Gaston RG, Peljovich AE, et al. Remodeling potential of phalangeal distal condylar malunions in children. J Hand Surg 2012;37:34–41.
16. Freeland AE, Orbay JL. Extraarticular hand fractures in adults: a review of new developments. Clin Orthop Relat Res 2006;445:133–45.
17. Henry M. Soft tissue sleeve approach to open reduction and internal fixation of proximal phalangeal fractures. Tech Hand Up Extrem Surg 2008; 12(3):161–5.
18. Seitz WH Jr, Fromison AI. Management of malunited fractures of the metacarpal and phalangeal shafts. Hand Clin 1988;4(3):529–36.
19. Birndorf MS, Daley R, Greenwald DP. Metacarpal fracture angulation decreases flexor mechanical efficiency in human hands. Plast Reconstr Surg 1997; 99(4):1079–83.
20. Gross MS, Gelberman RH. Metacarpal rotational osteotomy. J Hand Surg 1985;10:105–8.
21. Jawa A, Zucchini M, Lauri G, et al. Modified step-cut osteotomy for metacarpal and phalangeal rotational deformity. J Hand Surg 2009;34(2):335–40.
22. Manktelow RT, Mahoney JL. Step osteotomy: a precise rotation osteotomy to correct scissoring deformities of the fingers. Plast Reconstr Surg 1981; 68(4):571–6.
23. Pichora DR, Meyer R, Masear VR. Rotational step-cut osteotomy for treatment of metacarpal and phalangeal malunions. J Hand Surg 1991;16(3):551–5.
24. Trumble T, Gilbert M. In situ osteotomy for extraarticular malunion of the proximal phalanx. J Hand Surg 1998;23:821–6.

25. Ali A, Hamman J, Mass DP. The biomechanical effects of angulated boxer's fractures. J Hand Surg 1999;24:835–44.

26. Meunier MJ, Hentzen E, Ryan M, et al. Predicted effects of metacarpal shortening on interosseous muscle function. J Hand Surg 1998;29(4):689–93.

27. Low CK, Wong HC, Low YP, et al. A cadaver study of the effects of dorsal angulation and shortening of the metacarpal shaft on the extension and flexion ratios of the index and small fingers. J Hand Surg 1995; 20(5):609–13.

28. Strauch RJ, Rosenwasser MP, Lunt JG. Metacarpal shaft fractures: the effect of shortening on the extensor mechanism. J Hand Surg 1998;23: 519–23.

29. Westbrook AP, Davis TR, Armstrong D, et al. The clinical significance of malunions of fractures of the neck and shaft of the little finger metacarpal. J Hand Surg 2008;33B(6):732–9.

30. Agee J. Treatment principles for proximal and middle phalangeal fractures. Orthop Clin North Am 1992;23(1):35–40.

31. Coonrad RW, Pohlman MH. Impacted fractures in the proximal phalanx of the finger. J Bone Joint Surg Am 1969;51(7):1291–6.

32. Beekman RA, Abbot AE, Taylor NL, et al. Extensor mechanism slide for the treatment of proximal phalangeal joint extension lag: an anatomical study. J Hand Surg 2004;29(6):1063–8.

33. Vahey JW, Wegner DA, Hastings H III. Effect of proximal phalangeal fracture deformity on extensor tendon function. J Hand Surg 1998;23:673–81.

34. Buchler U, Gupta A, Ruf S. Corrective osteotomy for post-traumatic malunion of the phalanges in the hand. J Hand Surg 1996;21(1):33–42.

35. Potenza V, De Luna V, Maglione P, et al. Post-traumatic malunions of the proximal phalanx of the finger. Medium-term results in 24 cases treated by "in situ" osteotomy. Open Orthop J 2012;6:468–72.

36. Gould JS, Nicholson BG. Capsulectomy of the metacarpophalangeal and proximal interphalangeal joints. J Hand Surg 1979;4(5):482–6.

37. Hardy MA. Principles of metacarpal and phalangeal fracture management: a review of rehabilitation concepts. J Orthop Sports Phys Ther 2004; 34(12):781–99.

38. Chinchalkar SJ, Gan BS. Management of proximal interphalangeal joint fractures and dislocations. J Hand Ther 2003;16:117–28.

39. McClain RF, Steyers C, Stoddard M. Infections in open fractures of the hand. J Hand Surg 1991;16:108–12.

40. Gonzalez MH, Bach HG, Elhassan BT, et al. Management of open hand fractures. J Am Soc Surg Hand 2003;3(4):208–18.

41. Harder AT, An YH. The mechanisms of the inhibitory effects of non-steroidal anti-inflammatory drugs on bone healing: a concise review. J Clin Pharmacol 2003;43(8):807–15.

42. Thaller J, Walker M, Kline AJ, et al. The effect of nonsteroidal anti-inflammatory agents on spinal fusion. Orthopedics 2005;28(3):299–303.

43. Chow SP, Pun WK, So YC, et al. A prospective study of 245 open digital fractures of the hand. J Hand Surg 1996;16:137–40.

Outcomes of Hand Fracture Treatments

Paul C. Baldwin, MD, Jennifer Moriatis Wolf, MD*

KEYWORDS

- Hand • Outcomes • Metacarpal • Phalanges • Fracture • Recovery • Function

KEY POINTS

- Clinicians and researchers should use established and validated outcomes measures when assessing objective and subjective functional recovery.
- The 36-Item Short Form Health Survey is designed to assess the general health of a population and is therefore not specific to the function of the extremity or the hand.
- The Disabilities of the Shoulder, Arm, and Hand (DASH) questionnaire is a validated subjective outcomes measure of the upper extremity. Its use is well described in evaluating hand fracture outcomes, but concurrent injuries to the ipsilateral upper extremity as well as lower extremity injuries can negatively affect the reported DASH score.
- The Patient-rated Wrist Hand Evaluation is a reliable and validated outcomes measure that has been used to assess patients with hand fractures. It has been shown to be more responsive than the DASH when specifically evaluating patients with hand and wrist injuries.
- The Michigan Hand Questionnaire was specifically designed to subjectively evaluate the outcomes of patients with disorders of the hand. Although sensitive to detecting clinical changes in function, it has shown decreased correlation with overall patient disability.
- The Jebsen-Taylor Hand Function Test is a validated, objective measure of hand functional capacity and its use is well established in the analysis of numerous disorders of the hand and fingers.
- Physical examination is fundamental to predicting overall functional outcomes of the hand. However, normative values vary depending on age, gender, and hand dominance. Also, in certain situations the contralateral hand is not an accurate functional control.
- Radiographic assessment is an important aspect of the overall outcome following hand fractures, although radiographic findings do not always correlate with functional recovery.
- To date, a single, gold-standard outcomes assessment tool has yet to be identified. A combination of the currently established and validated outcome measurements may be required to comprehensively evaluate function, pain, disability, and treatment response.

INTRODUCTION

When evaluating outcome measures in medicine, the goal of any analysis should be to determine the beneficial or detrimental effect of a given intervention on a specific condition, disease, or injury. For an outcome measure to be helpful, it must be readily understood and administered and have been proved valid and consistent over a variety of demographic and cultural groups. The results of a reliable outcome measure should help predict the outcome of a treatment in a given patient population and guide future treatments for overall patient benefit.

The bones of the hand are the most commonly injured part of the body, with fractures of the phalanges and metacarpals (**Figs. 1–4**) accounting for

Department of Orthopaedic Surgery, New England Musculoskeletal Institute, University of Connecticut Health Center, 263 Farmington Avenue, Farmington, CT 06030, USA
* Corresponding author.
E-mail address: jmwolf@uchc.edu

Hand Clin 29 (2013) 621–630
http://dx.doi.org/10.1016/j.hcl.2013.08.013
0749-0712/13/$ – see front matter © 2013 Elsevier Inc. All rights reserved.

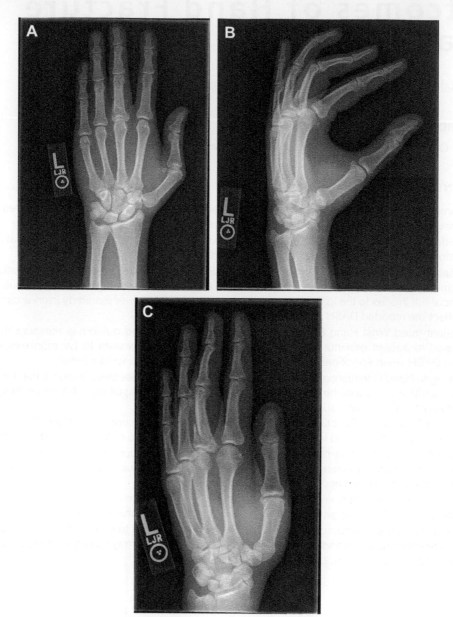

Fig. 1. Posteroanterior (*A*), lateral (*B*), and oblique (*C*) views of the hand showing a displaced fracture of the base of the middle finger proximal phalanx.

up to 10% of all fractures of the axial skeletal system.[1–4] Hand fractures are most commonly observed in men during the second and third decades of life, resulting from trauma or industry-related injuries in up to 50% of cases.[4] Most phalangeal and metacarpal fractures can be treated nonoperatively; however, certain fracture types warrant surgical intervention.[3,5,6] Numerous surgical techniques have been described in the treatment of phalangeal and metacarpal fractures. The specific technique used depends on the characteristics of the fracture and the preferences of the surgeon. Possible surgical treatment options include[6]:

- Closed reduction and percutaneous pin fixation
- External fixation
- Open reduction with internal fixation

The commonly used implant types for fixation include[6]:

- Kirschner wires (K wires)
- Composite wiring
- Intramedullary devices
- Interfragmentary fixation
- Plate and screw constructs (**Figs. 5** and **6**)

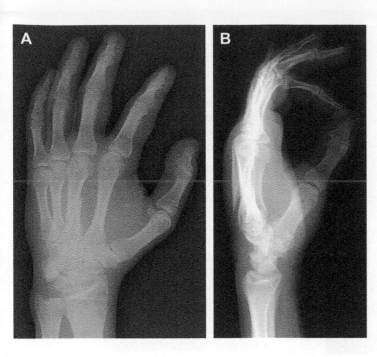

Fig. 2. Oblique (*A*) and lateral (*B*) radiographs showing a displaced fracture of the middle finger metacarpal mid-shaft.

Several outcome measures have been used to evaluate the results of the various treatment modalities for hand fractures. These include:

- Objective measures
- Patient-based subjective measures
- Radiographic assessments

At present, no single outcome measure is widely accepted as the gold standard by which to accurately predict function after treatment. In this article, an evidence-based evaluation of the advantages and disadvantages for each outcome measure and their practicality for use in clinical practice is provided.

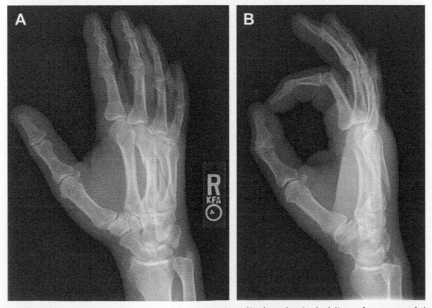

Fig. 3. Oblique (*A*) and lateral (*B*) radiographs demonstrating displaced spiral oblique fractures of the middle and ring metacarpals.

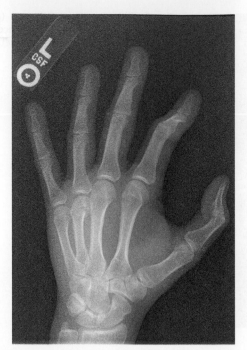

Fig. 4. Posteroanterior radiograph showing fracture of the ring metacarpal neck.

GENERAL PATIENT-REPORTED SUBJECTIVE OUTCOMES
The 36-Item Short Form Health Survey

The 36-Item Short Form Health Survey (SF-36) is a commonly used outcome measure used to evaluate the general health of a population. Originally developed in 1980 as a 108-item questionnaire for the insurance industry, it was designed for use in general population surveys, health population evaluations, research, and clinical practice.[7,8] Because the original survey was lengthy and difficult to use in clinical practice, the abbreviated SF-36 was created.

It focuses on 8 health concepts[7]:

- Limitations in physical activities because of health problems
- Limitations in social activities because of physical or emotional problems
- Limitations in usual role activities because of physical health problems
- Bodily pain
- General mental health (psychological distress and well-being)
- Limitations in usual role activities because of emotional problems
- Vitality (energy and fatigue)
- General health perceptions

The condensed version has proved to be highly reliable and reproducible in validation studies by Brazier and colleagues.[8] Given its relative ease of use and established validity, the SF-36 has been translated and validated in multiple languages and is commonly used as a reference standard when developing new outcome measures.

In the analysis of hand fracture treatment outcomes, Hornbach and Cohen[9] used a subset

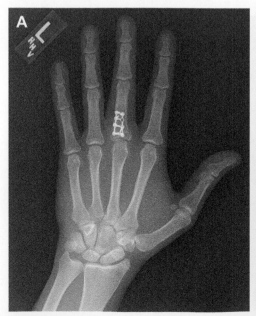

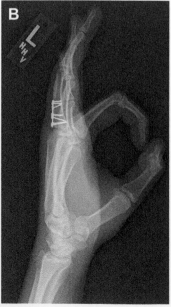

Fig. 5. Mini-plate and screw fixation of a fracture of the base of the proximal phalanx, shown in posteroanterior (*A*) and lateral (*B*) radiographs.

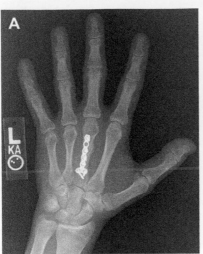
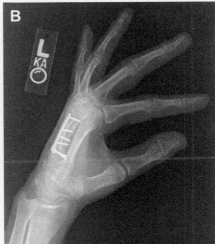

Fig. 6. Plate and screw fixation of the displaced metacarpal shaft fracture of the middle finger metacarpal, shown on posteroanterior (*A*) and lateral (*B*) radiographs.

analysis of the SF-36 in the postoperative evaluation of patients following closed reduction and percutaneous pinning (CRPP) of proximal phalanx fractures. In this study, analysis of the average SF-36 component scores showed no abnormalities, but individual subscales showed differences in patients with malrotation.

A Swedish study prospectively analyzed patients with injuries to the hand and forearm and the associated effects of these injuries on general health, function, health care costs, and societal costs using the SF-36 and the Disabilities of the Arm, Shoulder, and Hand (DASH) scores, with hand fractures representing 38% of all injuries in this study. Small to minimal differences were noted in physical and pain subsets and correlated with the results observed from the DASH scores.[10]

Although the SF-36 has proved to be a reliable and valid tool for outcome measures, it also has limitations. The SF-36, and its 108-item predecessor, were designed to assess the general health of a population and are therefore not specific to the extremity or the hand. As such, it has few questions that are affected by limitations of the upper extremity and is not ideal for analyzing local symptoms or function.[10,11] Medical, mental, and physical comorbidities that affect global health can negatively skew the overall SF-36 score of a patient with a hand injury.

EXTREMITY-SPECIFIC PATIENT-REPORTED SPECIFIC OUTCOMES
DASH Questionnaire

Created in 1996 by Hudak and colleagues,[12] the DASH questionnaire is a patient-rated outcomes measure that evaluates the upper extremity as a single functional unit.[13] The developers' goal was to provide a subjective means of evaluating patients' upper extremity outcomes distinct from objective data measures such as radiographic and physical examination findings. The questionnaire consists of 30-items with 5 possible responses for each item. The DASH is scored from 0 to 100, with 0 being no disability and 100 being maximum disability. Two optional 4-item scales measure the ability to play sports or a musical instrument, and the ability to work.[14] Since its inception in 1996, the DASH assessment has been validated as an outcome measure in multiple languages.[13–15]

Gummesson and colleagues[15] performed a longitudinal study of treatment effects to determine a clinically significant change in DASH outcome after surgical treatment of upper extremity problems. A difference of 19 points on the DASH corresponded with a change of much better or much worse. A difference of 10 points corresponded with changes that were somewhat better or somewhat worse. Gummesson and colleagues[15] concluded that a 10-point difference in the preoperative to postoperative DASH score signifies the value needed to observe the minimally important change, most specifically when applied to subacromial impingement and carpal tunnel syndrome.

The DASH questionnaire has been used extensively to measure patient-based outcomes after various hand injuries. Wong and colleagues[16] prospectively evaluated 146 patients with acute hand trauma, 28% of whom had hand fractures, using the DASH score at initial and 10-week follow-up. There was a statistically significant improvement in the DASH during the course of treatment with improvement averaging 31 points, and the amount of change correlated with return to work. Dumont and colleagues[17] prospectively analyzed the clinical and functional outcomes of 12 patients with 14 displaced, unstable metacarpal fractures that were treated with open reduction with internal fixation using absorbable plate and screw constructs. Average postoperative DASH scores obtained at 6, 12, and 26 weeks were 30, 13, and 3, respectively. These scores correlated with an improvement in the visual analog score (VAS) for pain over the course of treatment.

Ozer and colleagues[18] used the DASH as a primary outcomes measure in a prospective comparison of internal fixation versus intramedullary nail fixation in 52 patients with extra-articular metacarpal fractures. The postoperative DASH for the plate-and-screw construct was slightly better than that of the intramedullary nail fixation group, but the difference did not reach statistical significance. In a prospective, randomized controlled trial by Zyluk and colleagues[19] the DASH was used to analyze the functional outcomes of patients with phalangeal fractures. In this study, 22 patients were treated with either closed reduction and percutaneous K-wire pinning or closed reduction and immobilization, with 2-month and 6-month follow-up evaluations. For the operative group, the mean DASH scores at 2 months and 6 months were 25 and 7, respectively. The patients treated with closed reduction and immobilization showed mean DASH scores of 8 at 2 months and 3 at 6 months. Although a trend toward better DASH scores was observed for the nonoperative group at both follow-up evaluations, the difference between groups did not reach statistical significance.[19]

Functional outcomes following nonoperative treatment of hand fractures have also been evaluated using the DASH. In a prospective randomized trial, Hofmeister and colleagues[20] evaluated functional outcomes of patients with fifth metacarpal neck fractures who underwent treatment with closed reduction and immobilization using 2 different cast designs. Eighty-one active-duty military personnel received either a short-arm cast with volar outriggers (SAC-VOR) or a short-arm cast extended to the proximal interphalangeal (PIP) joint with a 3-point mold, placing the metacarpophalangeal (MCP) joints in extension (MCP-ext). Baseline DASH scores between the two groups were similar, as were all subsequent DASH scores over the following 3 months, although the DASH showed a trend toward less disability in the MCP-ext group compared with the SAC-VOR group.

The DASH provides upper extremity surgeons with a more specific outcomes measures tool for function of the limb, compared with general questionnaires such as the SF-36, but its application to hand fractures has limitations. The DASH evaluates the upper extremity as a single functional unit and provides a regional evaluation of the limb and is thus not specifically geared to hand function. In the presence of ipsilateral shoulder, elbow, or wrist disorders, the DASH scores could reflect an increase in disability, even in the presence of a highly functional hand.[11,21] There is a paucity of literature examining the effect of comorbid upper extremity disorders on hand injury functional outcomes. In addition, disabling conditions of the lower extremity can negatively affect DASH scores in patients with comorbid upper extremity disorders. Dowrick and colleagues[22] evaluated the DASH scores in 84 patients with upper extremity injuries, 73 patients with lower extremity injuries, and 49 control subjects, noting that patients with isolated upper and lower extremity injuries had statistically significantly higher DASH scores than the control group. It was concluded that any disability affecting the mobility and stability of the lower extremity can in turn cause limitations in upper extremity function and can be reflected in the DASH score.[22]

In addition, the general population normative DASH scores and the minimal numerical point value correlating with a clinically significant change in function may not apply to highly functioning individuals. In a study by Hsu and colleagues,[23] the validity of the DASH when applied to intercollegiate athletes was analyzed. The minimal numerical point value corresponding with a clinically significant change in the normal population could not be generalized to the athletes. Also, a ceiling effect pertained to the DASH scores in these athletes because they may obtain a normal DASH score before reaching their individual baseline physical function.

Patient-rated Wrist Evaluation and Patient-rated Wrist Hand Evaluation

The original Patient-rated Wrist Hand Evaluation (PRWE) was developed using a questionnaire in which physicians identified the factors they thought most indicative of patient recovery following wrist injury or surgery. These included pain intensity and frequency, frequently performed activities using either hand, and ability to perform activities of daily living.[24] On average, a subject can complete the PRWE in 4 minutes.[24] When used to evaluate patients with distal radius fractures and scaphoid nonunions, the PRWE showed excellent reliability. Validation of the survey was performed via comparison with specific components of the SF-36. A strong correlation between the SF-36 physical summary scores and PRWE scores was observed.[13]

Generated in 2004 as an offshoot of the PRWE, the Patient-rated Wrist Hand Evaluation (PRWHE) was developed as a more specific method of measuring functional outcomes in patients with hand disorders.[21] MacDermid and colleagues[21] compared it with the DASH, and the PRWHE was slightly more responsive for patients with wrist and hand injuries. In addition, with half as many items as the DASH, the PRWHE is shorter and more readily administered. A group of hand therapists supported this finding, stating that the PRWHE was simpler to use for both them and their patients. The PRWE is commonly used in the assessment of carpal tunnel syndrome, distal radius fractures, and other wrist based disorders, but the use of the more recently developed PRWHE has not been well described in evaluating hand fracture outcomes.[21]

The Michigan Hand Outcomes Questionnaire

The Michigan Hand Outcomes Questionnaire (MHQ) was developed in 1998 to specifically evaluate the overall health and function in patients with hand disorders. Originally consisting of 100 items, the current MHQ assessment tool represents a more focused and user-friendly 37-item survey that encompasses 6 domains[25,26]:

- Overall hand functioning
- Activity of daily living
- Pain
- Work performance
- Aesthetics
- Patient satisfaction with hand functioning

Cumulative scoring for the MHQ ranges from 0 to 100, with 0 representing minimal or worse function and 100 representing maximum function. The 37-item MHQ has undergone rigorous psychometric testing and showed high reliability and construct validity on each of the 6 domains, with the highest construct validity for activities of daily living. With high marks for reliability and validity, Chung and colleagues[27] reported the MHQ to be an excellent tool for assessing outcomes following hand surgery. Further testing of the MHQ by Chung and colleagues[28] showed that the instrument is responsive to the self-assessment of a patient's clinical change.

The MHQ has been used to analyze clinical outcomes following K-wire/traction device treatment of intra-articular PIP joint fractures. Theivendran and colleagues[29] reported that the average MHQ for 12 patients at mean follow-up of 24 weeks was 90, 6 points higher than the MHQ in another study of 7 patients with an average of 13.1 months' follow-up treated with a similar construct.[30,31] They attributed the high MHQ score of 90 to the dynamic nature of their construct, allowing for early mobilization and preventing excessive arthrofibrosis.

Although sensitive at detecting clinical changes in function, the MHQ has shown decreased correlation with overall patient disability compared with the DASH.[25] Other limitations of the MHQ include its length. At 37 items, it takes on average 15 minutes for a patient to complete the questionnaire.[32]

Jebsen-Taylor Hand Function Test

Developed in 1969, the Jebsen-Taylor Hand Function test (JTT) is a standardized and objective measure of hand function. It is composed of 7 subtests designed to provide a broad sampling of hand functional capacity[33]:

- Writing
- Simulation of page turning by turning over a 7.6 × 12.7 cm (3 × 5 inch) card
- Picking up small common objects
- Simulated feeding
- Stacking checkers
- Picking up large light objects
- Picking up large heavy objects

Over time, modifications of the JTT have been described. These modifications include eliminating the writing portion of the test, because this can depend on hand dominance, and administering the remaining 6 subtests with a strong enough correlation with activities of daily living and deformity to maintain the validity of the modified JTT.[34]

In a study by Hornbach and colleagues[9] the JTT was used to evaluate the clinical and functional outcomes of 11 patients with proximal phalanx fractures treated with CRPP using K wires. Abnormal JTT scores were seen with increasing PIP flexion contractures. Subjective evaluation with the VAS was satisfactory and only minimal functional compromise was reported.[9]

Advantages of the JTT include its ease of administration and validation in the assessment of multiple hand disorders. It can also be readily modified to exclude the written subtest when deemed appropriate. However, Davis Sears and Chung[34] found poor correlation between the JTT and patient-reported measures of disability, including patient satisfaction and domains that relate to activities of daily living, work, and function as assessed by the validated MHQ. In addition, the JTT was not as sensitive in detecting changes following hand surgery as the patient-reported responses obtained from the MHQ. They concluded that the JTT was a poor indicator of improvement and not a useful measure of the efficacy of treatments in hand surgery or of patient's ability to perform activities of daily living.

PHYSICAL EXAMINATION MEASURES OF OUTCOMES

Physical examination of the hand includes the arc of motion through full flexion to full extension of each joint. In addition, grip, key, and pinch testing are frequently performed using a dynamometer and pinch meter. These measured values are often reported as a percentage of the control values obtained from the unaffected contralateral side. However, concurrent disorders of the upper extremity and cervical spine, as well as hand dominance, can distort the measured values. Other factors within a given population, such as gender and age, can also cause variation in the normative values.

One way to measure digital range of motion is by calculation of the total active motion (TAM). TAM of a digit is defined as the sum of active flexion measurements at the MCP joint, PIP joint, and distal interphalangeal (DIP) joints minus the active extension deficits at the same three joints. Normal values for the TAM range from 260° to 270°.[35]

In a retrospective study by Faruqui and colleagues,[35] the postoperative TAM in patients undergoing percutaneous pinning of fractures in the proximal third of the proximal phalanx was analyzed. The proximal phalanx fractures were treated with either transarticular pinning or extra-articular cross-pinning fixation techniques. Mean postoperative TAM for the transarticular group and cross-pinning group were 201° and 198°, respectively. Motion at the PIP joint was most affected, with nearly half the patients from both groups losing greater than 20° of flexion.

Horton and colleagues[36] prospectively analyzed the functional outcomes of patients treated surgically for long oblique or long spiral fractures of the proximal phalanx. In this trial, 32 patients were randomized to receive treatment with CRPP with K wires or open reduction internal fixation with lag screws. Of the 32 patients enrolled, 28 were available for evaluation at a mean follow-up of 40 months. At final follow-up there was no statistically significant difference in active range of motion between the two groups with respect to PIP motion, DIP motion, and fingertip-to-palm distance. However, 3 of the patients treated with lag screw fixation showed decreased interphalangeal (IP) joint flexion

with the MCP joint extended, indicating intrinsic muscle tethering. In addition, 5 patients from both treatment groups showed weakness with abduction and adduction at final follow-up. In light of these minor findings, no statistically significant difference in hand grip and finger pinch strengths between the two groups was observed.

In a study by Shimizu and colleagues,[3] predictors of postoperative range of motion for comminuted periarticular metacarpal and phalangeal fractures treated with titanium plates were analyzed. Using the percentage TAM compared with the unaffected contralateral digit, they identified fracture location, soft tissue injury, and age as predictors of postoperative motion. Phalangeal fractures, associated soft tissue injuries, and increased age were all correlated with decreased percent TAM after surgery.

Grip and pinch values have been used for outcomes measurement, but normative means vary and depend on factors such as age, gender, fatigue, and hand dominance. Grip strength values vary from 5 kg for the nondominant hand in women more than 75 years of age to 73 kg for the dominant hand in men 24 to 34 years of age.[37] In an attempt to better define the observed variations across a given population, Walker and colleagues[38] analyzed the normal range of motion, pinch strength, and grip strength. Although men and women had similar range-of-motion profiles, men had 40% stronger pinch strength and double the grip strength of women. Mathiowetz and colleagues[39] reported that grip strengths were highest in the age range of 25 to 39 years, with a subsequent decline over time. Tip, key, and palmar pinch strength were stable from ages 20 to 59 years and then declined with age.

Omokawa and colleagues[2] prospectively analyzed the functional outcomes of patients treated for comminuted periarticular metacarpal and phalangeal fractures using a titanium plate system. Of the 51 patients enrolled, at the time of final follow-up postoperative TAM was excellent in 26 patients, good for 17, fair for 5, and poor for 3 patients. Average postoperative grip strength in these patients was 87% compared with the contralateral side. This study shows the direct correlation between grip strength and TAM and how, when possible, these measures should be combined to provide a complete objective function outcome analysis.

RADIOGRAPHIC MEASUREMENTS OF OUTCOME OF HAND FRACTURES

Radiographic evaluation is critical in the assessment of hand fracture outcomes. Serial radiographs are used to evaluate the alignment, bony healing, and hardware positioning of both operative and nonoperatively treated fractures.

Vahey and colleagues[40] evaluated radiographic alignment in a study of proximal phalanx fractures. Apex palmar angulated malunions resulted in skeletal shortening, extensor tendon lengthening, and PIP joint extensor lag. The radiographically measured apex palmar angulations of 16°, 27°, and 46° corresponded with extensor lags of 10°, 24°, and 66°, respectively. Other studies have substantiated this correlation, reporting a direct relationship between skeletal shortening and extensor lag.[41]

In nonoperatively treated hand fractures, radiographs are used to assess outcomes of specific treatments. Tavassoli and colleagues[42] performed a retrospective analysis of 3 casting techniques following closed reduction of extra-articular metacarpal fractures in 263 patients. In group 1, patients were immobilized with the MCP joint flexed but allowing full range of motion of the IP joints. Group 2 patients were casted with the MCP joint in extension with full range of motion of the IP joints permitted, and group 3 patients were treated with the MCP joint flexed and IP joints in extension. Anteroposterior and lateral radiographs were completed immediately following reduction and casting, at the 5-week follow-up after cast removal, and at the final 9-week follow-up appointment. Comparison of the radiographs for all 3 groups showed no statically significant difference in fracture alignment at any time point. At final follow-up, all 263 patients had radiographic evidence of healing and had returned to preinjury functional capacity.

SUMMARY

Numerous methods to evaluate outcome measures for hand fractures have been described and validated in the literature. These methods include patient-reported subjective measures, objective functional examination measures, a combination of both subjective and objective measures, and radiographic outcomes. There is no universally used outcome measure for hand fractures, although the optimal tool would be easily administered and comprehensive with regard to function, pain, disability, and responsive to surgery and over time. Unless a gold-standard outcomes assessment tool is identified, a combination of the currently established and validated outcome measurements may be required to obtain this information. The senior author has used the DASH score primarily in outcomes measurement, in addition to clinical and radiographic parameters. In addition, the SF-36 and Michigan hand questionnaire have been used to evaluate patient outcomes.

REFERENCES

1. Emmett JE, Breck LW. A review and analysis of 11,000 fractures seen in a private practice of orthopaedic surgery, 1937–1956. J Bone Joint Surg Am 1958;40(5):1169–75.
2. Omokawa S, Fujitani R, Dohi Y, et al. Prospective outcomes of comminuted periarticular metacarpal and phalangeal fractures treated using a titanium plate system. J Hand Surg Am 2008;33(6):857–63.
3. Shimizu T, Omokawa S, Akahane M, et al. Predictors of the postoperative range of finger motion for comminuted periarticular metacarpal and phalangeal fractures treated with a titanium plate. Injury 2012;43(6):940–5.
4. Egol KA, Koval KJ, Zuckerman JD, et al. Handbook of fractures. 4th edition. Philadelphia: Wolters Kluwer/Lippincott Williams & Wilkins Health; 2010. p. 305–23.
5. Pun WK, Chow SP, So YC, et al. A prospective study on 284 digital fractures of the hand. J Hand Surg Am 1989;14(3):474–81.
6. Freeland AE, Orbay JL. Extraarticular hand fractures in adults: a review of new developments. Clin Orthop Relat Res 2006;445:133–45.
7. Ware JE Jr, Sherbourne CD. The MOS 36-item short-form health survey (SF-36). I. Conceptual framework and item selection. Med Care 1992;30(6):473–83.
8. Brazier JE, Harper R, Jones NM, et al. Validating the SF-36 health survey questionnaire: new outcome measure for primary care. BMJ 1992;305(6846):160–4.
9. Hornbach EE, Cohen MS. Closed reduction and percutaneous pinning of fractures of the proximal phalanx. J Hand Surg Br 2001;26(1):45–9.
10. Rosberg HE, Carlsson KS, Dahlin LB. Prospective study of patients with injuries to the hand and forearm: costs, function, and general health. Scand J Plast Reconstr Surg Hand Surg 2005;39(6):360–9.
11. Schuind FA, Mouraux D, Robert C, et al. Functional and outcome evaluation of the hand and wrist. Hand Clin 2003;19(3):361–9.
12. Hudak PL, Amadio PC, Bombardier C. Development of an upper extremity outcome measure: the DASH (Disabilities of the Arm, Shoulder and Hand) [corrected]. The Upper Extremity Collaborative Group (UECG). Am J Ind Med 1996;29(6):602–8.
13. Changulani M, Okonkwo U, Keswani T, et al. Outcome evaluation measures for wrist and hand: which one to choose? Int Orthop 2008;32(1):1–6.
14. Atroshi I, Gummesson C, Andersson B, et al. The Disabilities of the Arm, Shoulder and Hand (DASH) outcome questionnaire: reliability and validity of the Swedish version evaluated in 176 patients. Acta Orthop Scand 2000;71(6):613–8.
15. Gummesson C, Atroshi I, Ekdahl C. The Disabilities of the Arm, Shoulder and Hand (DASH) outcome

questionnaire: longitudinal construct validity and measuring self-rated health change after surgery. BMC Musculoskelet Disord 2003;4:11.

16. Wong JY, Fung BK, Chu MM, et al. The use of Disabilities of the Arm, Shoulder, and Hand questionnaire in rehabilitation after acute traumatic hand injuries. J Hand Ther 2007;20(1):49–55 [quiz: 56].

17. Dumont C, Fuchs M, Burchhardt H, et al. Clinical results of absorbable plates for displaced metacarpal fractures. J Hand Surg Am 2007;32(4):491–6.

18. Ozer K, Gillani S, Williams A, et al. Comparison of intramedullary nailing versus plate-screw fixation of extra-articular metacarpal fractures. J Hand Surg Am 2008;33(10):1724–31.

19. Zyluk A, Budzynski T. Conservative vs operative treatment of isolated fractures of phalanges: results of the prospective, randomized study. Chir Narzadow Ruchu Ortop Pol 2009;74(2):74–8.

20. Hofmeister EP, Kim J, Shin AY. Comparison of 2 methods of immobilization of fifth metacarpal neck fractures: a prospective randomized study. J Hand Surg Am 2008;33(8):1362–8.

21. MacDermid JC, Tottenham V. Responsiveness of the Disability of the Arm, Shoulder, and Hand (DASH) and Patient-rated Wrist/Hand Evaluation (PRWHE) in evaluating change after hand therapy. J Hand Ther 2004;17(1):18–23.

22. Dowrick AS, Gabbe BJ, Williamson OD, et al. Does the Disabilities of the Arm, Shoulder and Hand (DASH) scoring system only measure disability due to injuries to the upper limb? J Bone Joint Surg Br 2006;88(4):524–7.

23. Hsu JE, Nacke E, Park MJ, et al. The Disabilities of the Arm, Shoulder, and Hand questionnaire in intercollegiate athletes: validity limited by ceiling effect. J Shoulder Elbow Surg 2010;19(3):349–54.

24. Ritting AW, Wolf JM. How to measure outcomes of distal radius fracture treatment. Hand Clin 2012; 28(2):165–75.

25. Horng YS, Lin MC, Feng CT, et al. Responsiveness of the Michigan Hand Outcomes Questionnaire and the Disabilities of the Arm, Shoulder, and Hand questionnaire in patients with hand injury. J Hand Surg Am 2010;35(3):430–6.

26. Naidu SH, Panchik D, Chinchilli VM. Development and validation of the hand assessment tool. J Hand Ther 2009;22(3):250–6 [quiz: 257].

27. Chung KC, Pillsbury MS, Walters MR, et al. Reliability and validity testing of the Michigan Hand Outcomes Questionnaire. J Hand Surg Am 1998;23(4):575–87.

28. Chung KC, Hamill JB, Walters MR, et al. The Michigan Hand Outcomes Questionnaire (MHQ): assessment of responsiveness to clinical change. Ann Plast Surg 1999;42(6):619–22.

29. Theivendran K, Pollock J, Rajaratnam V. Proximal interphalangeal joint fractures of the hand: treatment with an external dynamic traction device. Ann Plast Surg 2007;58(6):625–9.

30. Deshmukh SC, Kumar D, Mathur K, et al. Complex fracture-dislocation of the proximal interphalangeal joint of the hand. Results of a modified pins and rubbers traction system. J Bone Joint Surg Br 2004; 86(3):406–12.

31. Suzuki Y, Matsunaga T, Sato S, et al. The pins and rubbers traction system for treatment of comminuted intraarticular fractures and fracture-dislocations in the hand. J Hand Surg Br 1994;19(1):98–107.

32. Waljee JF, Kim HM, Burns PB, et al. Development of a brief, 12-item version of the Michigan Hand Questionnaire. Plast Reconstr Surg 2011;128(1):208–20.

33. Jebsen RH, Taylor N, Trieschmann RB, et al. An objective and standardized test of hand function. Arch Phys Med Rehabil 1969;50(6):311–9.

34. Davis Sears E, Chung KC. Validity and responsiveness of the Jebsen-Taylor Hand Function Test. J Hand Surg Am 2010;35(1):30–7.

35. Faruqui S, Stern PJ, Kiefhaber TR. Percutaneous pinning of fractures in the proximal third of the proximal phalanx: complications and outcomes. J Hand Surg Am 2012;37(7):1342–8.

36. Horton TC, Hatton M, Davis TR. A prospective randomized controlled study of fixation of long oblique and spiral shaft fractures of the proximal phalanx: closed reduction and percutaneous Kirschner wiring versus open reduction and lag screw fixation. J Hand Surg Br 2003;28(1):5–9.

37. Massy-Westropp N, Rankin W, Ahern M, et al. Measuring grip strength in normal adults: reference ranges and a comparison of electronic and hydraulic instruments. J Hand Surg Am 2004;29(3):514–9.

38. Walker PS, Davidson W, Erkman MJ. An apparatus to assess function of the hand. J Hand Surg Am 1978;3(2):189–93.

39. Mathiowetz V, Kashman N, Volland G, et al. Grip and pinch strength: normative data for adults. Arch Phys Med Rehabil 1985;66(2):69–74.

40. Vahey JW, Wegner DA, Hastings H 3rd. Effect of proximal phalangeal fracture deformity on extensor tendon function. J Hand Surg Am 1998;23(4):673–81.

41. Orbay JL, Touhami A. The treatment of unstable metacarpal and phalangeal shaft fractures with flexible nonlocking and locking intramedullary nails. Hand Clin 2006;22(3):279–86.

42. Tavassoli J, Ruland RT, Hogan CJ, et al. Three cast techniques for the treatment of extra-articular metacarpal fractures. Comparison of short-term outcomes and final fracture alignments. J Bone Joint Surg Am 2005;87(10):2196–201.

Index

Note: Page numbers of article titles are in **boldface** type.

Hand Clin 29 (2013) 631–634
http://dx.doi.org/10.1016/S0749-0712(13)00091-7
0749-0712/13/$ – see front matter © 2013 Elsevier Inc. All rights reserved.

hand.theclinics.com

United States Postal Service

Statement of Ownership, Management, and Circulation
(All Periodicals Publications Except Requestor Publications)

1. Publication Title	2. Publication Number	3. Filing Date
Hand Clinics	0 0 0 - 7 0 9	9/14/13

4. Issue Frequency	5. Number of Issues Published Annually	6. Annual Subscription Price
Feb, May, Aug, Nov	4	$390.00

7. Complete Mailing Address of Known Office of Publication (Not printer) (Street, city, county, state, and ZIP+4®)

Elsevier Inc.
360 Park Avenue South
New York, NY 10010-1710

Contact Person
Stephen R. Bushing
Telephone (Include area code)
215-239-3688

8. Complete Mailing Address of Headquarters or General Business Office of Publisher (Not printer)

Elsevier Inc., 360 Park Avenue South, New York, NY 10010-1710

9. Full Names and Complete Mailing Addresses of Publisher, Editor, and Managing Editor (Do not leave blank)
Publisher (Name and complete mailing address)

Linda Belfus, Elsevier, Inc., 1600 John F. Kennedy Blvd. Suite 1800, Philadelphia, PA 19103-2899
Editor (Name and complete mailing address)

Jennifer Flynn-Briggs, Elsevier, Inc., 1600 John F. Kennedy Blvd. Suite 1800, Philadelphia, PA 19103-2899
Managing Editor (Name and complete mailing address)

Adrianna Brigido, Elsevier, Inc., 1600 John F. Kennedy Blvd. Suite 1800, Philadelphia, PA 19103-2899

10. Owner (Do not leave blank. If the publication is owned by a corporation, give the name and address of the corporation immediately followed by the names and addresses of all stockholders owning or holding 1 percent or more of the total amount of stock. If not owned by a corporation, give the names and addresses of the individual owners. If owned by a partnership or other unincorporated firm, give its name and address as well as those of each individual owner. If the publication is published by a nonprofit organization, give its name and address.)

Full Name	Complete Mailing Address
Wholly owned subsidiary of	1600 John F. Kennedy Blvd, Ste. 1800
Reed/Elsevier, US holdings	Philadelphia, PA 19103-2899

11. Known Bondholders, Mortgagees, and Other Security Holders Owning or Holding 1 Percent or More of Total Amount of Bonds, Mortgages, or Other Securities. If none, check box. ☐ None

Full Name	Complete Mailing Address
N/A	

12. Tax Status (For completion by nonprofit organizations authorized to mail at nonprofit rates) (Check one)
The purpose, function, and nonprofit status of this organization and the exempt status for federal income tax purposes:
☐ Has Not Changed During Preceding 12 Months
☐ Has Changed During Preceding 12 Months (Publisher must submit explanation of change with this statement)

PS Form 3526, September 2007 (Page 1 of 3 (Instructions Page 3)) PSN 7530-01-000-9931 PRIVACY NOTICE: See our Privacy policy in www.usps.com

---

13. Publication Title	14. Issue Date for Circulation Data Below
Hand Clinics	August 2013

15. Extent and Nature of Circulation		14. Average No. Copies Each Issue During Preceding 12 Months	No. Copies of Single Issue Published Nearest to Filing Date
a. Total Number of Copies (Net press run)		1188	1028
b. Paid Circulation (By Mail and Outside the Mail)	(1) Mailed Outside-County Paid Subscriptions Stated on PS Form 3541. (Include paid distribution above nominal rate, advertiser's proof copies, and exchange copies)	715	665
	(2) Mailed In-County Paid Subscriptions Stated on PS Form 3541 (Include paid distribution above nominal rate, advertiser's proof copies, and exchange copies)		
	(3) Paid Distribution Outside the Mails Including Sales Through Dealers and Carriers, Street Vendors, Counter Sales, and Other Paid Distribution Outside USPS®	222	195
	(4) Paid Distribution by Other Classes Mailed Through the USPS (e.g. First-Class Mail®)		
c. Total Paid Distribution (Sum of 15b (1), (2), (3), and (4))	▶	937	860
d. Free or Nominal Rate Distribution (By Mail and Outside the Mail)	(1) Free or Nominal Rate Outside-County Copies Included on PS Form 3541	36	8
	(2) Free or Nominal Rate In-County Copies Included on PS Form 3541		
	(3) Free or Nominal Rate Copies Mailed at Other Classes Through the USPS (e.g. First-Class Mail)		
	(4) Free or Nominal Rate Distribution Outside the Mail (Carriers or other means)		
e. Total Free or Nominal Rate Distribution (Sum of 15d (1), (2), (3) and (4))	▶	36	8
f. Total Distribution (Sum of 15c and 15e)	▶	973	868
g. Copies not Distributed (See instructions to publishers #4 (page 83))	▶	215	160
h. Total (Sum of 15f and g)	▶	1188	1028
i. Percent Paid (15c divided by 15f times 100)		96.30%	99.08%

16. Publication of Statement of Ownership

☐ If the publication is a general publication, publication of this statement is required. Will be printed in the November 2013 issue of this publication. ☐ Publication not required

17. Signature and Title of Editor, Publisher, Business Manager, or Owner   Date

Stephen R. Bushing   September 14, 2013

Stephen R. Bushing – Inventory Distribution Coordinator

I certify that all information furnished on this form is true and complete. I understand that anyone who furnishes false or misleading information on this form or who omits material or information requested on the form may be subject to criminal sanctions (including fines and imprisonment) and/or civil sanctions (including civil penalties).

PS Form 3526, September 2007 (Page 2 of 3)

Moving?

Make sure your subscription moves with you!

To notify us of your new address, find your **Clinics Account Number** (located on your mailing label above your name), and contact customer service at:

Email: journalscustomerservice-usa@elsevier.com

800-654-2452 (subscribers in the U.S. & Canada)
314-447-8871 (subscribers outside of the U.S. & Canada)

Fax number: 314-447-8029

Elsevier Health Sciences Division
Subscription Customer Service
3251 Riverport Lane
Maryland Heights, MO 63043

ELSEVIER

Moving?

Make sure your subscription moves with you!

To notify us of your new address, find your Clinics Account Number (located on your mailing label above your name), and contact customer service at:

Email: JournalsCustomerService-usa@elsevier.com

800-654-2452 (subscribers in the U.S. & Canada)
314-447-8871 (subscribers outside of the U.S. & Canada)

Fax number: 314-447-8029

Elsevier Health Sciences Division
Subscription Customer Service
3251 Riverport Lane
Maryland Heights, MO 63043

*To ensure uninterrupted delivery of your subscription, please notify us at least 4 weeks in advance of move.

Printed and bound by CPI Group (UK) Ltd, Croydon, CR0 4YY

03/10/2024

01040366-0008